AF333195

NEUROSCIENCE RESEARCH PROGRESS

ENCEPHALITIS, ENCEPHALOMYELITIS AND ENCEPHALOPATHIES

SYMPTOMS, CAUSES AND POTENTIAL COMPLICATIONS

NEUROSCIENCE RESEARCH PROGRESS

Additional books in this series can be found on Nova's website
under the Series tab.

Additional e-books in this series can be found on Nova's website
under the e-book tab.

NEURODEGENERATIVE DISEASES - LABORATORY AND CLINICAL RESEARCH

Additional books in this series can be found on Nova's website
under the Series tab.

Additional e-books in this series can be found on Nova's website
under the e-book tab.

Neuroscience Research Progress

Encephalitis, Encephalomyelitis and Encephalopathies

Symptoms, Causes and Potential Complications

Andrew Ruiz
and
Douglas Fleming
Editors

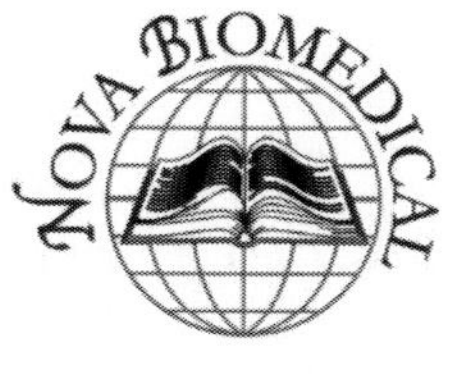

Nova Biomedical

New York

Copyright © 2013 by Nova Science Publishers, Inc.

All rights reserved. No part of this book may be reproduced, stored in a retrieval system or transmitted in any form or by any means: electronic, electrostatic, magnetic, tape, mechanical photocopying, recording or otherwise without the written permission of the Publisher.

For permission to use material from this book please contact us:
Telephone 631-231-7269; Fax 631-231-8175
Web Site: http://www.novapublishers.com

NOTICE TO THE READER

The Publisher has taken reasonable care in the preparation of this book, but makes no expressed or implied warranty of any kind and assumes no responsibility for any errors or omissions. No liability is assumed for incidental or consequential damages in connection with or arising out of information contained in this book. The Publisher shall not be liable for any special, consequential, or exemplary damages resulting, in whole or in part, from the readers' use of, or reliance upon, this material. Any parts of this book based on government reports are so indicated and copyright is claimed for those parts to the extent applicable to compilations of such works.

Independent verification should be sought for any data, advice or recommendations contained in this book. In addition, no responsibility is assumed by the publisher for any injury and/or damage to persons or property arising from any methods, products, instructions, ideas or otherwise contained in this publication.

This publication is designed to provide accurate and authoritative information with regard to the subject matter covered herein. It is sold with the clear understanding that the Publisher is not engaged in rendering legal or any other professional services. If legal or any other expert assistance is required, the services of a competent person should be sought. FROM A DECLARATION OF PARTICIPANTS JOINTLY ADOPTED BY A COMMITTEE OF THE AMERICAN BAR ASSOCIATION AND A COMMITTEE OF PUBLISHERS.

Additional color graphics may be available in the e-book version of this book.

Library of Congress Cataloging-in-Publication Data

ISBN: 978-1-62257-766-8

Library of Congress Control Number: 2012945367

Published by Nova Science Publishers, Inc. † New York

CONTENTS

PREFACE

Encephalopathies are disorders or diseases of the brain. In modern usage, encephalopathy does not refer to a single disease, but rather to a syndrome of global brain dysfunction which can be caused by many different illnesses. In this book, the authors discuss the symptoms, causes, and potential complications relating to encephalitis, encephalomyelitis and encephalopathies. Topics include HIV-1 associated neurocognitive disorder; nonconvulsive status epilepticus; the implications of sensitization for chronic fatigue syndrome; treatment of tick-borne encephalitis; the immunology of encephalomyelitis; neuromyelitis optica; viral encephalopathy and retinopathy in farmed fish; septic encephalopathy; and Japanese encephalitis.

Chapter 1 – HIV encephalopathy covers a range of HIV-related brain dysfunction. The most severe is HIV-associated Dementia (HAD), which is the most common cause of dementia in adults under 40. HAD has become less common since Highly Active AntiRetroviral Therapy (HAART) was introduced. Before the introduction of HAART, most HAD patients showed subcortical dementia, with predominant basal ganglia involvement, manifesting as psychomotor slowing, Parkinsonism, behavioral abnormalities and cognitive difficulties. HIV-1 enters the Central Nervous System (CNS) soon after it enters the body. In the CNS, it is largely impervious to HAART. As survival with chronic HIV-1 infection improves, the number of people harboring the virus in their CNS increases. The prevalence of HIV-associated neurocognitive disorder (HAND) therefore continues to rise, and less fulminant forms of HAND such as minor neurocognitive/motor disorder (MCMD) have become more common than their more fulminant predecessors. HAND remains a significant independent risk factor for AIDS mortality. It is also becoming clear that the brain is an important reservoir for the virus, and neurodegenerative and neuroinflammatory changes may continue despite the use of HAART.

Neurons themselves are rarely infected by HIV-1, and neuronal damage is felt to be mainly indirect. HIV-1 infects resident microglia, periventricular macrophages, leading to increased production of cytokines and to release of HIV-1 proteins, the most likely neurotoxins, among which are the envelope (Env) protein (gp120) and HIV-1 *trans*-acting protein Tat.

The authors used model systems in which recombinant gp120, or Tat, proteins are directly injected into the striatum. The neurotoxicity of such recombinant proteins is highly reproducible and can be used as a tool for testing novel therapeutic interventions. However, HIV-1 infection of the brain is a chronic process. This is in part the reason why the authors developed experimental models of chronic HIV-1 neurotoxicity based on recombinant SV40 (rSV40) vector-modified expression of gp120 or Tat, in the brain.

As HIV-1 infection of the brain lasts the lifetime of affected individuals, and as eradication of CNS HIV-1 is currently not possible, control of the damage caused by the virus may represent a useful approach to treatment. It is known that gp120 and Tat induce oxidative stress in the brain, leading to neuronal apoptosis/death. One way to limit the final damage could be by limiting oxidative stress-related neurotoxicity. The authors used SV40 vectors for gene delivery of transgenes to the brain. These vectors deliver long-term transgene expression to brain neurons and microglia, when administered by several different routes. Intracerebral injection of SV(SOD1) or SV(GPx1) carrying the antioxidant enzymes, Cu/Zn superoxide dismutase (SOD1) or glutathione peroxidase (GPx1) respectively, into the rat caudate putamen (CP), significantly protects neurons from apoptosis caused by subsequent inoculation of recombinant HIV-1 envelope glycoprotein, gp120 and Tat at the same location. Vector administration into the lateral ventricle (LV) or cisterna magna, particularly if preceded by intraperitoneal mannitol, protects from intra-CP gp120-induced neurotoxicity comparably to intra-CP vector administration. The safety of SV(SOD1) and SV(GPx1) delivered intra-CP has been demonstrated in rats and in Rhesus macaques monkeys, and resulting transgene expression is very durable.

These models should provide a better understanding of the pathogenesis of HIV-1 in the brain as well as offer new therapeutic avenues.

Chapter 2 – Nonconvulsive status epilepticus (NCSE) is a heterogeneous disorder with multiple subtypes that encompasses a variety of etiologies, electroencephalographic patterns, mental states, and prognoses. The term "nonconvulsive status epilepticus" has been used synonymously with complex partial status epilepticus (CPSE), absence status epilepticus (AS), and status epilepticus in comatose patients. It may present in the setting of metabolic disorders, neurotoxicity, acute cerebral lesions, and pre-existing epilepsy. Based on current estimates, NCSE constitutes about 25-50% of all cases of status epilepticus. Electroencephalogram (EEG) can be quite useful in diagnosing NCSE. However, the diagnosis is not always straight forward, particularly in the elderly and/or comatose patient, as clinical features and various periodic electroencephalographic patterns can be seen both in SE and in a variety of encephalopathic conditions. This has led to both under-recognition and misdiagnosis of NCSE. Although some subtypes of NCSE, such as absence status epilepticus, are easily treatable, others respond poorly to therapy. Given the unclear degree of morbidity and, at times, self-limiting course, debate exists over how aggressively clinicians should treat NCSE. Further work is needed to better classify NCSE subtypes and to determine which EEG patterns, in fact, represent NCSE, so that treatment paradigms and prognoses may be established for different subtypes of NCSE.

Chapter 3 – Many patients with chronic fatigue syndrome (CFS) have widespread pain which has a large role in patients' activity limitations. Central sensitization has been posited as an explanation of this pain in both Fibromyalgia (FM) and CFS. Repeated or sustained noxious stimulation can lead to central sensitization, which can cause the spinal cord to enter a "hyperexcitable" state. In this article, the authors will explore the relevance of the central sensitization theory for CFS, as well as link it to the kindling hypothesis that has been previously offered as one explanation for the etiology of CFS. The article also reviews the implications of this theory for both inflammatory markers and central nervous system involvement.

Chapter 4 – Comparative analysis of successful treatment based on induction of innate immunity, currently available drugs and up-to-date development of new principles to control virus infections may help to solve public health problems. Main criteria for anti-viral medicines should include not only selective inactivation of virus-specific proteins and/or nucleic acids but also minimal possible influence on host cellular biopolymers, prolonged action to avoid multiple frequent administrations as well as should take into consideration both innate resistance and immunity status of host organism. Despite long-term numerous efforts to develop specific and effective anti-viral medications beginning from the time of virus discovery there is no curative therapy for many viral infections including tick-borne encephalitis (TBE) till now. TBE is the most important flavivirus infection of the central nervous system (CNS) in Eurasia. The etiological agent, the TBE virus (TBEV) is transmitted to man by tick bytes. Geographic natural habitat of the TBEV appeared to be discontinuous and extended throughout southern part of Eurasian forest belt from Pacific to Atlantic ocean mainly within distribution areas of the virus vectors – ixodid ticks. In European endemic regions supportive treatment includes paracetamol, aspirin and other nonsteroidal anti-inflammatory drugs. In severe cases, some clinicians administer corticosteroids, although their use has not been validated. For patients with severe CNS symptoms intubation and ventilation are required to prevent coma or neuromuscular paralysis. In Russia TBE cure is based on the virus-specific immunoglobulin from donor blood sera, analogs of inteferons (viferon, reaferon-EC-lipint (human recombinant interferon α-1 and α-2b), interferon induction (by using larifan, neovir, tiloron, amixin, cycloferon, remantadin, ridosin, cameron, iodantipirin, enerion, mannitol, nootropil, pentoxifillin and others), as well as ribonuclease A from bovine pancreas. However, high molecular weight proteins such as immunoglobulins and RNases are not known to be able to penetrate into both host cells and enveloped viruses. Additionally for treatment of serious encephalitic manifestations artificial lung ventilation, panangin and glucose solutions can be used. In China oriental phytotherapy includes more than 10 elixirs with vitamins, microelements, as well as antiviral, antimicrobial, immunomodulation and anti-inflammatory effects, most of them are permitted to use in Russia. Numerous attempts to inhibit the TBEV reproduction by nucleoside analog ribavirin currently widely used for treatment of infections caused by plus-strand RNA-containing hepatitis C virus and poliovirus were not successful. Both aldehyde-containing and 4-N-exo-base-substituted photoreactive analogs of NTP, NDP and NMP could bind with RNA replicase subunits – the TBEV large nonstructural proteins NS3 and NS5 *in vitro* but their interaction did not completely inhibit the TBEV reproduction in infected cells.

New approach based on low molecular weight artificial ribonucleases - derivatives of aminoacids, short peptides, peptidomimetics and diazabicyclooctane (DABCO) has been suggested. Some of artificial RNases can serve as models of catalytic sites of natural RNases resulting in simple peptides or peptide-like molecules whereas others are based on the acceleration of RNA spontaneous hydrolysis due to the distortion of RNA secondary structure in the presence of polycationic molecules. In spite of complete cleavage of both viral and cellular RNA in the presence of the artificial RNases *in vitro* the degradation of the TBEV genome within extracellular virions and inside infected cells was not exhaustive. Further study should be aimed at development of specific affinity reagents with enhanced penetration into enveloped viruses or into infected cells.

Chapter 5 – The immune system is closely associated with the pathogenesis of encephalomyelitis and influences susceptibility to the disease. However, the pathogenetic mechanisms underlying encephalomyelitis are still unclear. Consequently, an effective therapy for this intractable disease is not yet available. Encephalomyelitis in humans most commonly manifests in the form of multiple sclerosis (MS). Experimental autoimmune encephalomyelitis (EAE) is a widely used animal model for human MS, although the relevance of the animal model to the human disease has been questioned by many neurologists.

In this chapter, the author focuses on the immunologic mechanisms underlying the development of encephalomyelitis. In the first half of this chapter, the author reviews the effector immune responses that induce encephalomyelitis and cause deterioration. This section covers both basic studies on the EAE animal model and clinical studies on MS patients. Oligopeptide fragments of myelin basic protein (MBP) and myelin oligodendrocyte glycoprotein (MOG) have been identified as antigens for T cell activation, and immunization of mice with these peptides induces encephalomyelitis. These observations confirm the involvement of T cells in the pathogenesis of this disease. Therefore, the author primarily focuses on T cell involvement, although many different types of cells are involved in the development of encephalomyelitis. In the second half of this chapter, he reviews the regulatory immune responses that are involved in the prevention or improvement of encephalomyelitis. Mature T cells that express the $\alpha\beta$-type T cell receptor (TCR) are classified as either CD4$^+$ or CD8$^+$. Regulatory T cells are thought to be part of both the CD4$^+$ and CD8$^+$ populations, although research on regulatory T cells during the last decade increasingly suggests that regulatory T cells are a part of the CD4$^+$ T cell population. In this section, the author describes both CD4$^+$ and CD8$^+$ regulatory T cells as new potential tools for overcoming not only encephalomyelitis but also other diseases caused by autoimmune reactions.

Chapter 6 – Neuromyelitis optica (NMO), also known as Devic's disease, is a chronic inflammatory disease of the central nervous system. NMO affects optic nerves and spinal cord of patients causing visual loss and myelopathy. Until recently, this disease had a poor prognosis and presented a number of clinical, diagnostic, and management challenges. Over the last decade NMO became a focus of intense research, which led to identification of a disease biomarker and introduction of novel diagnostic criteria. In this review, the authors discuss the most important clinical and management aspects of the disease. In addition, the authors analyze the current hypotheses related to the etiology and pathogenesis of NMO. In the conclusion of the review they outline several research directions that may be of future interest.

Chapter 7 – Viral encephalopathy and retinopathy (VER) in fish is caused by *betanodaviruses* leading to high destructive mortality rates within hatchery-reared larvae and juveniles of a wide variety of marine fish. The disease was also designated viral nervous necrosis (VNN) when first described in 1990. Pathogenesis of VER, in general, is related to the neuro-invasive nature of the virus and subsequent effect on tissues in the brain and retina. The virus localizes in the brain, spinal cord, and retina of the affected fish which exhibit erratic swimming patterns and a range of neurological abnormalities, including vacuolization and cellular necrosis in the central nervous system and retina. Histologically, lesions are observed in the brain, spinal cord and in the eyes of all diseased fish.

Similar to the insect *nodaviruses*, the genome of *betanodaviruses* consists of two single-stranded, positive-sense RNA molecules (RNA1 and RNA2) of about 3.0 and 1.4 kb in length, respectively. RNA1 encodes a non-structural protein of approximately 100 kDa the

RNA-dependent RNA polymerase (RdRP) also named protein A, that replicates the viral genome. Whereas RNA2 encodes the capsid protein precursor (CPp) which is about 42 kDa. Phylogenetically, viral isolates were examined into four clusters based on nucleotide sequences of the coat protein gene. The official virus species names are barfin flounder nervous necrosis virus (BFNNV), redspotted grouper nervous necrosis virus (RGNNV), striped jack nervous necrosis virus (SJNNV) and tiger puffer nervous necrosis virus (TPNNV). A novel subtype of *nodavirus* from turbot, *Psetta maxima* (L.), was recently described. Both vertical and horizontal transmissions of the disease have been suggested.

In recent years, great advances have been made in our understanding of teleost immunity, although it is still not as well understood as mammalian immunity. Innate or non-specific immunity is present as the first line of defence against pathogens, whereas the more specific active immunity takes a variable time to develop. At present, there are neither drugs nor vaccines available to prevent VNN in cultured fish. The control of the disease in based on the virus detection in infected animals.

Chapter 8 – Encephalopathy refers to a syndrome of global brain dysfunction. Septic encephalopathy shows a devastating neurological symptom. Here the authors introduce the *septic encephalopathy*, encephalopathy associated with sepsis. The pathogenesis of septic encephalopathy originates from the following order: (1) infection, (2) systemic inflammatory response syndrome (a whole-body inflammatory state), (3) multiple-organ dysfunction. These processes finally lead to be the symptoms of septic encephalopathy including mental confusion and delirium. The sequelas provoke the social issue. Accumulating body of studies suggest the hypothetical molecular mechanisms for patho-physiology of septic encephalopathy. The sensing of pathogen-associated molecular patterns such as lipopolysaccharides and peptidoglycans, and damage-associated molecular patterns such as endogenous DNAs and high mobility group box (HMGB) -1 by pattern recognition receptors drives a coordinated immune response. Sepsis is accompanied by a remarkable altered and imbalanced cytokine response (known as a cytokine storm), which burdens onto organs and results in multiple-organ dysfunctions. These processes finally result in septic encephalopathy. On the other hand, brain hemorrhage, edema, and ischemia were also found as complicated symptoms associated with sepsis. Hence, septic encephalopathy includes not only inflammatory symptoms but also neurovascular diseases. These neurovascular involvements may render the septic encephalopathy to be complicated diseases. Conversely, several kinds of trials have been tackled to control the immunological response in sepsis without successful. Recently, however, several lines of evidence suggest the validity that electrical stimulation of vagus nerve on the cervix after onset of sepsis may regulate the over-expressing cytokines and result in better prognosis. Hence, in this chapter, septic encephalopathy is discussed from molecular mechanisms to future therapeutic potential for the patho-physiology, respectively, in the following section: (1) causes, (2) symptoms, (3) potential complications in the future studies.

Chapter 9 – Encephalitis is defined as inflammation of the brain parenchyma and occasionally involving the leptomeninges. Various viruses more often affect the brain, the commonest being Japanese encephalitis (JE).

The first epidemic of Japanese Encephalitis was recorded in 1871 in Japan and since then it has been a recurrent feature. It was recognized as an Arbovirus infection and caused another major epidemic in Japan in 1924. This virus was isolated in 1935 and named Japanese 'B' and the mosquito transmission was proved in 1938. It is numerically the most important global cause of Arboviral encephalitis with an estimated 30,000 to 50,000 cases and about 15,000 deaths (30 to 50 %) per annum. Similar epidemics of JE have also been reported from Eastern Siberia and various Asian countries. Japanese B is the only virus so far confirmed to cause epidemics in India. The classification of viral encephalitis is as under.

In: Encephalitis, Encephalomyelitis and Encephalopathies   ISBN: 978-1-62257-766-8
Editors: Andrew Ruiz and Douglas Fleming   © 2013 Nova Science Publishers, Inc.

Chapter 1

HIV-1-ASSOCIATED NEUROCOGNITIVE DISORDER: ROLE OF OXIDATIVE STRESS AND PROTECTION BY GENE DELIVERY OF ANTIOXIDANT ENZYMES

Jean-Pierre Louboutin and David S. Strayer*
Department of Pathology, Anatomy and Cell Biology,
Thomas Jefferson University, Philadelphia, PA, US

ABSTRACT

HIV encephalopathy covers a range of HIV-related brain dysfunction. The most severe is HIV-associated Dementia (HAD), which is the most common cause of dementia in adults under 40. HAD has become less common since Highly Active AntiRetroviral Therapy (HAART) was introduced. Before the introduction of HAART, most HAD patients showed subcortical dementia, with predominant basal ganglia involvement, manifesting as psychomotor slowing, Parkinsonism, behavioral abnormalities and cognitive difficulties. HIV-1 enters the Central Nervous System (CNS) soon after it enters the body. In the CNS, it is largely impervious to HAART. As survival with chronic HIV-1 infection improves, the number of people harboring the virus in their CNS increases. The prevalence of HIV-associated neurocognitive disorder (HAND) therefore continues to rise, and less fulminant forms of HAND such as minor neurocognitive/motor disorder (MCMD) have become more common than their more fulminant predecessors. HAND remains a significant independent risk factor for AIDS mortality. It is also becoming clear that the brain is an important reservoir for the virus, and neurodegenerative and neuroinflammatory changes may continue despite the use of HAART.

Neurons themselves are rarely infected by HIV-1, and neuronal damage is felt to be mainly indirect. HIV-1 infects resident microglia, periventricular macrophages, leading to increased production of cytokines and to release of HIV-1 proteins, the most likely neurotoxins, among which are the envelope (Env) protein (gp120) and HIV-1 *trans*-acting protein Tat.

We used model systems in which recombinant gp120, or Tat, proteins are directly injected into the striatum. The neurotoxicity of such recombinant proteins is highly

---

* Email address: jplouboutin@hotmail.com. Phone number: 215-983-0457.

reproducible and can be used as a tool for testing novel therapeutic interventions. However, HIV-1 infection of the brain is a chronic process. This is in part the reason why we developed experimental models of chronic HIV-1 neurotoxicity based on recombinant SV40 (rSV40) vector-modified expression of gp120 or Tat, in the brain.

As HIV-1 infection of the brain lasts the lifetime of affected individuals, and as eradication of CNS HIV-1 is currently not possible, control of the damage caused by the virus may represent a useful approach to treatment. It is known that gp120 and Tat induce oxidative stress in the brain, leading to neuronal apoptosis/death. One way to limit the final damage could be by limiting oxidative stress-related neurotoxicity. We used SV40 vectors for gene delivery of transgenes to the brain. These vectors deliver long-term transgene expression to brain neurons and microglia, when administered by several different routes. Intracerebral injection of SV(SOD1) or SV(GPx1) carrying the antioxidant enzymes, Cu/Zn superoxide dismutase (SOD1) or glutathione peroxidase (GPx1) respectively, into the rat caudate putamen (CP), significantly protects neurons from apoptosis caused by subsequent inoculation of recombinant HIV-1 envelope glycoprotein, gp120 and Tat at the same location. Vector administration into the lateral ventricle (LV) or cisterna magna, particularly if preceded by intraperitoneal mannitol, protects from intra-CP gp120-induced neurotoxicity comparably to intra-CP vector administration. The safety of SV(SOD1) and SV(GPx1) delivered intra-CP has been demonstrated in rats and in Rhesus macaques monkeys, and resulting transgene expression is very durable.

These models should provide a better understanding of the pathogenesis of HIV-1 in the brain as well as offer new therapeutic avenues.

INTRODUCTION

HIV-1 enters the Central Nervous System (CNS) soon after it enters the body. There, it is largely impervious to highly active anti-retroviral therapeutic drugs (HAART). Human immunodeficiency virus (HIV) encephalopathy covers a range of HIV-related CNS dysfunction. The most severe is HIV-associated dementia (HAD), which is the most common cause of dementia in adults under 40 (Mattson et al., 2005). HAD was estimated to affect as many as 30% of patients with advanced AIDS (Major et al., 2000), but has become less common since HAART was introduced (McArthur et al., 1993). This reduction probably reflects better control of HIV in the periphery, since antiretroviral drugs penetrate the CNS poorly. Before the introduction of HAART, most neuroAIDS patients showed subcortical dementia, with predominant basal ganglia involvement, manifesting as psychomotor slowing, Parkinsonism, behavioral abnormalities and cognitive difficulties (Koutsilieri et al., 2002). As survival with chronic HIV-1 infection improves, the number of people harboring the virus in their CNS increases. The prevalence of HIV-associated neurocognitive disorder (HAND) therefore continues to rise, and less fulminant forms of HAND such as minor neurocognitive/motor disorder (MCMD) have become more common than their more severe predecessors. HAND remains a significant independent risk factor for AIDS mortality (Major et al., 2000; Mattson et al., 2005; McArthur et al., 2005; Nath and Sacktor, 2006; Ances and Ellis, 2007; Antinori et al., 2007). However, the number of HIV-infected individuals over 50 years of age is rapidly growing, including patients taking HAART (Ances and Ellis., 2007). It has been suggested that in 10 years, 50% of AIDS patients in the United States will be over the age of 50. Moreover, it is becoming clear that the brain is an important reservoir for the virus, and neurodegenerative and neuroinflammatory changes may continue despite HAART (Nath and Sacktor, 2006).

PATHOGENESIS OF HAND

1. HIV-1 Proteins Neurotoxicity

The principal manifestations of central nervous system in HIV infection result from neuronal injury and loss and from extensive damage to the dendritic and synaptic structures in the absence of neuronal loss. Neurons themselves are rarely infected by HIV-1, and neuronal damage is felt to be mainly indirect. In fact, the pathogenesis of HAND largely reflects the neurotoxicity of HIV-1 proteins (Rumbaugh et Nath, 2006). HIV-1 infects resident microglia, periventricular macrophages and some astrocytes (Gonzalez-Scarano and Martin-Garcia, 2005; Ranki et al., 1995), leading to increased production of cytokines and to release of HIV-1 proteins, the most likely neurotoxins, among which are the envelope (Env) proteins gp120 and gp41 and the nonstructural proteins Nef, Rev, Vpr and Tat (Kaul et al., 2001; van de Bovenkamp et al., 2002; Mattson et al., 2005; King et al., 2006).

The HIV-1 *trans*-acting protein Tat, an essential protein for viral replication, is a key mediator of neurotoxicity. Brain areas that are particularly susceptible to Tat toxicity include the CA3 region and the dentate gyrus of the hippocampus and the striatum. Tat is internalized by neurons primarily through lipoprotein related protein receptor (LRP) and by activation of NMDA receptor (Eugenin et al., 2003, 2006). It also interacts with several cell membrane receptors, including integrins, VEGF receptor in endothelial cells and possibly CXCR4 (Ghezzi et al., 2000).

Tat can directly depolarize neuron membranes, independently of Na^+ flux (Magnuson et al., 1995) and may potentiate glutamate- and N-methyl-D-aspartate (NMDA)-triggered calcium fluxes and neurotoxicity (Magnuson et al., 1995). It promotes excitotoxic neuron apoptosis (Bonavia et al., 2001; Haughey et al., 2001) by activating endoplasmic reticulum pathways to release intracellular calcium ($[Ca^{2+}]i$) (Norman et al., 2008). Consequent dysregulation of calcium homeostasis (Kruman et al., 1998; Nath et al., 2000; Bonavia et al., 2001) leads to mitochondrial calcium uptake, caspase activation and, finally, neuronal death. Tat also increases levels of lipid peroxidation (Haughey et al., 2004) by generating the reactive oxygen species (ROS) superoxide (O_2^-) and hydrogen peroxide (H_2O_2). It activates inducible nitric oxide synthase (iNOS) to produce nitric oxide (NO), which binds superoxide anion to form the highly reactive peroxynitrite (ONOO) (Bonfoco et al., 1995).

Tat neurotoxicity has been reported in cultured cells, but fewer studies have demonstrated its neurotoxic properties *in vivo* (Jones et al., 1998; Bansal et al., 2000; Aksenov, et al. 2001, 2003; Theodore et al., 2006).

Despite evidence that Tat has been detected in the striatum of patients with HIV encephalitis (Wiley et al., 1996; Hudson et al., 2000), it is difficult to know the exact levels of Tat generated. Althouh mRNA for Tat was detected by RT-PCR in brain extracts from half (Hudson et al., 2000) or more (Wiley et al., 1996) of patients with HIV encephalitis, protein levels could not be measured by ELISA (Hudson et al., 2000). There are important differences between the situation in the striatum of patients with AIDS and models where Tat is directly injected into the CP. In these models, Tat is localized initially in extracellular space following intra-CP injection, then it is internalized in neurons and in some microglial cells, while the sites of production are focal in patients with HAND (i.e., microglial cells and infected macrophages). Direct injection of Tat results in acute injury, while production of Tat is more protracted in the brain of patients with HAND. The lesions of HAND reflect chronic injury caused by ongoing production of Tat, as well as other susbstances, by HIV-1-infected cells.

The HIV-1 *env* gene codes for gp120 which is cleaved into two major envelope glycoproteins, gp120 and gp41. Soluble gp120 can induce apoptosis in a wide variety of cells including lymphocytes, cardiomyocytes and neurons (Garden et al., 2004; Xu et al., 2004). HIV-1 gp120 may be directly neurotoxic at high concentrations (Meucci et al., 1998). Gp120-induced apoptosis has been demonstrated in studies in cortical cell cultures, in rat hippocampal slices and by intracerebral injections *in vivo* (Regulier et al., 2004). Gp120 binds neuron cell membrane co-receptors (CCR3, CCR5 and CXCR4) and elicits apoptosis, apparently via G-protein-coupled pathways (Kruman et al., 1998; Kaul and Lipton, 1999). Soluble gp120 also increases glial cell release of arachidonate, which impairs neuron and astrocyte reuptake of glutamate (Lipton et al., 1993), leading to prolonged activation of NMDA receptor with consequent disruption of cellular Ca2+ homeostasis (Dreyer et al., 1990). This process involves generation of superoxide and peroxide species, with resultant oxidative stress, and leads to neuron cell death after mitochondrial permeabilization, cytochrome c release and activation of caspases and endonucleases (Major et al., 2000).

The trans-membrane protein gp41 is elevated in patients with HAD. *In vitro*, gp41 can induce neuronal death in the nanomolar range, requires the presence of astrocytes, suggesting indirect mechanisms, involving iNOS, NO formation, depletion of glutathione and disruption of mitochondrial function (Adamson et al., 1996, 1999).

Other HIV-1 proteins (Vpr, Nef, Rev) are also involved in HAND neuropathogenesis. HIV-1 viral protein r (Vpr) is thought to be important for effective viral replication in the early stages of the infection. Vpr is present as a soluble protein within the blood serum and the CSF of patients infected with HIV-1 (Hoshino et al., 2007; Levy et al., 1994, 1995) and accumulates within these compartments to increasing concentrations as disease progresses toward the later stages of disease. As an extracellular protein, HIV-1 Vpr has been shown to negatively affect the survival of brain-resident cells, especially neurons and astrocytes, which are the cell types most sensitive to local insult; they become dysfunctional and are gradually lost as patients infected with HIV-1 advance towards AIDS (Ferrucci et al.; submitted). Some studies have shown that Vpr can directly induce neuronal apoptosis (Patel et al., 2000; Sabbah and Roques, 2005), and that Vpr can deregulate calcium secretion in neural cells (Rom et al., 2009).

The non-structural protein Nef is required for the proper budding of virions from HIV-infected cells. *In vitro*, Nef can be lethal for astrocytes and neurons and can increase the expression of matrix metalloproteinases (MMPs) (Trillo-Pazos et al., 2000). Abundant Nef expression has been shown in astrocytes of HIV-1-infected patients with neuronal damage (Ranki et al., 1995; Saito et al., 1994).

The HIV-1 phosphoprotein Rev is involved in the nuclear export of unspliced viral mRNAs. Extracellular Rev has neurotoxic properties. These ones have been demonstrated in rodents by intracerebroventricular injection of a synthetic peptide spanning the basic region of Rev causing neuronal death (Mabrouk et al., 1991).

2. HIV-1 Proteins and Astrocytes

Astrocytes have a role in HAND (Li and al., 2007). Several HIV-1 proteins can influence the role of astrocytes in HAND. Astroglial infection is characterized by an initial small burst in viral production followed by a state of persistent infection with the presence of multiple spliced short transcripts (encoding primarily the Nef protein), inefficient translation of structural proteins (gag and env), and almost undetectable levels of viral genomic transcripts (Gorry et al., 1999). Astrocytes could represent a reservoir for HIV-1. During late stage HIV-1 disease, an increased frequency of infiltrating monocytes and CD4+ T cells may deliver neurotoxic factors, such as chemokines and viral proteins (Tat, Vpr, gp120, and Nef) (Giulian et al., 1990), which stimulates astroglia to secrete an elevated amount of glutamate, increasing the overall level of excitotoxicity. This sequence of events could play a significant role in astrocytic and neuronal dysregulation, leading to mild to severe neurocognitive impairment. Tat also induces NOS in human astroglia (Liu et al., 2002) and monocyte chemoattractant protein-1 (MCP-1) is induced in HIV-1 Tat-stimulated astrocytes (Conant et al., 1998). Tat expression in astrocytes leads to astrocytes activation and neuronal death (Zhou et al., 2004).

ANIMAL MODELS OF HAND

There are no perfect models for HAND. Several animal systems have been used to study the pathogenesis of HIV-1-induced neurological disease. Many of them are based on other lentiviruses (i,e., simian immunodeficiency virus infection of macaques, feline immunodeficiency virus infection of cats, Visna-Maedi virus infection in sheep) (Hurtrel et al., 1992; Thormar et al., 2005: Lackner and Veazey, 2007). However, only small percentages of animals develop neurological manifestations in these models and the costs for using these species may be high. Transgenic expression of gp120 in mice has been studied (Toggas et al., 1994), but the gp120 in that model is mainly expressed in astrocytes, whereas in humans HIV-1 chiefly infects microglial cells. Other models based on introduction of HIV-infected macrophages into the brains of SCID mice have been proposed, but they suffer from the fact of human macrophages delivered into a murine brain (Avgeropoulos et al., 1998). Some models of ongoing exposure to Tat have been developed. For example, GFAP-driven, doxycycline-inducible Tat transgenic mice have been useful for mechanistic studies of Tat contribution to HAND. However, the reported data concerning neuronal TUNEL positivity are still debated (Bruce-Keller et al., 2008).

We (Agrawal et al., 2006, 2012; Louboutin et al., 2007a) and others (Bansal et al., 2000; Nosheny et al., 2004) have used model systems in which recombinant gp120, or Tat, proteins are directly injected into the striatum. The neurotoxicity of such recombinant proteins is highly reproducible and can be used as an interesting tool for testing novel therapeutic interventions. Administration of recombinant proteins is useful in understanding the effects of HIV-1 gene products, and so their individual contribution to the pathogenesis of HAND. However, HIV-1 infection of the brain is a chronic process, and its study would benefit from a model system allowing longer term exposure to HIV-1 gene product.

This is in part the reason why we developed experimental models of chronic HIV-1 neurotoxicity based on recombinant SV40 (rSV40) vector-modified expression of gp120 (Louboutin et al., 2009a) or Tat (Agrawal et al., 2012) in the brain.

OXIDATIVE STRESS IN HAND

1. Role of Oxidative Stress in HAND

Oxygen is vital for all living cells whether neuronal or not, but on the other hand it is potentially dangerous in excess. Oxygen has a role in glucose breakdown in mitochondria through oxidative phosphorylation and generates energy currency of cell, i.e. ATP (Uttara et al., 2009). Under physiologic conditions, reactive oxygen species (ROS), which include superoxide (O_2^-), hydrogen peroxide (H_2O_2) and hydroxyl radical (OH-), are generated at low levels and play important roles in signaling and metabolic pathways (Broughton et al., 2009). Oxidative stress arises due to the disturbances of the balance in pro-oxidant/antioxidant homeostasis that further causes the generation of ROS which are potentially toxic for neurons. There are several reasons why the brain is more susceptible to ROS. Glial cells require more oxygen and glucose consumption to generate continuous ATP pool *in vivo* for normal functioning of the brain as it is one of the busiest organs, making them more susceptible to oxygen overload, and thus to free radicals generation (Uttara et al., 2009). Neurons are particularly susceptible to ROS because of their biochemical composition. Brain contains high levels of fatty acids, which are particularly susceptible to peroxidation and oxidative modification. Double bonds of unsaturated fatty acids are hot spots for attack by free radicals that initiate cascade to damage neighbouring unsaturated fatty acids (Butterfield et al., 2002). Membrane lipids can undergo oxidation, producing cytotoxic lipid peroxidation products like malondialdehyde (MDA) and 4-hydroxynonenal (4-HNE). Finally, brain is lower in antioxidant activity compared to other tissues and has higher levels of iron in some areas (Uttara et al., 2009).

ROS levels are controlled by endogenous antioxidant such as superoxide dismutases (SOD), glutathione peroxidase (GPx1), glutathione and catalase. The tripeptide glutathione (γ-L-glutamyl-L-cysteinylglycine, GSH) is the key low molecular thiol antioxidant involved in the defense of brain cells against oxidative stress. A decrease in GSH levels has been connected to physiological processes such as aging and neurological disorders like Alzheimer's disease, epilepsy, and Parkinson's disease (Banerjee et al., 2010). Although GSH is the primary molecule involved in detoxification of ROS in the body, antioxidant enzymes like GPx1, are also known to play a role in this process (Steiner et al., 2006). During detoxification of peroxides, the enzyme GPx1 converts GSH to GSSG (glutathione disulphide).

Interaction of ROS with other tissue components produces a variety of other radicals: following activation of iNOS, NO can bind superoxide anion to form the highly reactive peroxynitrite (Bonfoco et al., 1995). The latter may attack lipids, proteins and DNA, to enhance oxidant-related injury. Mitochondria are the primary source of ROS involved in many brain tissue injuries (i.e., hypoxia, excitotoxicity). Once generated, mitochondrial ROS influence the release of cytochrome c and other apoptotic proteins from the mitochondria into the neuronal cytosol, which leads to apoptosis (Broughton et al., 2009). For example, once released into the cytosol, cytochrome c forms a complex referred to as an apoptosome with procaspase-9, apoptotic protease activating factor 1 (APAF-1) and dATP. The formation of the apoptosome activates caspase-9 which then cleaves other procaspases. The activation of caspase-3 by this process, among other effectors, has multiple effects including proteolysis of an inhibitor of the caspase-activated DNase (Sims and Muyderman, 2010). Thus, a link between oxidative stress and activation of some caspases seems highly probable.

Abnormalities in oxidative metabolism have been reported in many nervous system diseases. These include neurodegenerative diseases (Parkinson's disease, Alzheimer's disease, Huntington's disease, amyotrophic lateral sclerosis and cerebellar degeneration) (Dexter et al., 1987; Rosen et al., 1993; Beal, 1995; Smith and Perry, 1995; Smith et al., 1995), vascular diseases (ischemia–reperfusion) (Cao et al., 1998) or toxic reactions (chronic alcoholism) (Montoliu et al., 1994), as well as aging (Smith et al., 1991).

Oxidative stress plays a role in the development of HAND as well (Mollace et al., 2001; Turchan et al., 2003). Oxidative stress in HIV-1 dementia has been documented by analyses of brain tissue, including increased levels of lipid peroxidation product (i.e., HNE) and the presence of oxidized proteins. Serum levels of GSH and GPx1 are decreased in HIV-1 patients while MDA levels are increased (Steiner et al., 2006). A characteristic of patients infected with HIV-1 in late stage disease is diffuse intracellular oxidation in the form of decreased availability of GSH, the main cellular antioxidant and redox buffer, and augmented lipid oxidation, which triggers a cascade of downstream signaling events.

Membrane-associated oxidative stress correlates with HIV-1 dementia pathogenesis and cognitive impairment (Mattson et al., 2005). HNE-positive neurons have been demonstrated in the brains of patients with HIV-1 encephalitis (Turchan et al., 2003; Haughey et al., 2004; Cutler et al, 2004). In the case of HIV-1 infection, Tat and gp120 can elicit such oxidative stress (Mattson et al., 2005; Agrawal et al; 2007). Such oxidative stress can induce apoptosis in cultured neurons (Kruman et al., 1997). It can also damage neurons and cause cognitive dysfunction *in vivo* (Bruce-Keller et al., 1998). Tat and gp120 induce ceramide production in cultured neurons by triggering sphingomyelinase activity via a mechanism that involves induction of oxidative stress by CXCR4 activation (Mattson et al., 2005). Oxidative stress can play a role in HAND in other ways. Circulating toxins in the CSF, derived from HIV-1-infected cells, may damage mitochondria, leading to release of cytochrome c and then to a cascade of events leading to apoptosis (Mollace et al., 2001; Turchan et al., 2003). HIV-1 gp120 and Tat can cause free radical production, possibly as part of the signal-transduction pathways they activate (Mattson et al., 2005; Agrawal et al., 2007).

It is still unclear whether oxidative stress is the primary initiating event associated with neurodegeneration. However, a growing body of evidence implicates it as being involved in at least the propagation of cellular injury that leads to neuron death (Andersen, 2004). Earlier reports support the hypothesis that oxidative modifications of macromolecular cell components (lipids, proteins and nucleic acids) may be an early step in the mechanism of Tat and gp120 neurotoxicity (Askenov et al., 2001, 2003).

2. Oxidative Stress Associated with Tat

Tat-induced protein oxidation is well documented (Aksenov, et al. 2001, 2003) but its effects on lipid peroxidation have also been reported. We recently demonstrated that Tat activates multiple signaling pathways. In one of these, Tat-induced superoxide acts as an intermediate, while the other utilizes peroxide as a signal transducer (Agrawal et al., 2007).

Tat-mediated neurotoxicity may be associated with increased oxidative modifications of proteins (Askenov et al., 2001). For example, increased protein carbonyl formation, a well-known marker of protein oxidative damage, occurred early after Tat injection and coincided with the earliest changes in the amount of degenerating striatal neurons (Askenov et al., 2003). When the number of degenerating neurons reaches its peak 1 day after Tat administration, protein oxidation in striatal extracts decreased back to control levels, probably because oxidized proteins are prone to proteolytic degradation (Askenov et al., 2003). There was a later increase in protein carbonyl levels 7 days after Tat injection, possibly caused by Tat-induced compromise astrocytic functions (Askenov et al., 2003). However, astrocytosis and associated changes in protein oxidation were not sufficient to cause an additional neuronal cell death (Askenov et al., 2003). Tat increase in levels of protein oxidation may result from Tat-mediated increase of the production of prooxidants, as Tat can trigger the production of inflammatory products, which, in turn, may cause an excess of ROS (Bruce-Keller et al., 2001; Askenov et al., 2003).

Tat can also mediate neurotoxicity through lipid peroxidation. There are few reports concerning MDA levels in the brain after Tat injection, and there are no data concerning late time points after inoculation. In one study, repeated intravenous injection of 50 ng Tat during 5 days decreases brain levels of GSH and GPx1 and increases levels of MDA (Banerjee et al., 2010). Pretreatment of the animals with thiol antioxidant N-acetylcysteine amide (NACA) increased the GSH levels significantly, indicating that the antioxidant NACA was able to partially abrogate oxidative stress induced damage in these animals. A significant decrease in the activity of GPx1 was observed in animals treated with Tat, as compared to the controls, indicating that the overwhelming oxidative stress induced by these toxins deplete the antioxidant enzyme in the brain. Animals pretreated with NACA had GPx-1 levels similar to that of the control.

In one study, we injected Tat into the striatum. We observed elevated MDA levels persisting one week after Tat administration (Figure 1). The sustained MDA levels might be due to the longterm neuroinflammation, because it is known that increased production of inflammatory products induced by Tat may cause an excess formation of ROS (Askenov et al., 2003). However, persisting elevated MDA levels were not associated with continuing apoptosis. These data resemble to the ones observed when an increase in protein carbonyl levels seen 7 days after Tat injection was not accompanied by neuron death (Askenov et al., 2003). The present study did not identify the reason(s) why the number of apoptotic neurons does not increase with time, despite the inflammatory response and astrocytosis on one hand, and the persisting lipid peroxidation on the other hand; the origin of the lack of neuron death despite persisting oxidative stress (either lipid peroxidation or protein oxidative damage) is not clear.

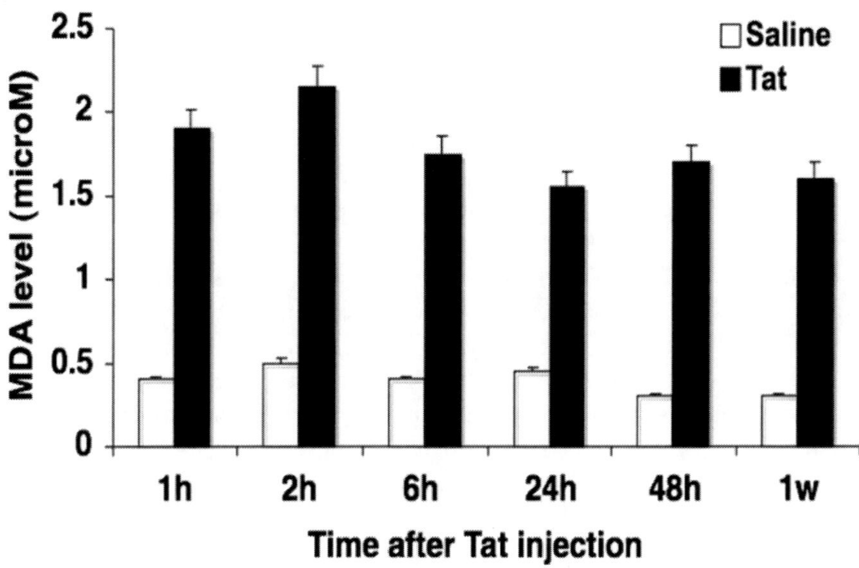

Figure 1. Lipid peroxidation after intra-CP injection of Tat. The HIV-1 nonstructural neurotoxic Tat protein was injected stereotaxically into the caudate-putamen (CP) according to the coordinates of Paxinos and Watson (1986). The levels of malondialdehyde (MDA), a lipid peroxidation product, were measured as previously reported (Louboutin et al., 2009a). Levels of MDA were significantly elevated after injection of Tat into the CP.

Tat is also known to trigger an increased production of inflammatory products, which in turn, may cause an excess formation of ROS (Bruce-Keller et al., 2001; Nath et al., 1999). Tat may induce superoxide and nitrite release in a microglial cell line (Bruce-Keller et al., 2001). An exposure of macrophages and astrocytes to Tat for few minutes *in vitro* is sufficient for sustained release of cytokines for several hours (Nath et al., 1999). Thus, Tat might promote oxidative stress and its consequences (i.e., neuron death) through activation of proinflammatory responses.

Numerous neurotoxic effects of Tat injection can be transient and can be observed only at early time points after its administration. Tat can decrease levels of GSH available to relieve oxidant stress (Banerjee et al., 2010). The presence of Tat in the striatum is short-lived after its injection. It is thus possible that after degradation of Tat, the levels of GSH are restored to normal levels. GSH could then protect neurons against ROS directly and indirectly, and could bind to lipid peroxidation products such as HNE, thereby providing neuroprotection (Steiner et al., 2006). Tat can also induce a lipid imbalance in neurons, resulting in an overproduction of sphingomyelin and ceramide, followed by increased levels of HNE (Steiner et al., 2006). Once Tat is degraded, the levels of ceramide and sphingomyelin return to control levels, limiting cellular dysfunction and death due to lipid imbalance. Tat can also trigger the expression of iNOS, leading to the overproduction of NO, which can react with superoxide anion to form peroxynitrite, a neurotoxic compound. NO can increase glutamate release from astrocytes, enhancing NMDA excitotoxicity (Steiner et al., 2006). If NO production can be increased shortly after Tat treatment, NO levels would decrease once Tat is degraded. Thus, if persisting increased MDA levels are observed one week after injection (possibly linked to continued neuroinflammation), they might not be enough, by themselves, to induce neuronal death at that time, because: 1) there is no direct interaction of Tat with neurons and no Tat-mediated dysregulation of calcium homeostasis one week after the injection; 2) some protective mechanisms (i.e, GSH) are probably restored at that time; 3) neurotoxic compounds like NO and peroxynitrite are probably not present at that time.

Oxidative stress is intimately linked with an integrated series of cellular phenomena, which all seem to contribute to neuronal death. Interaction between these various components is not necessarily a cascade but might be a cycle of events, of which oxidative stress is a major component (Andersen, 2004). Consequently, if one of the events, besides oxidative stress, is missing, neuronal death might be limited or not occur. Inhibition of oxidative stress therapeutically might act to 'break the cycle' of cell death. It might also suggest that a direct interaction of Tat with neurons is necessary for inducing early neuron death. However, it is difficult to directly answer the question whether Tat directly induces oxidative stress in neurons or promotes it through activation of proinflammatory responses. It remains plausible that direct interactions of Tat with neurons play the role of a triggering mechanism in the process of the development of oxidative stress and neurodegeneration (Askenov et al., 2003).

3. Gp120-induced Oxidative Stress

It has been previously shown that HIV-1 gp120 can cause lipid peroxidation and production of hydroxynonenal esters (Cutler et al., 2004), which can mediate oxidative stress-induced apoptosis of cultured neurons (Kruman et al., 1997) and can damage neurons and cause cognitive dysfunction in vivo (Bruce-Keller et al., 1998).

We showed that direct injection of recombinant gp120 into the striatum can induce lipid peroxidation attested by the measurement of MDA and the production of HNE (Figure 2) (Louboutin et al., 2010a). HNE was localized, not only in neurons, but also in endothelial cells and in astrocytes (not shown).

Experimental systems for studying the effects of gp120 and other HIV proteins on the brain have been limited to the acute effects of recombinant proteins *in vitro* or *in vivo*, or in chronic situation like simian immunodeficiency virus-infected monkeys. We described an experimental rodent model of ongoing gp120-induced neurotoxicity in which HIV-1 envelope gp120 is expressed in the brain using an SV40-derived gene delivery vector, SV(gp120) (Louboutin et al., 2009a). We previously demonstrated that SV40-derived vectors deliver long-term transgene expression to brain neurons and microglia, when administered by several different routes. rSV40s were employed in the current study because they transduce a wide range of cell types from humans and other mammals and deliver genes to cells in Go efficiently, including neurons, to achieve long-term transgene expression *in vitro* and *in vivo* (Strayer, 1999; Strayer et al., 1997, 2001). Moreover, they do not elicit immune response (McKee and Strayer, 2002). These vectors transduce > 95% of cultured human NT2-derived neurons, primary human neurons (Cordelier et al., 2003a,b) and microglia (Cordelier and Strayer, 2006) without detectable toxicity. When it is inoculated stereotaxically into the rat caudate putamen (CP), SV(gp120) caused a lesion in which neuron and other cell apoptosis continue for at least 12 weeks. Human immunodeficiency virus gp120 is expressed throughout this time, and some apoptotic cells are gp120 positive. MDA and HNE assays indicated that there was lipid peroxidation in these lesions (Figure 3). Similarly, protein oxidation was demonstrated by immunostaining for dinitrophenol (DNP) in brain cryosections, 1 week after injection of SV(gp120) (Figure 3). Thus, *in vivo* inoculation of SV(gp120) into the rat CP causes ongoing oxidative stress and apoptosis in neurons and may therefore represent a useful animal model for studying the pathogenesis and treatment of HIV-1 envelope-related brain damage.

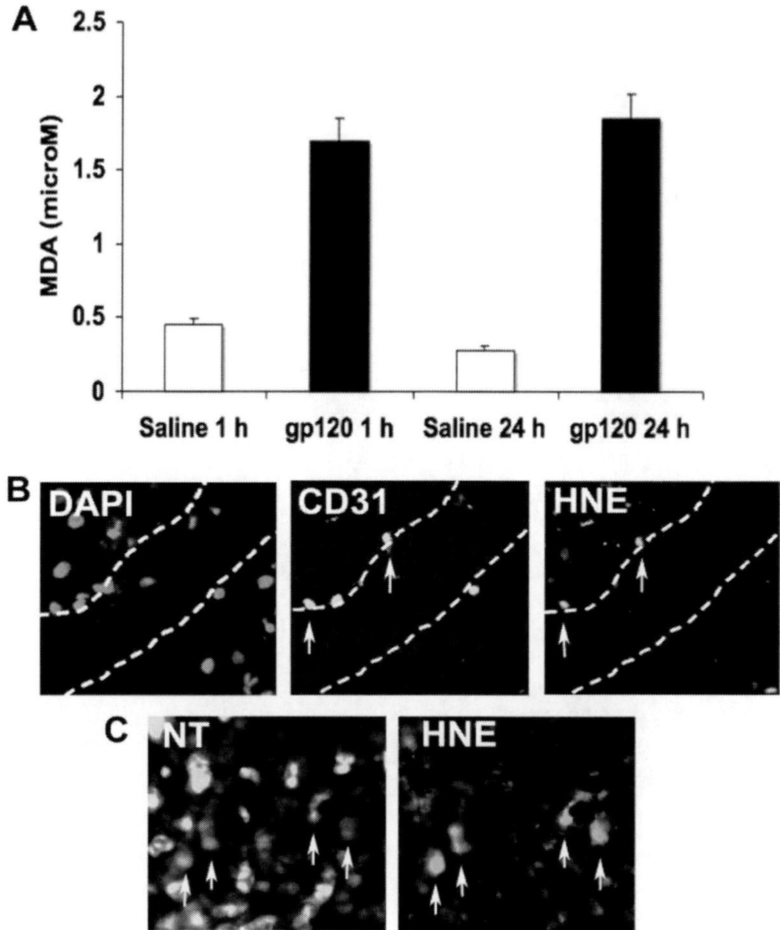

Figure 2. Lipid peroxidation after intra-CP injection of gp120. HIV-1 envelope glycoprotein gp120 (500 ng) was injected stereotaxically into the caudate-putamen (CP) according to the coordinates of Paxinos and Watson (1986). A. The levels of malondialdehyde (MDA), a lipid peroxidation product, were measured as previously reported (Louboutin et al., 2009a) and were significantly elevated. B,C. 4-hydroxynonenal esters (HNE), another product of peroxidation, was immunostained as previously reported (Rouger et al., 2001) and colocalized with endothelial cells immunopositive for CD31 (B, arrows), or cells positive for neurotrace, NT, a neuronal marker (C, arrows) (Morinville et al., 2004; Bigini et al., 2006; Louboutin et al., 2006, 2011c). Nuclei were stained by DAPI.

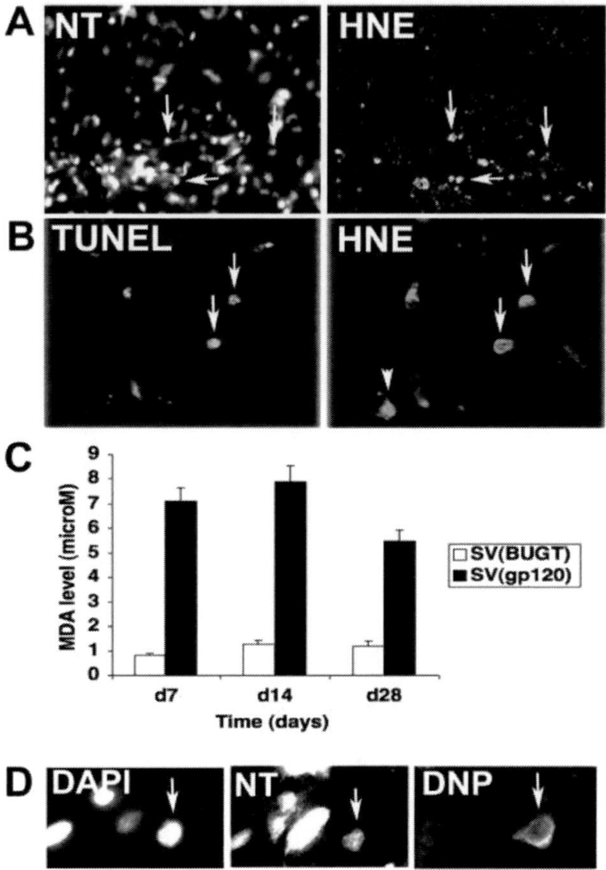

Figure 3. Oxidative stress in SV(gp120)-injected rats, a model of chronic exposure to gp120. In this model, HIV-1 envelope gp120 is expressed long term in the brain using an SV40-derived gene delivery vector, SV(gp120), injected into the caudate-putamen (CP). A. 4-hydroxynonenal esters (HNE), a product of peroxidation, was immunostained as previously reported (Rouger et al., 2001) and colocalized with cells positive for neurotrace, NT, a neuronal marker (arrows) (Morinville et al., 2004; Bigini et al., 2006; Louboutin et al., 2006, 2011c). B. Some of the HNE-positive cells were apoptotic, positive by TUNEL assay (arrows). Others were not (arrowhead). C. The levels of malondialdehyde (MDA), a lipid peroxidation product, were significantly elevated in SV(gp120) injected CPs, compared to the CPs injected with a control vector, SV(human bilirubin-uridine 5'-diphosphate-glucuronosyl-transferase) (BUGT), which was used here as negative control vector, with a non-toxic byproduct (Sauter et al., 2000). D. Protein oxidation was demonstrated by immunostaining for dinitrophenol (DNP), localized mainly in neurons positive for NT (arrows).

4. Oxidative Stress Associated with Vpr

Some recent studies have demonstrated the role of extracellular Vpr in impairing astrocytic metabolism by affecting the levels of the intracellular pools of both ATP and GSH, the main endogenous antioxidant molecule. Vpr-induced augmented production of ROS was related to an increase in the level of oxidized glutathione (GSSG) and a reduction in the overall GSH/GSSG ratio. This event was almost entirely suppressed by treatment with an anti-Vpr antibody or cotreatment with the antioxidant molecule N-acetyl-cysteine (NAC) (Ferrucci et al., submitted).

ANTIOXIDANT THERAPEUTIC APPROACHES IN HAND

1. Rationale and Therapeutic Options

As HIV-1 infection of the brain lasts the lifetime of affected individuals, and as eradication of CNS HIV-1 is currently not possible, control of the damage caused by the virus may represent a useful approach to treatment. This could entail limiting oxidative stress-related neurotoxicity.

A. Experimental Data

Antioxidant therapeutic options targeting oxidative stress can be artificially divided as targeting upstream and downstream pathways.

Upstream Antioxidant Therapy

Upstream preventive treatment is based on prevention of free radical generation, regulation of neuronal protein interaction with redox metals (i.e. Fe) and maintaining normal cellular metabolism. Our daily diet contains several natural antioxidants (lipoic acid, vitamins E and C, β-carotene). Antioxidant therapy involving endogenous enzymes and some anti-inflammatory drugs constitute upstream therapy in ROS generation and can prevent downstream neurodegeneration. Oxyradicals have a very short life and thus can be inactivated by antioxidants before they can inflict damage to proteins, lipids or nucleic acids. Two mechanisms can be described: inactivation of oxyradicals by dietary antioxidant like vitamin E, vitamin C, and replacement of esterified membrane phospholipids with polyunsaturated fatty acids by dietary supplementation with essential fatty acids (Uttara et al.; 2009).

Some components have been studied in models of HAND or can be useful in this context. Vitamin E can block the neurotoxicity induced by CSF of patients with HIV dementia (Turchan et al., 2003). Flavinoids are a group of compounds made by plants that have antioxidant and neuroprotective properties. This class of molecules has weak estrogen-receptor-binding properties and thus, do not have the side effects of estradiol. It has been described that diosgenin, a plant-derived estrogen present in yam and fenugreek can prevent neurotoxicity by HIV-1 proteins and by CSF from patients with HIV dementia (Turchan et al., 2003). Other interesting molecules include resveratrol, found in grape skins, red wine, and peanuts, as well as genistein and quercetin, found in soybeans. Polyphenols are a group of compounds with antioxidant properties. Among them, curcumin can induce stress response-protective genes, such as heme oxygenase 1 (HO-1), and can protect against heavy-metal insult to the brain and 6-OHDA in a model of Parkinson's disease, probably through reduction of lipid peroxidation and inhibition of iNOS, NF-kappaB and cyclooxygenase-2 (Steiner et al., 2006). Selenium is a key molecule in GPx1 metabolism. Some HIV-infected patients have low levels of selenium. Because selenium supplementation increases GPx1 activity, it might be beneficial in these patients. N-acetyl-L-cysteine (NAC) is a nutritional supplement precursor in the formation of the antioxidant glutathione in the body and its sulfhydryl group confers antioxidant effects and is able to reduce free radicals. NAC injected i.p. into rodents increases glutathione levels in the brain and protects the CNS against the damaging effects of hydroxyl radicals and lipid peroxidation product acrolein (Pocernich et al., 2000). However, NAC itself does not cross the BBB easily. In addition, bioavailability of NAC is very low because its carboxylic group loses its proton at physiological pH, making the compound negatively charged and consequently less permeable (Steiner et al., 2006). N-acetylcysteine amide (NACA), a modified form of NAC, where the carboxyl group has been replaced by an amide group, has been found to be more effective in neurotoxic cases because of its ability to permeate cell membranes and the blood-brain barrier (BBB). Treatment of animals injected intravenously with gp120, Tat and methamphetamine METH by NACA significantly rescued the animals from oxidative stress. Further, NACA-treated animals had significantly less BBB permeability as compared to the group treated with gp120+Tat+METH alone, indicating that NACA can protect the BBB from oxidative stress-induced damage in gp120, Tat and METH exposed animals (Banerjee et al., 2010).

Downstream Antioxidant Therapy

The therapeutic coverage of post oxidative stress events can be done by downstream antioxidant therapy. Non steroidal anti-inflammatory drugs (NSAIDS) limit the infiltration of macrophages and can reduce the inflammatory cascade induced by oxidative stress. CPI-1189, a nitrone related compound, is supposed to regulate the pro-inflammatory cytokine cascade of genes in primary glial cells (Uttara et al., 2009). Minocycline is a tetracycline-derived compound that demonstrated neuroprotective profile in several models of neurodegeneration. The molecule has significant anti-inflammatory actions and can easily cross the BBB. *In vitro* data show that minocycline protected mixed neuronal cultures in an oxidative stress assay and has effective antioxidant properties with radical-scavenging potency similar to that of vitamin E (Kraus et al., 2005). Furthermore, minocycline treatment suppressed viral load in the brain, decreased the expression of CNS inflammatory markers and reduced the severity of encephalitis in a SIV model of HIV dementia (Zink et al., 2005). A chemical moiety that resembles vitamin E in its chemical structure is the female sex hormone estrogen (estradiol) that contains a phenolic free radical scavenging site and acts as an antioxidant. It actually has the capability to prevent an upstream neurodegeneration and downstream the oxidative overload (Uttara et al., 2009). Estrogen replacement may result in improvement of cognitive function in several neurodegenerative disorders and conversely estrogen deficiency has been considered as a risk factor in some of them. Estradiol can protect against the neurotoxic effects of HIV-1 proteins in human neuronal cultures, probably by protecting the neuronal mitochondria in a receptor-independent manner (Turchan et al., 2003). However, estradiol has well known side effects in women (potential risk of developing breast or uterine cancer), and cannot be used in men or children because of feminizing effects (Steiner et al., 2006). It has been shown that several novel antioxidants (ebselen, diosgenin) can protect *in vitro* against neurotoxicity induced by CSF from patients with HV dementia (Turchan et al., 2003).

It is likely that neuroprotective therapies should benefit from multiple and combination approaches targeting different aspects and pathways of the oxidative-stress insult. For example, coupling a potent antioxidant with a compound that modifies downstream signaling pathways (i.e., minocycline) could provide a synergistic neuroprotective effects, at lower doses (and thus with less toxicity) that each molecule could achieve alone. The combination of HAART with an antioxidant compound and a molecule involved in downstream antioxidant therapy could be a promising avenue in the treatment of HAND (Steiner et al., 2006). However, it should be reminded that one of the challenges in designing antioxidants to protect the CNS against ROS is the crossing of the BBB.

B. Clinical Trials

A few antioxidants have been tried in small prospective controlled studies in HAND. However, the findings have all been relatively disappointing so far. Selegiline (L-deprenyl), which mechanism of action is speculative, albeit it might decrease the production of ROS and serve as an anti-apoptotic factor, was used in 2 double-blind controlled studies in the pre-HAART era. The first trial involving patients with minor cognitive and motor dysfunction (MCMD) showed improvement in verbal learning and trends for improvement in recall (Consortium D, 1998; Sacktor et al., 2000). The second study was a smaller study in patients with MCMD and HIV dementia and showed significant improvement in delayed recall. However, other tests were not improved. A slight improvement was noted in patients treated with OPC-14117, a lipophilic compound structurally similar to vitamin E that acts as an antioxidant by scavenging superoxide radicals (Consortium D, 1997). CPI-1189, a lipophilic antioxidant that scavenges superoxide anion radicals and block the neurotoxicity of gp120 and TNF-alpha (Pulliam et al., 2001), showed no effect on neurocognition in patients with MCMD and HIV dementia (Clifford et al., 2002).

2. Gene Delivery of Antioxidant Enzymes in HAND

A. Introduction

In order to deliver potent antioxidant compounds to the brain, we used gene transfer of antioxidant enzymes. Gene transfer of antioxidant enzymes has been studied in numerous models of neurological disorders by using diverse viral vectors (Watanabe et al., 2003; Hoehn et al., 2003; Ridet et al., 2006). We used rSV40 vectors to deliver SV(SOD1) or SV(GPx1) carrying the antioxidant enzymes Cu/Zn superoxide dismutase (SOD1) or glutathione peroxidase (GPx1) respectively, into the rat caudate putamen (CP). The safety of SV(SOD1) and SV(GPx1) delivered intra-CP has been demonstrated in rats and in Rhesus macaques monkeys, and resulting transgene expression is very durable (Louboutin et al., 2011a). Transgene expression of antioxidant enzymes can also be achieved through intravenous injection (Louboutin et al., 2010b).

Mitochondria are a major site of production of superoxide in normal cells and probably contribute to increased oxidative stress in numerous diseases. Overexpression of mitochondrial Mn^{2+}-superoxide dismutase results in moderate reductions in infarction in temporary ischemia. Glutathione, the major water-soluble antioxidant, is localized in both the cytosol and the mitochondria. Mice overexpressing the cytosolic enzyme $Cu^{2+}Zn^{2+}$-superoxide dismutase develop smaller infarcts than wild-type ones, with a decrease in multiple events associated with mitochondrially mediated apoptosis, including the release of cytochrome c (Sims and Muyderman, 2010). It is thus possible that cytosolic overexpression of antioxidant enzymes delivered by SV40-derived vectors can mitigate the apoptotic events linked to mitochondria.

B. Gene Delivery of Antioxidant Enzymes Mitigates Oxidative Stress in Animal Models of HAND

We studied acute exposure to Tat by injecting recombinant Tat protein into the CP. Acute Tat exposure induced lipid peroxidation. Prior administration of recombinant SV40 vectors carrying antioxidant enzymes SOD1 or GPx1 protected from Tat-induced oxidative injury (Figure 4).

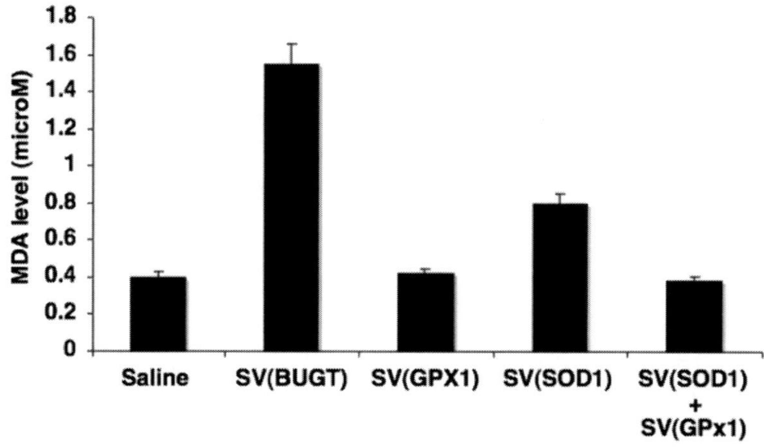

Figure 4. Tat-induced oxidative stress is mitigated by rSV40 vectors-mediated gene delivery of antioxidant enzymes. Prior administration of recombinant SV40 vectors carrying the antioxidant enzymes Cu/Zn superoxide dismutase (SOD1) or glutathione peroxidase (GPx1), SV(DOD1) and SV(GPx1) respectively, into the rat caudate putamen (CP), reduced Tat-induced lipid peroxidation, as measured by the levels of malondialdehyde (MDA). SV(BUGT) was used as a control vector. Note that the reduction in MDA levels was greater when SV(SOD1) and SV(GPx1) were injected together.

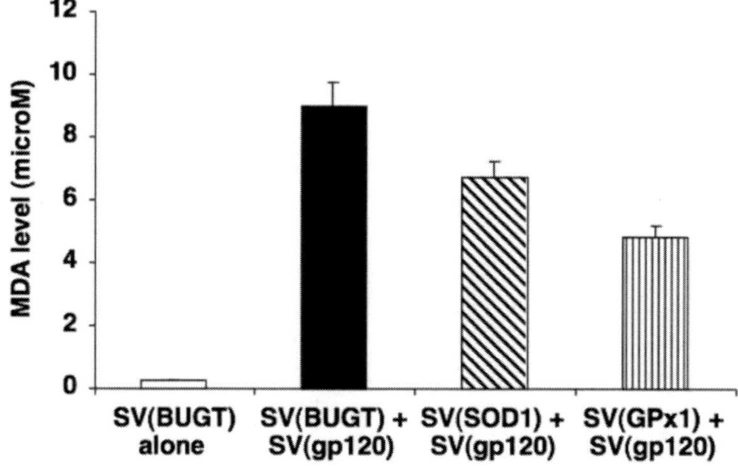

Figure 5. Gene transfer of antioxidant enzymes reduces SV(gp120)-induced lipid peroxidation. Prior administration of recombinant SV40 vectors carrying the antioxidant enzymes Cu/Zn superoxide dismutase (SOD1) or glutathione peroxidase (GPx1) respectively, into the rat caudate putamen (CP), was protective against SV(gp120)-induced lipid peroxidation, as measured by the levels of malondialdehyde (MDA). SV(BUGT) was used as a control vector.

Prior administration of recombinant SV40 vectors carrying antioxidant enzymes, SOD1 or GPx1, was similarly protective against SV(gp120)-induced oxidative injury (Figure 5).

C. Protection Against gp120-elicited Apoptosis and Neuronal Loss by SV40-mediated Gene Delivery of Antioxidant Enzymes

Gp120-induced Apoptosis of Striatal Neurons

Intracerebral injection of SV(SOD1) or SV(GPx1) into the rat caudate putamen (CP), induces long-lasting transgene expression and significantly protects neurons from apoptosis (Figure 6) and neuronal loss caused by subsequent inoculation of recombinant HIV-1 envelope glycoprotein, gp120 at the same location (Agrawal et al., 2006; Louboutin et al., 2007a,b; Louboutin et al., 2009b). Vector administration into the lateral ventricle (LV) (Louboutin et al., 2007b) or cisterna magna (CM) (Louboutin et al., 2012a), particularly if preceded by intraperitoneal mannitol, protects from intra-CP gp120-induced neurotoxicity comparably to intra-CP vector administration (Figure 7).

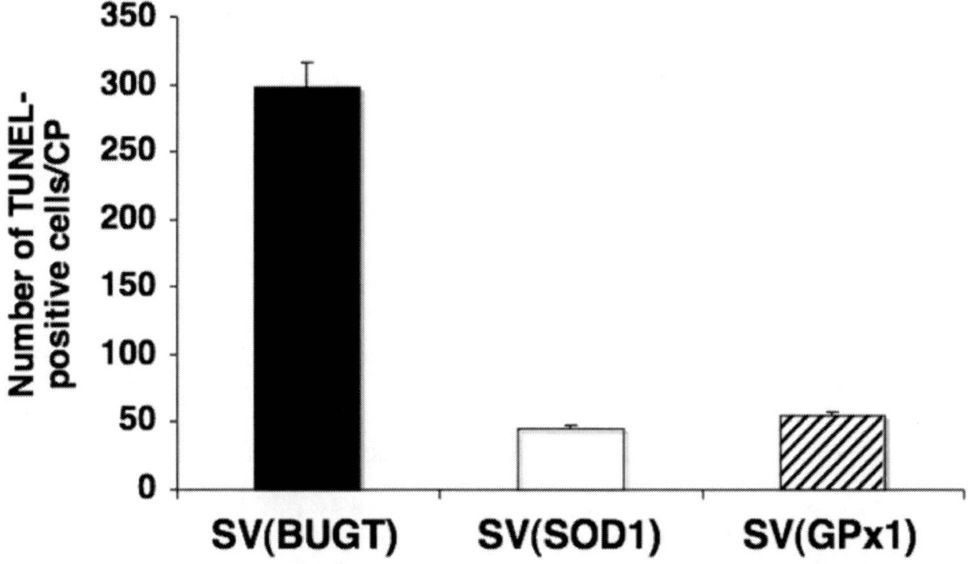

Figure 6. SV40-mediated gene delivery of antioxidant enzymes protects against gp120-induced apoptosis. SV(SOD1) and SV(GPx1) were injected into the CP one month before the inoculation of gp120 into the same structure. Brains were harvested one day after gp120 challenge and analyzed for apoptotic cells by TUNEL assay. Apoptotic cells were counted using morphometric methods (Mandel et al., 1998; Louboutin et al., 2006) after TUNEL assay. Significantly less TUNEL-positive, apoptotic, neurons were enumerated in CPs injected with SV(SOD1) and SV(GPx1), compared to CPs injected with a control vector, SV(BUGT).

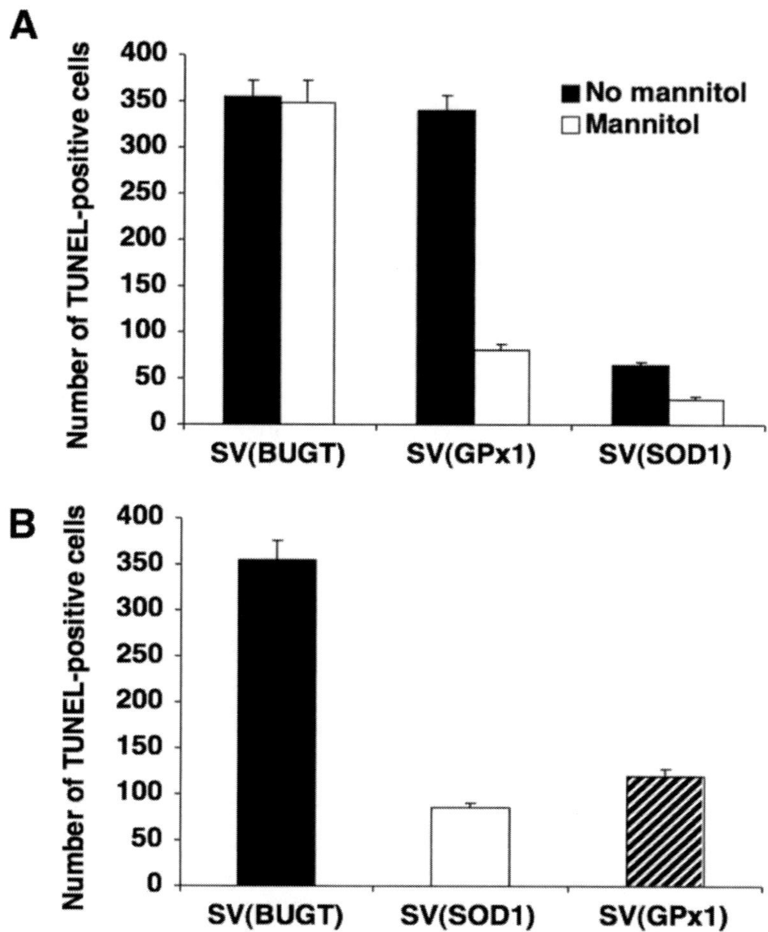

Figure 7. Intraperitoneal injection of mannitol increases gene delivery and protection efficiency after administration of SV(SOD1) and SV(GPx1) into the lateral ventricle (LV) and Cisterna Magna (CM). Mannitol was injected i.p. before the administration of SV(SOD1), SV(GPx1) or a control vector, SV(BUGT), either into the LV or the CM. Gp120 was injected into the CP one month later and TUNEL assay was performed on brain sections harvested one day after gp120 inoculation. A. There were significantly less apoptotic cells when administration of SV(SOD1) and SV(GPx1) was preceded by injection of mannitol. B. Significantly less TUNEL-positive less were enumerated in the CPs of rats whose CM has been injected by SV(SOD1) or SV(GPx1), compared to rats administered with SV(BUGT).

Antioxidant Enzymes Gene Delivery Mitigates SV(gp120)–induced Apoptosis

SV(SOD1) and SV(GPx1) were administered into the CP one month before the injection of SV(gp120) in the same structure. Gene delivery of antioxidant enzymes protected against apoptosis in this animal model of protracted exposure to gp120 (Figure 8).

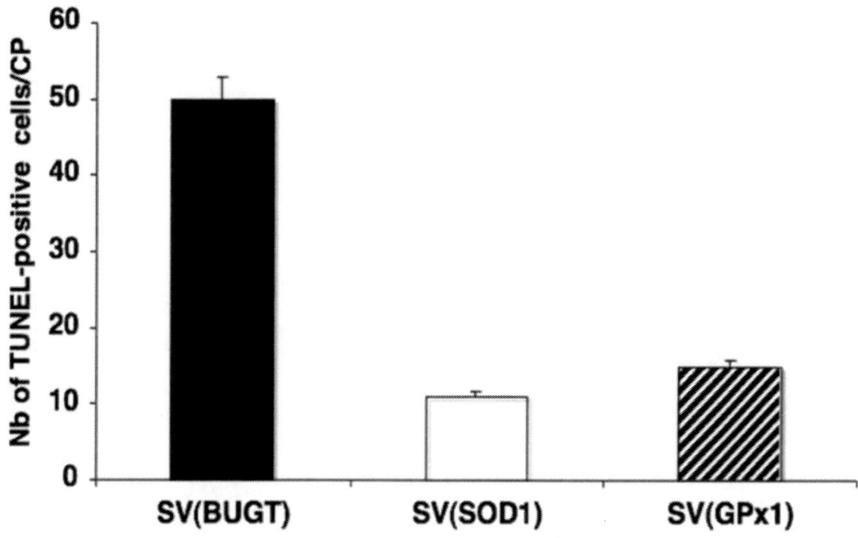

Figure 8. Gene delivery of SOD1 and GPx1 mitigates SV(gp120)-induced apoptosis. SV(SOD1), SV(GPx1) or SV(BUGT), a control vector, were administered into the CP one month before the inoculation of SV(gp120) into the same structure. One week thereafter, brains were harvested, TUNEL assay was performed, and TUNEL-positive cells were enumerated. Significantly less apoptotic cells were seen in the CPs injected with SV(SOD1) or SV(GPx1) compared to the CPs administered with SV(BUGT).

Role of ROS in gp120-induced Loss of Dopaminergic Neurons

We also examined the role of ROS in the loss of dopaminergic neurons (DNs) from the substantia nigra (SN) in HAD. The frequency of Parkinson-like symptomatology, and DN loss, in HAD is often attributed to nonspecific DN fragility to oxidative stress. Cultured DN were more sensitive to ROS than non-dopaminergic neurons (RN): DN underwent apoptosis at far lower H_2O_2 concentrations than RN. Gene delivery of GPx1, which detoxifies H_2O_2, largely protected both neuron types. HIV-1 envelope, gp120, which elicits oxidative stress in neurons, caused apoptosis more readily in DN than in RN. However, unlike apoptosis caused by H_2O_2, gp120-induced DN apoptosis was specific: DNs were specifically more sensitive than RN to receptor-mediated [Ca(2+)](i) fluxes triggered by gp120. Gp120-induced Ca(2+) signaling in both neuron types was inhibited by GPx1 or SOD1, implicating superoxide and peroxide in ligand (gp120)-induced signaling upstream of Ca(2+) release from intracellular stores. *In vivo*, rats given 10 ng of gp120 stereotaxically showed rapid DN loss within the SN, while loss of RN in the SN and CP was slower and required > or =100 ng of gp120. Furthermore, gp120 injected into the CP was transported axonally retrograde to the SN, causing delayed DN loss there. This, too, was prevented by SOD1 or GPx1. DNs are therefore specifically hypersensitive to gp120-induced apoptosis, signaling for which involves ROS intermediates. These findings may help explain why DN loss and Parkinson's-like dysfunction predominate in HAD (Sardar et al., 1996; Ramachandran et al., 1997; Mirsattari et al., 1998) and may apply to other neurodegenerative diseases involving the SN (Agrawal et al., 2010).

D. Gene Delivery of Antioxidant Enzymes Inhibits HIV-1 gp120-induced Expression of Caspases

Caspases are implicated in neuronal death in neurodegenerative and other Central Nervous System (CNS) diseases. The caspases family of proteases is conserved from nematodes through mammals. They are central to apoptotic death and are expressed as inactive zymogens that become cleaved during apoptosis (Ribe et al., 2008). Initiator caspases (among them caspases 8 and 9) autoactivate and self-process upon recruitment to adaptor proteins. Then, they proceed to cleave and thereby activate the executioner/effector caspases (among them caspases 3 and 6). Activated executioner/effector caspases proceed to process key structural and nuclear proteins and thereby cause the disassembly and death of the cell (Madden and Cotter, 2008). Two major caspases pathways have been described: the intrinsic pathway is initiated by cytochrome c release from the mitochondrion while the extrinsic pathway is initiated by the binding of ligands to plasma-membrane death receptors (Sims and Muyderman, 2010).

Intrinsic apoptosis pathway is required for fetal and postnatal brain development, but is downregulated through the suppression of the expression of one of its key mediator, caspase-3 (Madden and Cotter, 2008). During stroke and neurodegenerative diseases, some caspases are upregulated in the brain (Ribe et al., 2008). Cerebral ischemia triggers both the intrinsic and extrinsic pathways of apoptosis (Broughton et al., 2009; Sims and Muyderman, 2010). Mounting evidence suggests the involvement of caspases in the disease process associated with neurodegenerative diseases such as Alzheimer's disease (AD) (Rohn, 2010) and amyotrophic lateral sclerosis (ALS) (Madden and Cotter, 2008).

The involvement of caspases in HIV-1 neurotoxicity has been documented *in vitro* and *in vivo*. Higher levels of caspase-3 and caspase-6 have been shown in the brains of patients with HAD (Petito and Roberts, 1995; James et al., 1999; Kaul et al., 2001; Noorbakhsh et al., 2010). Both HIV-1 neurotoxins gp120 and Tat significantly increase caspase-3 activation in striatal neurons *in vitro*. However, gp120 acts in large part through the activation of caspase(s), while Tat-induced neurotoxicity is also accompanied by activating an alternative pathway involving endonuclease G (Singh et al., 2004). Tat can induce both caspases 3/7 and 9 in hippocampal cell cultures (Askenov et al., 2009). Increased expression of caspase-3 has been shown in neurons following exposure to Tat (Bonavia et al., 2001; Kruman and Mattson, 1999; Kruman et al., 1998; Singh et al., 2004) and to gp120 (Nosheny et al., 2006, 2007; Bachis et al., 2006; Ahmed et al., 2009). In HIV-1 transgenic mice, Tat induction increased the percentage of neurons expressing caspase-3 (Bruce-Keller et al., 2008). Caspase-3-positive cells were also observed in a model of protracted exposure to gp120, SV(gp120) (Louboutin et al., 2009a).

However, so far, no study was focused on the expression of different caspases following gp120 injection. We studied the effect of gp120 on different caspases (3, 6, 8, 9) expression. Caspases production increased in the rat CP 6h after gp120 injection into the same structure. The expression of caspases peaked by 24h. Caspases colocalized mainly with neurons. There was a relationship with the concentration of gp120 injected. Both initiator (caspases 8 and 9) and effector/executioner (caspases 3 and 6) were increased after gp120 injection. We showed that about 70% of caspase-8- and 9-positive cells were TUNEL-positive while about 60% of caspase-3- and 6-positive cells were TUNEL-positive one day after intra-CP injection of gp120 (Louboutin et al., 2012b). These results suggest that not all caspases-positive cells undergo apoptosis, at least as assessed by the methods used here and/or at the time points we considered. It is also possible that apoptosis will occur in the remaining caspases-positive cells at later time points. Gp120-induced caspase-3 activity may also be causing nonlethal neuron injury. As previously noted (Bruce-Keller et al., 2008), if cell death in response to caspase-3 depends on total enzyme activity within a cell, the caspase-3 activity detected may be below the threshold required to initiate neuron death. This is difficult to determine based on immunocytochemistry. It has also been shown that activated caspase-3 rapidly degrades itself (Cribbs et al., 2004).

As previously described, a link between oxidative stress and activation of some caspases seems highly probable. Prior gene delivery of the antioxidant enzymes SOD1 or GPx1 into the CP before injecting gp120 there reduced levels of gp120-induced caspases, recapitulating the effect of antioxidant enzymes on gp120-induced apoptosis observed by TUNEL (Figure 9). Thus, HIV-1 gp120 increased caspases expression in the CP. Prior antioxidant enzyme treatment mitigated production of these caspases, probably by reducing ROS levels. While the present study strongly implicates caspases 3, 6, 8 and 9, additional studies are needed to determine the relative contribution of the various caspases to neuronal demise in HAND.

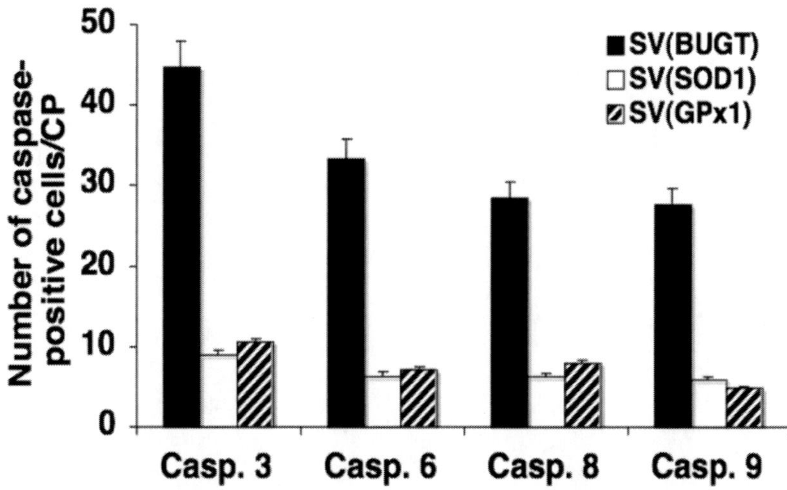

Figure 9. Reduction of gp120-induced caspases expression by gene delivery of antioxidant enzymes. SV(SOD1), SV(GPx1) or a control vector, SV(BUGT) were injected into the CP one month before inoculation of gp120. Expression of different caspases was then analyzed by immunocytochemistry one day after gp120 injection into the CP. Prior gene delivery of the antioxidant enzymes SOD1 or GPx1 into the CP before injecting gp120 there reduced levels of gp120-induced caspases, recapitulating the effect of antioxidant enzymes on gp120-induced apoptosis observed by TUNEL. SV(BUGT) had no effect.

E. Gp120-mediated Abnormalities of the Blood-Brain Barrier Are Mitigated by SV(SOD1) and SV(GPx1)

Reduction of MMPs Levels

Reactive oxygen species are important in the pathogenesis of HIV-induced CNS injury (Sacktor et al., 2004) and can be induced in brain endothelial cells by HIV-1 gp120 and Tat (Ullrich et al., 2000; Price et al., 2005, 2006). Although damage to the BBB has been documented in patients with HIV-related encephalopathy (Petito and Cash, 1992; Power et al., 1993; Avison et al., 2004), the exact mechanism by which this injury occurs is still debated (Toneatto et al., 1999; Huang et al., 1999; Dallasta et al., 1999; Banks et al., 1999, 2001, 2005; Cioni et al., 2002; Annunziata et al., 2003; Kanmogne et al., 2005, 2007; Eugenin et al., 2006). We used animal models of HAND to characterize abnormalities of the BBB in this context. Exposure to gp120, whether acute (by direct intra-CP injection) or chronic (using SV(gp120), an experimental model of ongoing production of gp120) disrupted the BBB, and led to leakage of vascular contents into the area of gp120 exposure. Gp120 was directly toxic to brain endothelial cells and gp120-mediated BBB abnormalities were related to lesions of brain microvessels (Louboutin et al., 2010c). Abnormalities of the BBB may reflect the activity of proteolytic enzymes, particularly matrix metalloproteinases (MMPs). MMPs are a family of neutral proteases that are grouped according to their protein structures. MMP-2 and MMP-9 are considered gelatinases (Clark *et al.*, 2008), and are enzymatically activated by the cleavage of precursor propeptides. These target laminin, a major BBB component, and attack the tight junctions between endothelial cells and BBB basal laminae. MMP-2 and MMP-9 were upregulated following intra-CP gp120-injection. Gp120 greatly dimished total CP content of laminin and tight junction proteins. Reactive oxygen species have been reported to activate MMPs. Injecting gp120 into the CP induced lipid peroxidation, assessed by increased MDA levels. One product of gp120-triggered lipid peroxidation, HNE, was immunolocalized to vascular endothelial cells. Moreover, gene transfer of antioxidant enzymes using recombinant SV(SOD1) and SV(GPx1) protected against gp120-induced BBB abnormalities (Figure 10). BBB injury has also been linked to NMDA, which upregulates the proform of MMP-9 and increases MMP-9 gelatinase activity (Manabe et al., 2005). Using the NMDA receptor (NMDAR-1) inhibitor, memantine, we observed partial protection from gp120-induced BBB injury (Louboutin et al., 2010a).

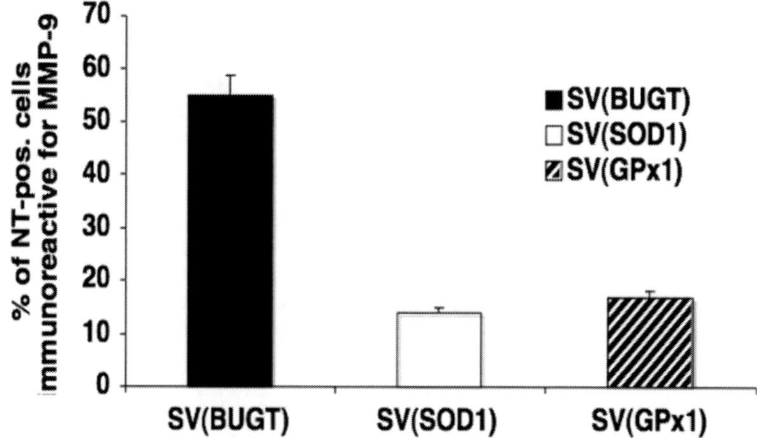

Figure 10. Neuronal expression of MMP-9 is decreased by SV(SOD1) and SV(GPx1). CPs received either SV(SOD1), SV(GPx1), or the control vector, SV(BUGT), then brains were challenged one month later by gp120 with the brains being harvested one day after gp120 inoculation. Matrix metalloproteinase MMP-9 expression was studied by immunocytochemistry one day after gp120 injection. Neuronal cells, positive for NT, and immunopositive for MMP-9 were enumerated. Significantly less MMP-9-positive neurons were counted in the CPs injected with SV(SOD1) or SV(GPx1) compared to the CPs administered with SV(BUGT).

MMPs are upregulated in different neurological diseases and models of CNS injury (Rosenberg, 2002; Gu et al. 2002; Yong et al., 2001; Lo et al., 2002; Gursoy-Ozdemir et al., 2004; Zozulya et al., 2007; Haorah et al., 2008). Various factors, such as ROS, NO, and proteases such as plasmin and stromelysin-1, are involved in MMP activation and upregulation in CNS injury (Asahi et al., 2000; Gasche et al., 2001; Kim et al., 2003). MMPs have been reported in the cerebrospinal fluid of HIV-1 infected patients (Sporer et al., 1998; Liuzzi et al., 2000) as well as in models of HIV-1 encephalopathy (Marshall et al., 1998; Toschi et al., 2001; Conant et al., 2004; Russo et al., 2007). In rapidly progressing simian immunodeficiency virus-infected monkeys, MMP-9 levels correlate with motor and cognitive deficits (Berman et al., 1999). Moreover, cerebrospinal fluid levels of the urokinase-type plasminogen activator receptor, which plays an important role in degradation of extracellular matrix, and hence BBB injury, are elevated in patients with HIV dementia (Cinque et al., 2004).

Restoring the Balance between MMPs and TIMPs

Relatively little is known about the roles of ROS and oxidative stress in the balance between MMPs and their endogenous tissue inhibitors (TIMPs). More than 20 MMPs and four TIMPs act together to control tightly temporally restricted, focal proteolysis of extracellular matrix (ECM) (Dzwonek *et al.*, 2004). Once activated, MMPs are subject to inhibition by specific TIMPs that bind MMPs non-covalently (Dzwonek *et al.*, 2004). Tissue destruction by MMPs is regulated by TIMPs and TIMPs prevent excessive MMP-related degradation of extracellular matrix components. The balance between MMPs and TIMPs is linked to ECM remodeling and imbalance between TIMPs and MMPs can lead to excessive degradation of matrix components as in rheumatoid arthritis. Tumor metastasis and angiogenesis may also reflect such imbalances.

In the myocardium, ROS activate MMPs, decrease TIMPs levels and collagen synthesis (Siwik and Colucci, 2004). A relationship between oxidative damage, MMP production and BBB disruption has been found in some lesions of the striatum (Kim et al., 2003). We reported above that prior gene transfer of antioxidant enzymes mitigates gp120-induced MMP-9 production and BBB leakiness (Louboutin *et al.*, 2010a). We studied the effect of gp120 on TIMP1- and TIMP-2 production. TIMP-1 and TIMP-2 levels increased 6h after gp120 injection into rat CP. TIMP-1 and TIMP-2 colocalized mainly with neurons (92 and 95% respectively). By 24h, expression of these protease inhibitors diverged, as TIMP-1 levels remained high but TIMP-2 subsided. Gene delivery of the antioxidant enzymes SOD1 or GPx1 into the CP before injecting gp120 there reduced levels of gp120-induced TIMP-1 and TIMP-2, recapitulating the effect of antioxidant enzymes on gp120-induced MMP-2 and MMP-9 (Figure 11). A significant correlation was observed between MMP/TIMP upregulation and BBB leakiness. Thus, HIV-1 gp120 upregulated TIMP-1 and TIMP-2 in the CP. Prior antioxidant enzyme treatment mitigated production of these TIMPs, probably by reducing MMP expression. This might be explained by reduced ROS generation, either as effectors of damage or as signaling intermediates, or both, by antioxidant gene transfer with subsequent decrease in MMP expression. Moreover, there was a significant correlation between gp120-related BBB disturbances and MMP/TIMP upregulation. Following prior antioxidant gene delivery, a relationship was also seen between the reduction in Evans Blue (EB) extravasation and MMP-9/TIMP-1 decreased production (Louboutin et al., 2011b).

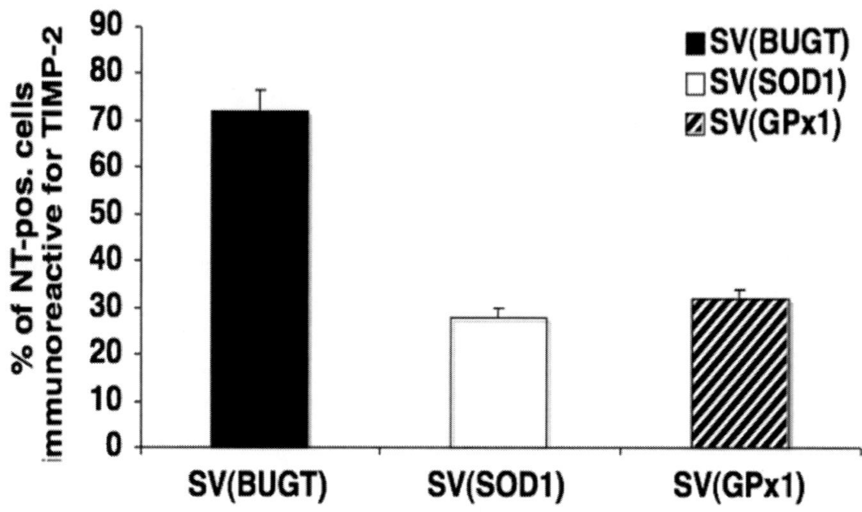

Figure 11. Reduction of gp120-induced TIMP-2 levels by gene delivery of antioxidant enzymes. Gene delivery of the antioxidant enzymes SOD1 or GPx1 into the CP one month before injecting gp120 there reduced levels of gp120-induced TIMP-2. SV(BUGT) had no effects.

Thus, MMPs and their inhibitors, TIMPs, are upregulated in response to oxidative stress produced in a rat model of HIV encephalopathy. In this setting, increase TIMPs may counterbalance the increase in MMPs. The centrality of ROS to this process is demonstrated by the fact that prior gene delivery of antioxidant enzymes mitigates production of TIMPs, possibly by reducing MMP expression. These results suggest that gp120-related oxidative stress induces MMP upregulation, potentially which triggers TIMP production.

F. SV40-mediated Gene Delivery of Antioxidant Enzymes Reduces gp120-induced Neuroinflammation

If neuron loss (Bansal et al., 2000; Nosheny et al., 2004; Louboutin et al., 2007a, 2009b) and astrogliosis (Bansal et al.,2000) have been described in animals receiving gp120 directly into their brains, a temporal relationship between neuronal degeneration, astrocytic reaction, proinflammatory cytokine production and microglial proliferation remained to be established. Rat CPs were challenged with 100–500 ng HIV-1BaL gp120, with or without prior rSV40-delivered SOD1 or GPx1. CD11b-positive microglia were increased 1 day post-challenge; Iba-1- and ED1-positive cells peaked at 7 days and 14 days respectively. Astrocyte infiltration was maximal at 7–14 days. MIP-1alpha was produced immediately, mainly by neurons. ED1- and GFAP-positive cells correlated with neuron loss and gp120 dose. We also tested the effect of more chronic gp120 exposure on neuroinflammation using an experimental model of continuing gp120 exposure. SV(gp120), a recombinant SV40-derived gene transfer vector was inoculated into the rat CP, leading to chronic expression of gp120, ongoing apoptosis in microglia and neurons, and oxidative stress. Increase in microglia and astrocytes was seen following intra-CP SV(gp120) injection, suggesting that continuing gp120 production increased neuroinflammation. SV(SOD1) or SV(GPx1) significantly reduced MIP-1alpha and limited neuroinflammation following gp120 administration into the CP (Figure 12), as well as microglia and astrocytes proliferation after injection of SV(gp120) in the striatum. Thus, gp120-induced CNS injury, neuron loss and inflammation may be mitigated by antioxidant gene delivery (Louboutin et al., 2010d).

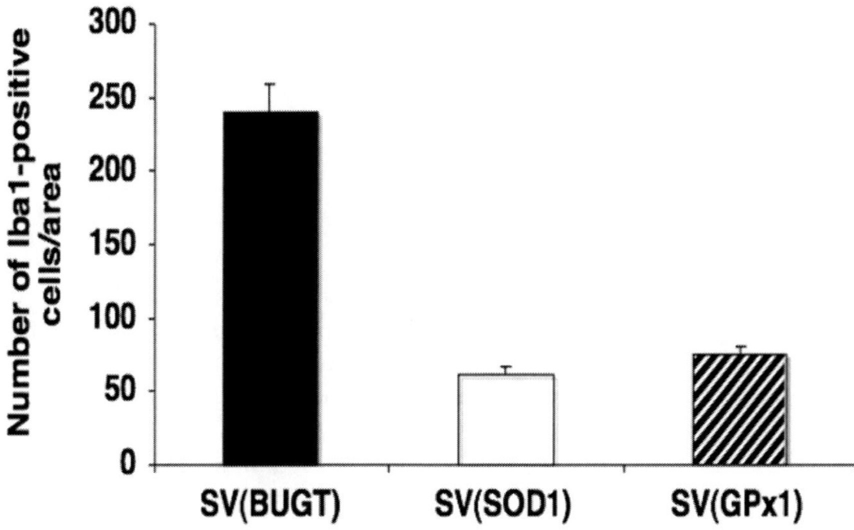

Figure 12. Neuroinflammation caused by gp120 was decreased by prior gene delivery of antioxidant enzymes. Rat CPs were challenged with HIV-1 gp120 following prior rSV40-mediated delivery of SOD1 or GPx1. Microglial cells were immunostained for Iba-1. Iba-1- positive cells were enumerated 7 days after gp120 injection. SV(SOD1) or SV(GPx1) significantly limited neuroinflammation following gp120 administration into the CP.

Free radical production may be accompanied by elevated expression of MIP-1 alpha contributing to microglial recruitment and delayed neuronal death in several models of CNS injury (Chan et al., 1984, 1991; Gasche et al., 2001; Aoki et al., 2002; Wang et al., 2008). The radical scavengers, like vitamin E analogs may inhibit free radicals and MIP-1 alpha production, and recruitment of microglia in the injured area (Wang et al., 2008). In models of ischemia/reperfusion injury, transgenic mice that overexpressed antioxidant enzymes, such as SOD-1 and GPx1 showed less upregulation of MIP-1 alpha and MCP-1 and less neuron loss and inflammation (Ishibashi et al., 2002; Nishi et al., 2005). Our findings extend the principle of antioxidant protection from neuroinflammation to HIV-related injury, and suggest that rSV40 antioxidant gene delivery may be therapeutically applicable in the case of ongoing injury and neuroinflammation such as HAND.

HIV-1 envelope gp120 induces neuroinflammation when injected in the rat CP. Gp120-induced neuroinflammation correlates with neuron loss. An increase in expression of MIP-1alpha may play a role in this phenomenon, as well as ROS, as evidenced by the protective effects of rSV40-delivered antioxidant enzymes. The participation of other chemokines/cytokines in gp120-induced lesions *in vivo* remains to be established. The modulation of the interaction between these chemokines/cytokines and their ligands needs to be investigated.

G. Neuroprotection against Tat-induced Brain Injury by SV(SOD1) and SV(GPx1)

Tat activates multiple signaling pathways, in one of which superoxide acts as an intermediate, while the other utilizes peroxide (Agrawal et al., 2007). Tat elicits lipid peroxidation (induced by generation of ROS), one of the elements leading to cell death. In culture, SV(SOD1) and SV(GPx1) not only increase levels of antioxidant enzymes and decrease lipid peroxidation but also have an effect on Tat-induced cytosol calcium fluxes (Agrawal et al., 2007). Neuroprotection from apoptosis caused by Tat requires detoxification of both O_2^- and H_2O_2 via SOD1 and GPx1. Combining SV(SOD1) and SV(GPx1) provides such protection.

We studied acute exposure by injecting recombinant Tat protein into the CP. Ongoing Tat expression, which more closely mimicks HIV-1 infection of the brain, was studied by delivering Tat-expression over time using an SV40-derived gene delivery vector, SV(Tat). Both acute and chronic Tat exposure induced lipid peroxidation and neuronal apoptosis. Prior administration of recombinant SV40 vectors carrying antioxidant enzymes SOD1 or GPx1 protected from Tat-induced oxidative injury and apoptosis (Figure 13). Thus, injection of recombinant HIV-1 Tat and the expression vector, SV(Tat), into the rat CP cause respectively acute or ongoing apoptosis and oxidative stress in neurons and may represent useful animal models for studying the pathogenesis and, potentially, treatment of HIV-1 Tat-related damage (Agrawal et al., 2012).

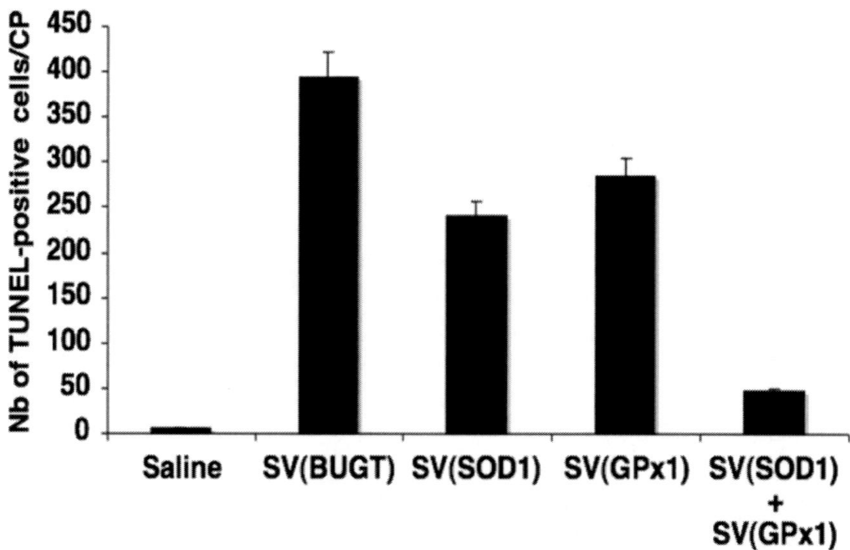

Figure 13. Protection against Tat-induced apoptosis by SV(SOD1) and SV(GPx1). rSV40 vectors were injected into the CP one month before inoculation of Tat in the same structure. Brains were harvested two days after Tat challenge and analyzed for apoptotic cells using TUNEL assay. Prior administration of recombinant rSV40 vectors carrying antioxidant enzymes SOD1 or GPx1 protected from Tat-induced apoptosis.

CONCLUSION

HIV-1-associated neurocognitive disorder (HAND) is an increasingly common, progressive disease characterized by neuronal loss and progressively deteriorating CNS function. HIV-1 gene products, particularly gp120 and Tat, elicit ROS that lead to oxidant injury, cause neuron apoptosis, as well as subsequent consequences (e.g. neuroinflammation, abnormalities of the BBB). Understanding of, and developing therapies for, HAND requires accessible models of the disease. We have devised experimental approaches to studying the acute and chronic effects of gp120 and Tat on the CNS. These approaches to gp120 and Tat administration may therefore represent useful animal models for studying the pathogenesis and treatment of HIV-1 gp120- and Tat-related damage. Gene delivery of antioxidant enzymes by recombinant SV40-derived vectors protects against gp120 and Tat-induced oxidative stress and neuronal apoptosis, opening new avenues for potential therapeutics of HAND.

ACKNOWLEDGEMENTS

This work was supported by NIH grants MH70287, MH69122 and AH48244 to DS.

REFERENCES

Adamson, DC; Wildemann, B; Sasaki, MD; *et al*. Immunologic NO synthase elevation in severe AIDS dementia and induction by HIV-1 gp41. *Science* 1996; 274: 1917-20.

Adamson, DC; Kopnisky, KL; Dawson, TM; *et al*. Mechanisms and structural determinants of HIV-1 coat protein, gp41-induced neurotoxicity. *J. Neurosci.* 1999; 19: 64-71.

Ahmed, F; McArthur, L; De Bernardi, M; *et al*. Retrograde and anterograde transport of HIV protein gp120 in the nervous system. *Brain Behav. Immun.* 2009; 23: 355-64.

Ances, BM; Ellis, RJ. Dementia and neurocognitive disorders due to HIV-1 infection. *Semin. Neurol.* 2007; 27: 86-92.

Andersen, JK. Oxidative stress in neurodegeneration: cause or consequence? *Nat. Med.* 2004; 5: S18-S25.

Agrawal, L; Louboutin, JP; Reyes, BAS; *et al*. Antioxidant enzyme gene delivery to protect from HIV-1 gp120-induced neuronal apoptosis. *Gene Ther.* 2006; 13: 1645-1656.

Agrawal, L., Louboutin, JP; Strayer DS. Preventing HIV-1 Tat-induced neuronal apoptosis using antioxidant enzymes: mechanistic and therapeutic implications. *Virology* 2007; 363: 462-72.

Agrawal, L., Louboutin, JP; Marusich, E; *et al*. Dopaminergic neurotoxicity of HIV-1 gp120: reactive oxygen species as signaling intermediates. *Brain Res.* 2010; 1306: 116-30.

Agrawal, L; Louboutin, JP; Reyes, BAS; *et al*. HIV-1 Tat neurotoxicity: a model of acute and chronic exposure, and neuroprotection by gene delivery of antioxidant enzymes. *Neurobiol. Dis.* 2012; 45: 657-70.

Annunziata, P. Blood-brain barrier changes during invasion of the central nervous system by HIV-1. Old and new insights into the mechanism. *J. Neurol.* 2003; 250: 901-06.

Antinori, A; Arendt, G; Becker, JT; *et al.* Updated research nosology for HIV-associated neurocognitive disorders. *Neurology* 2007; 69: 1789-99.

Aoki, T; Sumii, T; Mori, T; *et al.* Blood–brain barrier disruption and matrix metalloproteinase-9 expression during reperfusion injury: mechanical versus embolic focal ischemia in spontaneously hypertensive rats. *Stroke* 2002; 33: 2711–17.

Asahi, M; Asahi, K; Jung, J-C; *et al.* Role for matrix metalloproteinase 9 after focal cerebral ischemia: effects of gene knockout and enzyme inhibition with BB-94. *J. Cereb. Blood Flow Metab.* 2000; 20: 1681-89.

Askenov, MY; Hasselrot, U; Bansal, AK; *et al.* Oxidative damage induced by the injection of HIV-1 Tat protein in the rat striatum. *Neurosci. Lett.* 2001; 305: 5-8.

Askenov, MY; Hasselrot, U; Wu, G; *et al.* Temporal relationship between HIV-1 Tat-induced neuronal degeneration, OX-42 immunoreactivity, reactive astrocytosis, and protein oxidation in the rat striatum. *Brain Res.* 2003; 987: 1-9.

Askenov, MY; Askenova, MV; Mactutus, CF; *et al.* Attenuated neurotoxicity of the transactivation-defective HIV-Tat protein in hippocampal cell cultures. *Exp. Neurol.* 2009; 219: 586-90.

Avison, MJ; Nath, A; Greene-Avison, R; *et al.* Neuroimaging correlates of HIV-associated BBB compromise. *J. Neuroimmunol.* 2004; 157: 140-46.

Avgeropoulos, N; Kelley, B; Middaugh, L; *et al.* SCID mice with HIV encephalitis develop behavioral abnormalities. *J. Acquir. Immune Defic. Syndr.* 1998; 18: 13-20.

Bachis, A; Aden, SA; Nosheny, RL; *et al.* Axonal transport of human immunodeficiency virus type 1 envelope protein glycoprotein 120 is found in association with neuronal apoptosis. J. Neurosci. 2006; 26: 6771-80.

Banerjee, A; Zhanq, X; Manda, KR; *et al.* HIV proteins (gp120 and Tat) and methamphetamine in oxidative stress-induced damage in the brain: potential role of the thiol antioxidant N-acetylcysteine amide. *Free Rad. Biol. Med.* 2010; 48: 1388-98.

Banks, WA; Ibrahimi, F; Farr, SA; *et al.* Effects of wheatgerm agglutinin and aging on the regional brain uptake of HIV-1 gp120. *Life Sci.* 1999; 65: 81-89.

Banks, WA; Freed, EO; Wolf, KM, *et al.* Transport of human immunodeficiency virus type 1 pseudoviruses across the blood-brain barrier: role of envelope proteins and adsorptive endocytosis. *J. Virol.* 2001; 75: 4681-91.

Banks, WA; Robinson, SM; Nath, A. Permeability of the blood-brain barrier to HIV-1 Tat. *Exp. Neurol.* 2005; 193: 218-27.

Bansal, AK; Mactutus, CF; Nath, A; *et al.* Neurotoxicity of HIV-1 proteins gp120 and Tat in the rat striatum. *Brain Res.* 2000; 879: 42-49.

Beal, MF. Aging, energy, and oxidative stress in neurodegenerative diseases. *Ann. Neurol.* 1995; 38: 357-66.

Berman, NE; Marcario, JK; Yong, C; *et al.* Microglial activation and neurological symptoms in the SIV model of neuroAIDS: association with MHC-II and MMP-9 expression with behavioral deficits and evoked potential changes. *Neurobiol. Dis.* 1999; 6: 486-98.

Bigini, P; Gardoni, F; Barbera, S; *et al.* Expression of AMPA and NMDA receptor subunits in the cervical spinal cord of wobbler mice. *BMC Neurosci.* 2006; 7: 71.

Bonavia, R; Bajetto, A; Barbero, S; *et al.* HIV-1 Tat causes apoptosis death and calcium homeostasis alterations in rat neurons. *Biochem. Biophys. Res. Commun.* 2001; 288: 301-8.

Bonfoco, E; Krainc, D; Ankarcrona, M; *et al.* Apoptosis and necrosis: two distinct events induced, respectively, by mild and intense insults with N-methyl-D-aspartate or nitric oxide/superoxide in cortical cell cultures. *Proc. Natl. Acad. Sci. USA* 1995; 92: 7162-66.

Broughton, BRS; Reutens, DC; Sobey CG. Apoptotic mechanisms after cerebral ischemia. *Stroke* 2009; 40: e331-e339.

Bruce-Keller, AJ; Li, YJ; Lovell, MA; *et al.* 4-Hydroxynonenal, a product of lipid peroxidation, damages cholinergic neurons and impairs visuospatial memory in rats. *J. Neuropathol. Exp. Neurol.* 1998; 57: 257-67.

Bruce-Keller, AJ; Barger, SW; Moss, NI; *et al.* Proinflammatory and pro-oxidant properties of Tat in a microglial cell line: attenuation by 17b-estradiol. *J. Neurochem.* 2001; 78: 1315-24.

Bruce-Keller, AJ; Turchan-Cholewo, J; Smart, EJ; *et al.* Morphine causes rapid increases in glial activation and neuronal injury in the striatum of inducible HIV-1 Tat transgenic mice. *Glia* 2008; 56: 1414-27.

Butterfield, DA; Castegna, A; Lauderback, CM; *et al.* Evidence that amyloid β-peptide induced lipid peroxidation and its sequelae in Alzheimer's disease brain contribute to neuronal death. *Neurobiol. Aging* 2002; 23: 655-64.

Cao, W; Carney, JM; Duchon, A; *et al.* Oxygen free radicals involvement in ischemia and reperfusion of the brain injury to brain. *Neurosci. Lett.* 1998; 88: 233-38.

Chan, PH; Schmidley, JW; Fishman, RA; *et al.* Brain injury, edema, and vascular permeability changes induced by oxygen-derived free radicals. *Neurology* 1984; 34: 315–20.

Chan, PH; Yang, GY; Carlson, E; *et al.* Cold-induced brain edema and infarction are reduced in transgenic mice overexpressing CuZn-superoxide dismutase. *Ann. Neurol.* 1991; 29: 482–86.

Cinque, P; Nebuloni, M; Santovito, ML; *et al.* The urokinase receptor is overexpressed in the AIDS dementia complex and other neurological manifestations. *Ann. Neurol.* 2004; 55: 687-94

Cioni, C; Annunziata, P. Circulating gp120 alters the blood-brain barrier permeability in HIV-1 gp120 transgenic mice. *Neurosci. Lett.* 2002; 330: 299-301.

Clark, IM; Swingler, TE; Sampieri, CL; *et al.* The regulation of matrix metalloproteinases and their inhibitors. *Int. J. Biochem. Cell Biol.* 2008; 40: 1362-78.

Clifford, DB; McArthur, JC; Schifitto, G; *et al.* A randomized clinical trial of CPI-1189 for HIV-associated cognitive-motor impairment. *Neurology* 2002; 59: 1568-73.

Conant, K; Garzino-Demo, A; Nath, A; *et al.* Induction of monocyte chemoattractant protein-1 in HIV-1 Tat-stimulated astrocytes and elevation in AIDS dementia. *Proc. Nat. Acad. Sci. USA* 1998; 95: 3117-21.

Conant, K; St Hillaire, C; Anderson, C; *et al.* Human immunodeficiency virus type 1 Tat and methamphetamine affect the release and activation of matrix-degrading proteinases. *J. Neurovirol.* 2004; 10: 21-28.

Consortium D. Safety and tolerability of the antioxidant OPC-14117 in HIV-associated cognitive impairment: the Dana Consortium on the therapy of HIV dementia and related cognitive disorders. *Neurology* 1997; 49: 142-46.

Consortium D. A randomized, double-blind, placebo-controlled trial of deprenyl and thioctic acid in human immunodeficiency virus-associated cognitive impairment: Dana

Consortium on the therapy of HIV dementia and related cognitive disorders. *Neurology* 1998; 50: 645-51.

Cordelier, P; Calarota, SA; Pomerantz, RJ; *et al.* Inhibition of HIV-1 in the central nervous system by IFN-alpha2 delivered by an SV40 vector. J. Interferon Cytokine Res. 2003a; 23: 477-88.

Cordelier, P; Van Bockstaele, E; Calarota, SA; *et al.* Inhibiting AIDS in the central nervous system: gene delivery to protect neurons from HIV. *Mol. Ther.* 2003b; 7: 801-10.

Cordelier, P; Strayer, DS. Using gene delivery to protect HIV-susceptible CNS cells: inhibiting HIV replication in microglia. *Virus Res.* 2006; 118: 87-97.

Cribbs, DH; Poon, WW; Rissman, RA; *et al.* Caspase-mediated degeneration in Alzheimer's disease. *Am. J. Pathol.* 2004; 165: 353-55.

Cutler, RG; Haughey, NJ; Tammara, A; *et al.* Dysregulation of sphingolipids and sterol metabolism by ApoE4 in HIV dementia. *Neurology* 2004; 63: 626-30.

Dallasta, LM; Pisarov, LA; Esplen, JE; *et al.* Blood-brain barrier tight junction disruption in human immunodeficiency virus-1 encephalitis. *Am. J. Pathol.* 1999; 155: 1915-27.

Dexter, DT; Carter, CJ; Wells, FR; *et al.* Basal lipid perxidation in substantia nigra is increased in Parkinson's disease. *J. Neurochem.* 1987; 52: 381–89.

Dreyer, EB; Kaiser, PK; Offermann, JT; *et al.* HIV-1 coat protein neurotoxicity prevented by calcium channel antagonists. *Science* 1990; 248: 364-67.

Dzwonek, J; Rylski, M; Kaczmarek, L. Matrix metalloproteinases and their endogenous inhibitors in neuronal physiology of the adult brain. *FEBS Lett.* 2004; 567: 129-35.

Eugenin, EA; D'Aversa, TG; Lopez, L; *et al.* MCP-1 (CCL2) protects human neurons and astrocytes from NMDA or HIV-tat-induced apoptosis. *J. Neurochem.* 2003; 85: 1299-311.

Eugenin, EA; Osiecli, K; Lopez, L; *et al.* CCL2/monocyte chemoattractant protein-1 mediates enhanced transmigration of human immunodeficiency virus (HIV)-infected leukocytes across the blood-brain barrier: a potential mechanism of HIV-CNS invasion and neuroAIDS. *J. Neurosci.* 2006; 26: 1098-1106.

Ferrucci, R; Nonnemacher, MR; Cohen EA; *et al.* Extracellular human immunodeficiency 1 virus type 1 viral protein R causes reductions in astrocytic ATP and glutathione levels compromising the antioxidant reservoir (submitted).

Garden, GA; Guo, W; Jayadev, S; *et al.* HIV associated neurodegeneration requires p53 in neurons and microglia. *FASEB J.* 2004; 18: 1141-43.

Gasche, Y; Copin, J-C; Sugawara, T; *et al.* Matrix metalloproteinases inhibition prevents oxidative stress-associated blood-brain barrier disruption after transient focal cerebral ischemia. *J. Cereb. Blood Flow Metab.* 2001; 21: 1393-1400.

Ghezzi, S; Noolan, DM; Aluigi, MG; *et al.* Inhibition of CXCR-3-dependent HIV-1 infection by extracellular HIV-1 Tat. *Biochem. Byophys. Res. Commun.* 2000; 270: 992-6.

Giulian, D; Vaca, K; Noonan, CA. Secretion of neurotoxins by mononuclear phagocytes infected with HIV-1. *Science* 1990; 250: 1593-96.

Gonzalez-Scarano, F; Martin-Garcia, J. The neuropathogenesis of AIDS. *Nat. Rev. Immunol.* 2005; 5: 69-81.

Gorry, PR, Howard, JL, Churchill, MJ, *et al.* 1999. Diminished production of human immunodeficiency virus type 1 in astrocytes results from inefficient translation of gag, env, and nef mRNAs despite efficient expression of Tat and Rev. *J. Virol.* 1999; 73: 352-61.

Gu, Z; Kaul, M; Yan, B; *et al*. S-nitrosylation of matrix metalloproteinases: signaling pathway to neuronal cell death. *Science* 2002; 297: 1186-90.

Gursoy-Ozdemir, Y; Qiu, J; Matsuoka, N; *et al*. Cortical spreading depression activates and upregulates MMP-9. *J. Clin. Invest.* 2004; 113: 1447-55.

Haorah, J; Schall, K; Ramirez, S; *et al*. Activation of protein kinases and matrix metalloproteinases causes blood-brain barrier injury: novel mechanisms for neurodegeneration associated with alcohol abuse. *Glia* 2008; 56: 78-88.

Haughey, NJ; Nath, A; Mattson, MP. HIV-1 tat through phosphorylation of NMDA receptors potentiates glutamate excitotoxicity. *J. Neurochem.* 2001; 78: 457-67.

Haughey, NJ; Cutler, RG; Tamara, A; *et al*. Perturbation of sphingolipid metabolism and ceramide production in HIV-dementia. *Ann. Neurol.* 2004; 5: 257-67.

Hoehn, B; Yenari, MA; Sapolsky, RM; *et al*. Glutathione peroxidase overexpression inhibits cytochrome C release and proapoptotic mediators to protect neurons from experimental stroke. *Stroke* 2003; 34: 2489-94.

Hoshino, S; Sun, B; Konishi, M; *et al*. Vpr in plasma of HIV type 1-positive patients is correlated with the HIV type 1 RNA titers. *AIDS Res. Hum. Retroviruses* 2007; 23: 391-97.

Huang, MB; Hunter, M; Bond, VC. Effect of extracellular human immunodeficiency virus type 1 glycoprotein 120 on primary human vascular endothelium cell cultures. *AIDS Res. Hum. Retroviruses* 1999; 15: 1265-77.

Hudson, L; Liu, J; Nath, A; *et al*. Detection of the human immunodeficiency virus regulatory protein tat in CNS tissues. *J. Neurovirol.* 2000; 6: 144-55.

Hurtrel, M; Ganiere, JP; Guelfi, JF; *et al*. Comparison of early and late feline immunodeficiency virus encephalopathies. *AIDS* 1992: 6: 399-406.

Ishibashi, N; Prokopenko, O; Weisbrot-Lefkowitz, M; *et al*. Glutathione peroxidase inhibits cell death and glial activation following experimental stroke. *Brain Res. Mol. Brain Res.* 2002; 109: 34–44.

James, HJ; Sharer, LR; Zhang, Q; *et al*. Expression of caspase-3 in brains from paediatric patients with HIV-1 encephalitis. *Neuropathol. Appl. Neurobiol.* 1999; 25: 380-86.

Jones, M; Olafson, K; Del Bigio, MR; *et al*. Intraventricular injection of human immunodeficiency virus type 1 (HIV-1) tat protein causes inflammation, gliosis, apoptosis, and ventricular enlargment. *J. Neuropathol. Exp. Neurol.* 1998; 57: 563-70.

Kanmogne, GD; Primeaux, C; Grammas, P. HIV-1 gp120 proteins alter tight junction protein expression and brain endothelial cell permeability: implications for the pathogenesis of HIV-associated dementia. *J. Neuropath. Exp. Neurol.* 2005; 64: 498-505.

Kanmogne, GD; Schall, K; Leibhart, J; *et al*. HIV-1 gp120 compromises blood-brain barrier integrity and enhance monocyte migration across blood-brain barrier: implication for viral neuropathogenesis. *J. Cereb. Blood Flow Metab.* 2007; 27: 123-34.

Kaul, M; Lipton, SA. Chemokines and activated macrophages in HIV gp120-induced neuronal apoptosis. *Proc. Natl. Acad. Sci. USA* 1999; 96: 8212-16.

Kaul, M; Garden, GA; Lipton, SA. Pathways to neuronal injury and apoptosis in HIV-associated dementia. *Nature* 2001; 410: 988-94.

Kim, GW; Gasche, Y; Grzeschik, S; *et al*. Neurodegeneration in striatum induced by the mitochondrial toxin 3-nitropropionic acid: role of matrix metalloproteinase-9 in early blood-brain barrier disruption? *J. Neurosci.* 2003; 23: 8733-42.

King, JE; Eugenin, EA; Buckner, CM; *et al.* HIV Tat and neurotoxicity. *Microbes Infect.* 2006; 8: 1347-57.

Koutsilieri, E; Sopper, S; Scheller, C; *et al.* Parkinsonism in HIV dementia. *J. Neural Transm.* 2002; 109: 767-75.

Kraus, RL; Pasieczny, R; Lariosa-Willingham, K; *et al.* Antioxidant properties of minocycline: neuroprotection in an oxidative stress assay and direct radical-scavenging activity. *J. Neurochem.* 2005; 94: 819-27.

Kruman, II; Bruce-Keller, AJ; Bredesen, D; *et al.* Evidence that 4-hydroxynonenal mediates oxidative stress-induced neuronal apoptosis. *J. Neurosci.* 1997; 17: 5089-100.

Kruman, II; Nath, A; Mattson, MP. HIV-1 protein Tat induces apoptosis of hippocampal neurons by a mechanism involving caspase activation, calcium overload, and oxidative stress. *Exp. Neurol.* 1998; 154: 276-88.

Kruman, II; Mattson, MP. Pivotal role of mitochondrial calcium uptake in neural cell apoptosis and necrosis. *J. Neurochem.* 1999; 72: 529-40.

Lackner,AA; Veazey, RS. Current concepts in AIDS pathogenesis: Insights from the SIV/macaque model. *Annu. Rev. Med.* 2007; 58: 461-76.

Levy, DN; Refaeli, Y; MacGregor, RR; *et al.* Serum Vpr regulates productive infection and latency of human immunodeficiency virus type 1. *Proc. Natl. Acad. Sci. U S A* 1994; 91, 10873-77.

Levy, DN; Refaeli, Y; Weiner, DB. Extracellular Vpr protein increases cellular permissiveness to human immunodeficiency virus replication and reactivates virus from latency. *J. Virol.* 1995; 69: 1243-52.

Li, J; Bentsman, G; Potash, MJ; *et al.* 2007. Human immunodeficiency virus type 1 efficiently binds to human fetal astrocytes and induces neuroinflammatory responses independent of infection. *BMC Neurosci.* 2007; 8: 31.

Lipton, SA; Choi, YB; Pan, ZH; *et al.* A redox-based mechanism for the neuroprotective and neurodestructive effects of nitric oxide and related nitrosocompounds. *Nature* 1993; 364: 626-32.

Liu, X; Jana, M; Dasgupta, S; *et al.* Human immunodeficiency virus type 1 (HIV-1) Tat induces nitric-oxide synthase in human astroglia. *J. Biol. Chem.* 2002; 277: 39312-19.

Liuzzi, GM; Mastroianni, CM; Santacroce, MP; *et al.* Increased activity of matrix metalloproteinases in the cerebrospinal fluid of patients with HIV-associated neurological diseases. *J. Neurovirol.* 2000; 6: 156-63

Lo, EH; Wang, X; Cuzner, MI. Extracellular proteolysis in brain injury and inflammation: role for plasminogen activators and matrix metalloproteinases. *J. Neurosci. Res.* 2002; 69: 1-9.

Louboutin, JP; Liu, B; Reyes, BAS; *et al.* Rat bone marrow progenitor cells transduced in situ by rSV40 vectors differentiate into multiple CNS cell lineages. *Stem Cells* 2006; 24: 2801-09.

Louboutin, JP; Agrawal, L; Reyes, BAS; *et al.* Protecting neurons from HIV-1 gp120-induced oxidant stress using both localized intracerebral and generalized intraventricular administration of antioxidant enzymes delivered by SV40-derived vectors. *Gene Ther.* 2007a; 14: 1650-61.

Louboutin, JP; Reyes, BAS; Agrawal, L; *et al.* Strategies for CNS-directed gene delivery: *in vivo* gene transfer to the brain using SV40-derived vectors. *Gene Ther.* 2007b; 14: 939-49.

Louboutin, JP; Agrawal, L; Reyes, BAS; *et al*. A rat model of human immunodeficiency virus 1 encephalopathy using envelope glycoprotein gp120 expression delivered by SV40 vectors. *J. Neuropathol. Exp. Neurol.* 2009a; 68: 456-73.

Louboutin, JP; Agrawal, L; Reyes, BAS; *et al*. HIV-1 gp120 neurotoxicity proximally and at a distance from the point of exposure: Protection by rSV40 delivery of antioxidant enzyme. *Neurobiol. Dis.* 2009b; 34: 462-76.

Louboutin, JP; Agrawal, L; Reyes, BAS; *et al*. HIV-1 gp120-induced injury to the blood-brain barrier: role of metalloproteinases 2 and 9 and relationship to oxidative stress. *J. Neuropathol. Exp. Neurol.* 2010a; 69: 801-16.

Louboutin, JP; Chekmasova, AA; Marusich, E; *et al*. Efficient CNS gene delivery by intravenous injection. *Nature Meth.* 2010b; 7: 905-07.

Louboutin, JP; Reyes, BAS; Agrawal, L.; *et al*. Blood-brain barrier abnormalities caused by exposure to HIV-1 gp120- Protection by gene delivery of antioxidant enzymes. *Neurobiol. Dis.* 2010c; 38: 313-25.

Louboutin, JP; Reyes, BAS; Agrawal, L; *et al*. HIV-1 gp120-induced neuroinflammation: relationship to neuron loss and protection by rSV40-delivered antioxidant enzymes. *Exp. Neurol.* 2010d; 221: 231-45.

Louboutin, JP; Marusich, E; Fisher-Perkins, J; *et al*. Gene transfer to the Rhesus monkey brain using SV40-derived vectors is durable and safe. *Gene Ther.* 2011a; 18: 682-91.

Louboutin, JP; Reyes, BAS; Agrawal, L.; *et al*. HIV-1 gp120 upregulates matrix metalloproteinases and their inhibitors in a rat model of HIV encephalopathy. *Eur. J. Neurosci.* 2011b; 34: 2015-23.

Louboutin, JP; Chekmasova, A; Marusich, E; *et al*. Role of CCR5 and its ligands in the control of vascular inflammation and leukocyte recruitment required for acute excitotoxic seizure induction and neural damage. *FASEB J.* 2011c; 25: 737-53.

Louboutin, JP; Reyes, BAS; Agrawal, L; *et al*. Intracisternal rSV40 administration provides effective pan-CNS transgene expression. *Gene Ther.* 2012a; 19: 114-18..

Louboutin, JP; Reyes, BAS; Agrawal, L.; *et al*. Gene delivery of antioxidant enzymes inhibits HIV-1 gp120-induced expression of caspases. *Neuroscience* 2012b; in press.

Mabrouk, K; Van Rietschoten, J.; Vives, E; *et al*. Lethal neurotoxicity in mice of the basic domains of HIV and SIV Rev proteins. Study of these regions by circular dichroism. *FEBS Lett.* 1991; 289: 13-17.

McArthur, JC; Hoover, DR; Bacellar, H; *et al*. Dementia in AIDS patients: incidence and risk factors. Multicenter AIDS Cohort Study. *Neurology* 1993; 43: 2245–52.

McArthur, JC; Brew, BJ; Nath, A. Neurological complications of HIV infection. *Lancet Neurol.* 2005; 4: 543-55.

McKee, HJ; Strayer, DS. Immune responses against SIV envelope glycoprotein, using recombinant SV40 as a vaccine delivery vector. *Vaccine* 2002; 20: 3613-25.

Madden, SD; Cotter, TG. Cell death in brain development and degeneration: control of caspase expression may be key! *Mol. Neurobiol.* 2008; 37: 1-6.

Magnuson, DS; Knudsen, BE; Geiger, JD; *et al*. Human immunodeficiency virus type 1 tat activates non-N-methyl-o-aspartate excitatory amino receptors and causes neurotoxicity. *Ann. Neurol.* 1995; 37: 373-80.

Major, EO; Rausch, D; Marra, C; *et al*. HIV-associated dementia. *Science* 2000; 288: 440-42.

Manabe, S; Gu, Z; Lipton, SA. Activation of matrix metalloproteinase-9 via neuronal nitric oxide synthase contributes to NMDA-induced retinal ganglion cell death. *Invest. Ophtalmol. Vis. Sci.* 2005; 46: 4747-53.

Mandel, RJ; Rendahl, KG; Spratt, SK; *et al.* Characterization of intrastriatal recombinant adeno-associated virus-mediated gene transfer of human tyrosine hydroxylase and human GTP-cyclohydrolase I in a rat model of Parkinson's disease. *J. Neurosci.* 1998; 18: 4271-84.

Marshall, DCL; Wyss-Coray, TW; Abraham, CR. Induction of matrix metalloproteinase-2 in human immunodeficiency virus-1 glycoprotein 120 transgenic mouse brains. *Neurosci. Lett.* 1998; 254: 97-100.

Mattson, MP; Haughey, NJ; Nath, A. Cell death in HIV dementia. *Cell Death Diff.* 2005; 12: 893-904.

Meucci, O; Fatatis, A; Simen, AA; *et al.* Chemokines regulate hippocampal neuronal signalling and gp120 neurotoxicity. *Proc. Natl. Acad. Sci. USA* 1998; 95: 14500–505.

Mirsattari, SM; Power, C; Nath, A. Parkinsonism with HIV infection. *Mov. Disord.* 1998; 13: 684-89.

Mollace, V; Nottet, HS; Clayette, P; *et al.* Oxidative stress and neuroAIDS: triggers, modulators and novel antioxidants. *Trends Neurosci.* 2001; 24: 411-16.

Montoliu, C; Valles, S; Renau-Piqueras, J; *et al.* Ethanol-induced oxygen radical formation and lipid peroxidation in rat brain: effect of chronic alcohol consumption. *J. Neurochem.* 1994; 63: 1855–62.

Morinville, A; Cahill, CM; Aibak, H; *et al.* Morphine-induced changes in delta opioid receptor trafficking are linked to somatosensory processing in the rat spinal cord. *J. Neurosci.* 2004; 24: 5549-59.

Nath, A; Conant, K; Chen, P; *et al.* Transient exposure to HIV-1 Tat protein results in cytokine production in macrophages and astrocytes: A hit and run phenomenon. *J. Biol. Chem.* 1999; 274: 17098-102.

Nath, A; Haughey, NJ; Jones, M; *et al.* Synergistic neurotoxicity by human immunodeficiency virus proteins tat and gp120: protection by memantine. *Ann. Neurol.* 2000; 47: 186-94.

Nath, A; Sacktor, N. Influence of highly active antiretroviral therapy on persistence of HIV in the central nervous system. *Curr. Opin. Neurol.* 2006; 19: 358-61.

Nishi, T; Maier, CM; Hayashi, T; *et al.* Superoxide dismutase 1 overexpression reduces MCP-1 and MIP-1 alpha expression after transient focal cerebral ischemia. *J. Cereb. Blood Flow Metab.* 2005; 25: 1312–24.

Noorbakhsh, F; Ramachandran, R; Barsby, N; *et al.* MicroRNA profiling reveals new aspects of HIV neurodegeneration: caspase-6 regulates astrocyte survival. *FASEB J.* 2010; 24: 1799-812.

Norman, JP; Perry, SW; Reynolds, HM; *et al.* HIV-1 Tat activates neuronal ryanodine receptors with rapid induction of the unfolded protein response and mitochondrial hyperpolarization. *PLoS ONE* 2008; 3: e3731

Nosheny, RL; Bachis, A; Acquas, E; *et al.* Human immunodeficiency virus type 1 glycoprotein gp120 reduces the levels of brain-derived neurotrophic factor in vivo: potential implication for neuronal cell death. *Eur. J. Neurosci.* 2004; 20: 2857-64.

Nosheny, RL; Bachis, A; Aden, SA; *et al.* Intrastriatal administration of human immunodeficiency virus-1 glycoprotein 120 reduces glial cell-line derived neurotrophic factor levels and causes apoptosis in the substantia nigra. *J. Neurobiol.* 2006; 66: 1311-21.

Nosheny, RL; Ahmed, F; Yakoviev, A; *et al.* Brain-derived neurotrophic factor prevents the nigrostriatal degeneration induced by human immunodeficiency virus-1 glycoprotein 120 *in vivo. Eur. J. Neurosci.* 2007; 25: 2275-84.

Patel, CA; Mukhtar, M; Pomerantz, RJ. HIV-1 Vpr induces apoptosis in human neuronal cells. *J. Virol.* 2000; 74: 9717-26.

Paxinos G, Watson C. The Rat Brain in Stereotaxic Coordinates. 2nd ed. New York, NY: Academic Press; 1986.

Petito, CK; Cash, KS. Blood-brain barrier abnormalities in the acquired immunodeficiency syndrome: immunohistochemical localization of serum proteins in postmortem brain. *Ann. Neurol.* 1992; 32: 658-66.

Petito, CK; Roberts, B. Evidence of apoptotic cell death in HIV encephalitis. *Am. J. Pathol.* 1995; 146: 1121-30.

Pocernich, CB; La Fontaine, M; Butterfield, DA. In-vivo glutathione elevation protects against hydroxyl free radical-induced protein oxidation in rat brain. *Neurochem. Int.* 2000; 36: 185-91.

Power, C; Kong, PA; Crawford, TO; *et al.* Cerebral white matter changes in acquired immunodeficiency syndrome dementia: alterations of the blood-brain barrier. *Ann. Neurol.* 1993; 34: 339-50.

Price, TO; Ercal, N; Nakaoke, R; *et al.* HIV-1 viral proteins gp120 and Tat induce oxidative stress in brain endothelial cells. *Brain Res* 2005; 1045: 57-63.

Price, TO; Uras, F; Banks, WA; *et al.* A novel antioxidant N-acetylcysteine amide prevents gp120- and Tat-induced oxidative stress in brain endothelial cells. *Exp. Neurol.* 2006; 201: 193-202.

Pulliam, L; Irwin, I; Kusdra, L; *et al.* CPI-1189 attenuates effects of suspected neurotoxins associated with AIDS dementia: a possible role for ERK activation. *Brain Res.* 2001; 893: 95-103.

Ramachandran, G; Glickman, L; Levenson, J; *et al.* Incidence of extrapyramidal syndromes in AIDS patients and a comparison group of medically ill patients. *J. Neuropsychiatry Clin. Neurosci.* 1997; 9: 579-83.

Ranki, A; Nyberg, M; Ovod, V; *et al.* Abundant expression of HIV Nef and Rev proteins in brain astrocytes in vivo is associated with dementia. *AIDS* 1995; 9: 1001-8.

Regulier, EG; Reiss, K; Khalili, K; *et al.* T-cell and neuronal apoptosis in HIV infection: implications for therapeutic intervention. *Int. Rev. Immunol.* 2004; 23: 25-59.

Ribe, EM; Serrano-Saiz, E; Akpan, N; *et al.* Mechanisms of neuronal death in disease: defining the models and the players. *Biochem. J.* 2008; 415: 165-82.

Ridet, JL; Bensadoun, JC; Deglon, N; *et al.* Lentivirus-mediated expression of glutathione peroxidase: neuroprotection in murine models of Parkinson's disease. *Neurobiol. Dis.* 2006; 21: 29-34.

Rohn, TT. The role of caspases in Alzheimer's disease: potential novel therapeutic opportunities. *Apoptosis* 2010; 15: 1403-09.

Rom, I; Deshmane, SL; Mukerjee, R; *et al.* HIV-1 Vpr deregulates calcium secretion in neural cells. *Brain Res.* 2009; 1275: 81-86.

Rosen, DR; Siddique, T; Patterson, D; *et al.* Mutations in Cu/Zn superoxide dismutase are associated with familial amyotrophic lateral sclerosis. *Nature,* 1993; 362: 59–62

Rosenberg, GA. Matrix metalloproteinases in neuroinflammation. *Glia* 2002; 39: 279-91.

Rouger, K; Louboutin, JP; Villanova, M; *et al.* X-linked vacuolated myopathy: TNF-alpha and IFN-gamma expression in muscle fibers with MHC class I on sarcolemma. *Am. J. Pathol.* 2001; 158: 355-59.

Rumbaugh, JA; Nath, A. Developments in HIV neuropathogenesis. *Curr. Pharm. Des.* 2006; 12: 1023-44.

Russo, R; Siviglia, E; Gliozzi, M; *et al.* Evidence implicating matrix metalloproteinases in the mechanism underlying accumulation of IL-1□ and neuronal apoptosis in the neocortex of HIV/gp120-exposed rats. *Int. Rev. Neurobiol.* 2007; 82: 407-21.

Sabbah, EN; Roques, BP. Critical implication of the (70-96) domain of human immunodeficiency virus type 1 Vpr protein in apoptosis of primary rat cortical and striatal neurons. J. *Neurovirol.* 2005; 11: 489-502.

Sacktor, N; Schifitto, G; McDermott, MP; *et al.* Transdermal seleginine in HIV-associated cognitive impairment: pilot, placebo-controlled study. *Neurology* 2000; 54: 233-35.

Sacktor, N; Haughey, N; Cutler, R; *et al.* Novel markers of oxidative stress in actively progressive HIV dementia. *J. Neuroimmunol.* 2004; 157: 176-84.

Saito, Y; Sharer, LR; Epstein, LG; *et al.* Overexpression of nef as a marker for restricted HIV-1 infection of astrocytes in postmortem pediatric central nervous tissues. *Neurology* 1994; 44: 474-81.

Sardar, AM; Czudek, C; Reynolds, GP. Dopamine deficits in the brain: the neurochemical basis of parkinsonism symptoms in AIDS. *Neuroreport* 1996; 7: 9-12.

Sauter, BV; Parashar, B; Chowdhury, NR; *et al.* A replication-deficient rSV40 mediates liver-directed gene transfer and a long-term amelioration of jaundice in gunn rats. *Gastroenterology* 2000; 119: 1348-57.

Sims, NR; Muyderman, H. Mitochondria, oxidative metabolism and cell death in stroke. *Biochim. Biophysis. Acta* 2010; 1802: 80-91.

Singh, IN; Goody, RJ; Dean, C; *et al.* Apoptotic cell death of striatal neurons induced by human immunodeficiency virus-1 Tat and gp120: Differential involvement of caspase-3 and endonuclease G. *J. Neurovirol.* 2004; 10: 141-51.

Siwik, DA, Colucci, WS. Regulation of matrix metalloproteinases by cytokines and reactive oxygen/nitrogen species in the myocardium. *Heart Fail. Rev.* 2004; 9: 43-51.

Smith, CD; Carney, JM; Starke-Reed, PE; *et al.* Excess brain protein oxidation and enzyme dysfunction in normal aging and in Alzheimer's disease. *Proc. Natl. Acad. Sci. USA* 1991; 88: 10540-43.

Smith, MA; Perry, G. Free radical damage, iron, and Alzheimer's disease. *J. Neurol. Sci.* 1995; 134: 92-94.

Smith, MA; Sayre, LM; Monnier, VM; *et al.* Radical ageing in Alzheimer's disease. *Trends Neurosci.* 1995; 18: 172-76.

Sporer, B; Paul, R; Koedel, U; *et al.* Presence of matrix metalloproteinase-9 activity in the cerebrospinal fluid of human immunodeficiency virus-infected patients. *J. Infect. Dis.* 1998; 178: 854-57.

Steiner, J; Haughey, N; Li, W; *et al.* Oxidative stress and therapeutic approaches in HIV dementia. *Antioxid. Redox Sign.* 2006, 8: 2089-100.

Strayer, DS; Kondo, R; Milano, J; *et al.* Use of SV40-based vectors to transduce foreign genes to normal human peripheral blood mononuclear cells. *Gene Ther.* 1997; 4: 219-25.

Strayer, DS. Gene therapy using SV40-derived vectors: what does the future hold? *J. Cell Physiol.* 1999; 181: 375-84.

Strayer, DS; Lamothe, M; Wei, D; *et al.* Generation of recombinant SV40 vectors for gene transfer. SV40 protocols. In: Raptis L, ed. *Methods in Molecular biology.* Humana Press, Totowa, NJ, 2001; vol. 165, pp. 103-117.

Theodore, S; Cass, WA; Maragos, WF. Methamphetamine and human immunodeficiency virus protein Tat synergize to destroy dopaminergic terminals in the rat striatum. *Neuroscience* 2006; 137: 925-35.

Thormar, H. Maedi-Visna virus and its relationship to human deficiency virus. *AIDS Rev.* 2005; 7: 233-45.

Toggas, SM; Masliah, E; Rockenstein, EM; *et al.* Central nervous system damage produced by expression of the HIV-1 coat protein gp120 in transgenic mice. *Nature* 1994; 367: 188-93.

Toneatto, S; Finco, O; van der Putten, H; *et al.* Evidence of blood-brain barrier alteration and activation in HIV-1 gp120 transgenic mice. *AIDS* 1999; 13: 2343-48.

Toschi, E; Barillari, G; Sgadari, C; *et al.* Activation of matrix-metalloproteinase-2 and membrane-type-1-matrix-metalloproteinase in endothelial cells and induction of vascular permeability in vivo by human immunodeficiency virus-1 Tat protein and basic Fibroblast Growth Factor. *Mol. Biol. Cell* 2001; 12: 2934-46.

Trillo-Pazos, G.; McFarlane-Abdulla, E; Campbell, IC; *et al.* Recombinant nef HIV-IIIB protein is toxic to human neurons in culture. *Brain Res.* 2000; 864: 315-26.

Turchan, J; Pocernich, CB; Gairola, C; *et al.* Oxidative stress in HIV demented patients and protection ex vivo with novel antioxidants. *Neurology* 2003; 60: 307-14.

Ullrich, CK; Groopman, JE; Ganju, RK. HIV-1 gp120- and gp160-induced apoptosis in cultured endothelial cells is mediated by caspases. *Blood* 2000; 96: 1436-42.

Uttara, B; Singh, AV; Zamboni, P; *et al.* Oxidative stress and neurodegenerative diseases: a review of upstream and downstream antioxidant therapeutic options. *Curr. Neuropharmacol.* 2009; 7: 65-74.

van de Bovenkamp, M; Nottet, HS; Pereira, CF. Interactions of human immunodeficiency virus-1 proteins with neurons: possible role in the development of human immunodeficiency virus-1 associated dementia. *Eur. J. Clin. Invest.* 2002; 32: 619-27.

Wang, HK; Park, UJ; Kim, SY; *et al.* Free radical production in CA1 neurons induces MIP-1alpha expression, microglial recruitment, and delayed neuronal death after transient forebrain ischemia. *J. Neurosci.* 2008; 28, 1721–27.

Watanabe, Y; Chu, Y; Andresen, JJ; *et al.* Gene transfer of extracellular superoxide dismutase reduces cerebral vasospasm after subarachnoid hemorrhage. *Stroke* 2003; 34: 434-40.

Wiley, CA; Baldwin, M; Achim, CL. Expression of HIV regulatory and structural mRNA in the central nervous system. *AIDS* 1996; 10: 843-47.

Xu, Y; Kulkosky, J; Acheampong, E; *et al.* HIV-1-mediated apoptosis of neuronal cells: proximal molecular mechanisms of HIV-1-induced encephalopathy. *Proc. Natl. Acad. Sci. USA* 2004; 101: 7070–75.

Yong, VW; Power, C; Forsyth, P; *et al.* Metalloproteinases in biology and pathology of the central nervous system. *Nat. Rev. Neurosci.* 2001; 2: 502-11.

Zhou, BY; Liu, Y; Kim, B; *et al.* Astrocyte activation and dysfunction and neuron death by HIV-1 tat expression in astrocytes. *Mol. Cell. Neurosci.* 2004; 27: 296-305.

Zinc, MC; Uhrlaub, J; DeWitt, J; *et al.* Neuroprotective anti-human immunodeficiency virus activity of minocycline. *JAMA* 2005; 293: 2003-11.

Zozulya, AL; Reinke, E; Baiu, DC; *et al.* Dendritic cell transmigration through brain microvessel endothelium is regulated by MIP-1α chemokine and matrix metalloproteinases. *J. Immunol.* 2007; 178: 520-29.

In: Encephalitis, Encephalomyelitis and Encephalopathies   ISBN: 978-1-62257-766-8
Editors: Andrew Ruiz and Douglas Fleming   © 2013 Nova Science Publishers, Inc.

Chapter 2

NONCONVULSIVE STATUS EPILEPTICUS

Kenneth Imerman[1] and Rama Maganti[1]
[1]Barrow Neurological Institute/St Joseph's Hospital and
Medical Center, Phoenix, AZ, US

ABSTRACT

Nonconvulsive status epilepticus (NCSE) is a heterogeneous disorder with multiple subtypes that encompasses a variety of etiologies, electroencephalographic patterns, mental states, and prognoses. The term "nonconvulsive status epilepticus" has been used synonymously with complex partial status epilepticus (CPSE), absence status epilepticus (AS), and status epilepticus in comatose patients. It may present in the setting of metabolic disorders, neurotoxicity, acute cerebral lesions, and pre-existing epilepsy. Based on current estimates, NCSE constitutes about 25-50% of all cases of status epilepticus. Electroencephalogram (EEG) can be quite useful in diagnosing NCSE. However, the diagnosis is not always straight forward, particularly in the elderly and/or comatose patient, as clinical features and various periodic electroencephalographic patterns can be seen both in SE and in a variety of encephalopathic conditions. This has led to both under-recognition and misdiagnosis of NCSE. Although some subtypes of NCSE, such as absence status epilepticus, are easily treatable, others respond poorly to therapy. Given the unclear degree of morbidity and, at times, self-limiting course, debate exists over how aggressively clinicians should treat NCSE. Further work is needed to better classify NCSE subtypes and to determine which EEG patterns, in fact, represent NCSE, so that treatment paradigms and prognoses may be established for different subtypes of NCSE.

1. INTRODUCTION

Nonconvulsive status epilepticus (NCSE), a subset of status epilepticus (SE), is simply described as a change in mental status and behavior, without major motor signs, associated with continuous epileptiform features on the electroencephalogram. But for the simplicity of the description, NCSE is, in fact, a heterogeneous disorder with multiple subtypes that span a variety of etiologies, electroencephalographic patterns, mental states, and prognoses.

In the early 1800s, French and English physicians referred to status epilepticus by several names, including *furor epilepticus*; *epileptic mania, epileptic delirium*, and *fureur epileptique*. By the mid-1800s, the term *petit mal intellectual* was also used [1]. However, it was not until the introduction of EEG that distinctions between the different forms of status epilepticus could be determined. Subsequently, conditions without overt motor signs could, for the first time, be identified as epileptic. The first description of absence status was given by William Lennox in 1945. Complex partial status epilepticus was subsequently described by Gastaut in 1956 [1]. The understanding of nonconvulsive status has evolved over the last 50 years with descriptions of "spike–wave stupor" by Niedermeyer and Khalifeh [2] and the differences in "subtle versus overt" status epilepticus described by Treiman and colleagues [3].

Today, NCSE is a common yet still under-recognized condition, particularly in critically ill and comatose patients. Delay in diagnosis and treatment may be associated with increased mortality and morbidity. Therefore, prompt identification of the condition and administration of appropriate treatment is paramount. However, arriving at effective treatment strategies has proved challenging. Firstly, there is still no universally accepted definition. Secondly, there is disagreement on the electroencephalographic features that are consistent with NCSE and confusion on how aggressively NCSE should be treated, especially in patients who are critically ill and/or comatose. Even prognosis varies widely from subtype to subtype.

In this chapter, we will discuss the nosology and definitions of NCSE as well as epidemiology with regard to various age groups. We then outline several classification schemes that can and have been used to distinguish subtypes, including a classification based on etiology. We shall then outline the pathophysiology and neuropsychological consequences of the disorder, and identify various EEG patterns associated with NCSE. Finally, we will discuss several principles of treatment for NCSE.

2. Nosology and Definitions

A variety of terms have been used in the current literature to denote NCSE, including minor status epilepticus, spike–wave stupor, epileptic twilight state, epilepsia minores continua, petit mal, impulsive-petit mal status, and dialeptic status epilepticus [4]. None of the terms encompasses all the features of NCSE, which can be varied. For example, petit mal status may simply denote absence status epilepticus. Spike–wave stupor has been used to denote a specific EEG pattern [2]. Subtle convulsive status is a term used to describe status epilepticus with subtle clinical features of myoclonic jerks or nystagmus in association with electrographic discharges [3]. Epileptic twilight state is a term used in the setting of complex partial status epilepticus [5]. Dialeptic status is a term that incorporates semiology into classification [6]. None of the preceding terms are universal, as the condition encompasses diverse clinical, etiological, and EEG features, and thus the term NCSE is currently accepted terminology with the understanding that there are many subtypes. The definition of NCSE cannot rely on clinical symptoms alone because those symptoms may range from subtle encephalopathy and subtle clinical signs to a frank comatose state.

Moreover, clinical symptoms may be indistinguishable from those of other nonepileptic disorders, for example, transient global amnesia [7]. Definitions cannot rely simply on EEG criteria because there are no EEG patterns that are pathognomonic of NCSE, which can range from continuous ictal discharges that may be focal or generalized to rhythmic and periodic patterns of undetermined significance. Definitions cannot be based on duration alone either.

Most epidemiological studies of status epilepticus have specified a duration of 30 minutes, though this is somewhat arbitrary. Response to treatment can be considered a part of the definition, though lack of immediate response to treatment does not necessarily exclude the diagnosis. From a practical standpoint, a working definition should consist of all of the aforementioned aspects. Thus, NCSE can be defined as a condition with a prolonged state of impaired consciousness or altered sensorium associated with continuous paroxysmal activity or electrographic discharges on the EEG.

3. EPIDEMIOLOGY

The incidence of NCSE varies according to age and subtype. Because of this variation, general population-based incidence rates for NCSE are difficult to obtain. Moreover, existing studies use different diagnostic criteria and definitions for NCSE. Because studies rarely address the incidence and prevalence of NCSE directly, it must therefore be inferred.

That being understood, incidence rates for status epilepticus (of all types) vary in epidemiological studies from 9.9/100,000 per year in adults to 54.2/100,000 per year in the elderly [8-12]. Cumulative incidence of status epilepticus, which includes both convulsive and nonconvulsive status, has been studied both in Europe and in the United States. European studies show incidence rates from 9.9/100,000 in French-speaking Switzerland [10] to 10.7 in Bologna, Italy [12] and 17.1 in Germany [11]. In the United States, two studies examined the incidence of status epilepticus. In a cohort from Rochester, MN, the incidence rate was 18.3/100,000 [9], and in another prospective study in Richmond, VA, rates were higher at 41/100,000 per year [8]. The causes underlying such variation are not clear, though differences in case ascertainment may account for it. The incidence of both convulsive and nonconvulsive status in these studies has a bimodal distribution, with the highest incidence in children less than 1 year of age and in the elderly over the age of 60.

Several studies have examined NCSE in the critically ill. Knake et al. [11] point out that NCSE constitutes about 25–50% of all cases of status epilepticus. In a prospective study of comatose patients in the ICU without overt clinical signs, Towne et al. [13] found that 8% of patients had NCSE on the basis of the EEG. Others have reported prevalences of 31 and 38% for NCSE in comatose adults in ICU. In another prospective study, Litt et al. [14] showed that about 0.5% (24 of 4559 patients over 2 years) of elderly admitted to the medical ICU have NCSE. In the neurological ICU, the prevalence may be higher, with 22 of 210 (10.5%) patients having NCSE either on an emergent EEG or following continuous EEG monitoring [15].

The prevalence of nonconvulsive seizures (not necessarily NCSE) may be even higher. Claassen et al. [16] found that 18% of patients who underwent continuous EEG monitoring in the ICU had nonconvulsive seizures. Furthermore, estimates of prevalence for NCSE in the elderly are much higher than those in young adults. Epidemiological studies from both

Europe and the United States report a much higher prevalence of status epilepticus in the population over age 60. Age-adjusted prevalence rates averaged 54.5/100,000 in the German study [11], though this included both convulsive and nonconvulsive status epilepticus. In the Rochester cohort as well, the incidence of status was much higher in elderly over the age of 65 (>50/100,000) and children under 1 year of age compared with adults younger than 65 [9]. Finally, the incidence rate for patients over 60 for status epilepticus of all types is 15/100,000 per year in Finland [10].

Data on the epidemiology of NCSE in children are much sparser, and there is a lack of any large-scale prospective studies. Most reports are based on continuous EEG recordings in the pediatric/neonatal ICU, with incidence rates ranging from 10 to 34%. In one study [17] among critically ill children, 24 of 117 (20.5%) had NCSE on continuous EEG recording. Tay et al. [18] found that over a 2-year period, 19 of 195 children who had continuous EEG recordings in the pediatric ICU had evidence of NCSE. However, it is not clear if all studies used the same definition of NCSE, and moreover, there was selection bias.

4. CLASSIFICATION

If the definition of altered mental status and continuous epileptiform activity on the EEG with no overt clinical signs is used, NCSE may be classified in several ways.

Age-based classification: includes NCSE in neonates, in children, in adults, and in the elderly. Classification based on age, however, is not perfect, as there may be overlap of conditions across age groups. Clinical classification: this system, based on International League Against Epilepsy seizure types, is used most often and groups patients into those with focal NCSE and those with generalized NCSE (Figure 1). Generalized NCSE may be further subdivided into absence status (ASE), atypical absence, and de novo late absence status epilepticus. Focal NCSE may be further subdivided into simple partial, complex partial, and subtle NCSE. Semiological presentations and clinical features may be varied as described below. Etiological classification: Proposed by Maganti and colleagues [19], NCSE may be divided into those with acute brain injury, those with metabolic disorders, and those with preexisting epilepsy with or without an epileptic encephalopathy. However, etiological classification may be complicated by the fact that knowledge of the etiology may not be as immediately available as clinical signs or EEG patterns. This classification scheme will be revisited when we discuss etiology below.

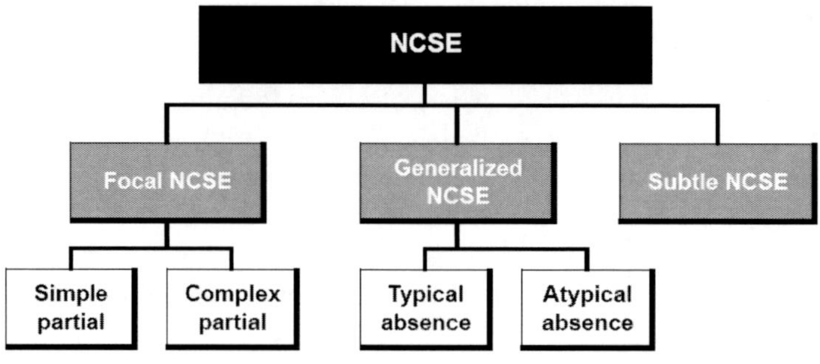

Figure 1. Clinical classification of NCSE [19].

4.1. Clinical Classification

4.1.1. Absence Status Epilepticus

Absence status epilepticus (ASE) is seen in patients with idiopathic generalized epilepsy or may occur de-novo and has a characteristic EEG pattern [20,21]. Clinically, patients present with varying degrees of confusion and slowing of mental functions. The patients are typically not comatose; however, ASE can be punctuated by generalized tonic–clonic seizures that lead to fluctuation in mental status. Though some patients appear cognitively "normal," they are clearly different from their baseline. Some exhibit automatic behavior and others have minor motor findings, such as rhythmic blinking of the eyes or subtle clonic twitching [21,22]. Duration may range from minutes to days. Atypical ASE may be difficult to distinguish from typical ASE as both have similar clinical features.

4.1.2. Simple Partial Status Epilepticus and Complex Partial Status Epilepticus

As with their discrete seizure counterparts, simple partial status epilepticus (SPSE) is characterized by a prolonged focal seizure without impairment of consciousness, whereas complex partial status epilepticus (CPSE) is accompanied by disturbance of awareness. Both are associated with a focal lesion or disturbance that may be acute or chronic. For the purposes of this chapter, SPSE refers only to those patients with nonconvulsive ictal phenomena, for example, prolonged aphasia and olfactory, gustatory, psychic, acoustic, autonomic, sensory, or visual symptoms. CPSE is characterized by confusion and clouding of consciousness of variable degree and may be associated with automatic behavior [21,22].

4.1.3. Subtle Status Epilepticus

Subtle status epilepticus (SSE), as described by Treiman et al. [3], occurs as a natural progression of untreated or insufficiently treated convulsive status epilepticus in which motor phenomena are exhausted. However, in some patients, minor motor findings may still be apparent, such as rhythmical twitching of facial muscles, ocular muscles, or distal extremities, though these patients are invariably comatose. The definition and clinical classification can be confusing because in most patients, convulsive status epilepticus, if untreated, eventually evolves into NCSE.

Similarly, focal status epilepticus may evolve into a generalized pattern. Thus, classification may change within the same patient at different times. Therefore, there is no current classification of NCSE that completely encompasses all aspects of the disease, and both the definition and classification are constantly evolving.

4.2. Nonconvulsive Status Epilepticus and Coma

NCSE in coma presents its own difficulties because it does not fit neatly into the categories listed above, and these patients, in contrast with patients with subtle status epilepticus who, at an earlier time, exhibit overt convulsive activity, may present with no clinical signs other than a comatose state. Just as with other types of SE, the EEG may show generalized or lateralized epileptiform discharges. However, Bauer and Trinka [23] have proposed that what is referred to as NCSE in coma may, indeed, be a distinct condition.

 Kenneth Imerman and Rama Maganti

Table 1. Etiological classification of NCSE [19]

Metabolic / medical disorders	Acute cerebral lesions	Preexisting epilepsy w/wo encephalophathy	Critically ill and comatose patients
Metabolic • Hypoglycemia • Hyperglycemia • Nonketotic hyperosmolar coma • Hyponatreima • Hypocalcemia • Hepatic encephalopathy • Uremia **Medical** • Hypertensive encephalopathy • Posterior reversible encephalopathy syndrome (PRES) • Systemic lupus erythematosus **Drugs / Drug related** • Antibiotics – cephalosporins, imipenam, fluoroquinolones, penicillins, isoniazid, gatifloxacin, ofloxacin • CNS – olanzapine, Clozaril, Lithium, TCA • Serotonin syndrome • Neuroleptic malignant syndrome • Chemo - ifosfamide • Illicit drugs – cocaine, amphetamines, heroin, phencyclidine • Alcohol withdrawal	• Ischemic stroke • Subarachnoid hemorrhage • Intracerebral hemorrhage • Dural sinus thrombosis • CNS tumors • Traumatic brain injury • Demyelinating disease • Vasculitides (SLE) • CNS infection	• Localization-related epilepsy AND idiopathic generalized epilepsy • Pediatric epilepsy syndromes: Ohtahara, West, Lennox-Gastaut, Dravet, Continuous spike-wave during slow-wave sleep	**Children** • Exacerbation of preexisting epilepsy • Perinatal infarcts • Hypoxic-ischemic encephalopathy • Intracerebral hemorrhage • Trauma **Young adult (18-65 years old)** • Ischemic cerebral infarcts • Hypoxic/anoxic encephalopathy • Discontinuation of AEDs • Metabolic abnormalities **Elderly** • Hypoxic-ischemic encephalopathy • Other • Post cardiac arrest • Sepsis • Drugs • Hyponatremia

They coined the terms *coma with lateralized epileptiform discharges* (coma-LED) and *coma with generalized epileptiform* (Coma-GED), and have suggested that the epileptiform discharges observed reflect an end-stage *coma*, associated with the underlying etiology, rather than late stage status epilepticus, as is the case with SSE.

Maganti and colleagues proposed an etiological classification for NCSE including NCSE in metabolic disorders, NCSE in acute cerebral lesions, NCSE in those with preexisting epilepsy with or without epileptic encephalopathy, and NCSE in coma [19]. The advantage of an etiological classification is that it can include all subtypes of NCSE.

5. NCSE AND OTHER DISORDERS

5.1. NCSE in Metabolic/Medical Disorders

A number of metabolic disorders may be associated with NCSE (Table 1). These include hypoglycemia, hyperglycemia, and nonketotic hyperosmolar coma, which are associated with both generalized and focal NCSE, though patients may present early in the course with discrete seizures [25]. Hyponatremia and hypocalcemia are electrolyte abnormalities that may be associated with seizures and NCSE [26]. Status epilepticus has also been observed in patients with hepatic encephalopathy [27,28] and in patient on dialysis with uremia [29,30]. Hypertensive encephalopathy and posterior reversible encephalopathy syndrome (PRES) may also be associated with NCSE and coma [27,28]. NCSE has been observed with medical disorders such as systemic lupus erythematosus [31]. Several medications, including cephalosporin antibiotics [32,33], fluoroquinolones [34], penicillins, and isoniazid, may be associated with NCSE. Psychotropic medications, such as antipsychotics and lithium [35], and complications associated with usage of psychotropic medications, such as serotonin syndrome and neuroleptic malignant syndrome [36], may be associated with NCSE. Finally, illicit drug use and alcohol withdrawal may present with NCSE, as well (Table 1).

5.2. NCSE in Acute Cerebral Lesions

Among acute cerebral lesions, ischemic stroke, subarachnoid hemorrhage, intracerebral hemorrhage, dural sinus thrombosis, brain tumors, and traumatic brain injury are the most common causes of NCSE. Other causes that occur infrequently include demyelinating diseases [37] and vasculitides such as systemic lupus erythematosus [31]. Several studies have examined the prevalence of status epilepticus in patients with cerebrovascular disorders. In a large series, over a 2-year period, Velioglu et al. [38] reported that 1.4% of patients with prior stroke presented with status epilepticus. Similar results were reported by others, who found that 0.7 to 1.1% of patients with any stroke present with status epilepticus [39,40]. Also, among patients with subarachnoid hemorrhage (SAH), who often have persistent mental status changes, evidence indicates that NCSE may be more common than previously reported. Little et al. [41] reported that 19 of 389 patients (2.8%) with SAH due to ruptured aneurysm had NCSE on continuous EEG monitoring. Claassen et al. [42] reported a higher incidence of NCSE of 13% in 108 patients with SAH. Differences in the threshold for continuous EEG monitoring may account for some of the difference. In a neurological ICU, other common causes of NCSE include dural sinus thrombosis, central nervous system infections, and prior epilepsy [15]. Traumatic brain injury is another frequent cause of NCSE, reported in about 21% of cases [43,44] (Table 1).

5.3. NCSE in Preexisting Epilepsy with or without Encephalopathy

NCSE may occur in patients with preexisting epilepsy. Both patients with localization-related syndromes and those with idiopathic generalized syndromes can present with status epilepticus. Indeed, Children with epilepsy more often have episodes of status epilepticus. In a recent study, 36% of episodes of status epilepticus occurred in children with preexisting epilepsy [45,46]. In patients with prior epilepsy, NCSE is encountered more often in localization-related epilepsies (simple partial and complex partial) than in idiopathic generalized epilepsies (IGEs). Among patients with IGEs, absence, atypical absence, and myoclonic status can be observed. A number of the pediatric epilepsy syndromes, particularly those with cognitive disabilities (termed epileptic encephalopathies) may be associated with NCSE during their course. These syndromes include Ohtahara syndrome, West syndrome, Lennox–Gastaut syndrome, Dravet syndrome, and epilepsy with continuous spike–wave activity during slow wave sleep. In children with these syndromes, however, the EEGs at baseline may show continuous or nearly continuous electrographic activity that fluctuates in severity. Therefore, the diagnosis of NCSE may be controversial.

5.4. NCSE in Critically Ill and in Comatose Patients

The etiology of NCSE in patients who are comatose and/or critically ill may vary with the age of the patient (Table 1). In children, NCSE in coma is most commonly due to exacerbation of preexisting epilepsy and less often due to perinatal infarcts and hypoxic–ischemic encephalopathy [45]. Within this study, in children less than 1 year of age, the most commonly associated conditions were perinatal infarcts, hypoxic–ischemic encephalopathy, and intracerebral hemorrhages. Trauma was the least common cause. In young adults (ages 18–65), however, ischemic cerebral infarcts and hypoxic or anoxic encephalopathy were most common. Discontinuation of antiepileptic drugs, metabolic abnormalities, and brain tumors were the other causes [8,13]. In the elderly, however, etiology differs in that hypoxic–ischemic encephalopathy is the most common cause. Litt et al. [14] showed that 41.5% of patients (10 of 24) had NCSE following cardiac arrest. Other etiologies included metabolic problems such as sepsis, drugs, hyponatremia, and cerebrovascular causes such as stroke and subarachnoid hemorrhage.

6. PATHOPHYSIOLOGY AND CONSEQUENCES OF NCSE

NCSE may be associated with neuronal loss as well as cognitive/behavioral consequences. Based on the currently available literature, there are several unresolved issues: 1) it is difficult to exactly assess the full spectrum of consequences associated with status epilepticus in humans, 2) it is difficult to extrapolate data from animal studies to humans, and 3) it is not clear if the neuronal changes associated with NCSE are similar in animals and humans with prior epilepsy compared with those who have de novo NCSE.

Evidence of neuronal damage associated with NCSE comes mostly from animal studies. The earliest studies examined the effects of status epilepticus in baboons with GCSE [47], which showed neuronal loss both in hippocampi and in neocortical regions. Later, animal models for NCSE were developed in vivo and in vitro. Pathological changes reported in animal models of complex partial NCSE include neuronal loss in the hippocampus and mossy fiber sprouting [48]. Neuronal loss was demonstrated in extrahippocampal structures as well [49], and the pathological changes observed were similar to those seen in human temporal lobe epilepsy [48].

At a theoretical level, seizures become self-sustaining through an imbalance of neuronal transmission characterized by a predominance of excitation over inhibition [50]. A number of mechanisms have been proposed including activation of glutamate receptors (NMDA type) [51], influx of calcium ions [52], mitochondrial dysfunction, reactive oxygen and nitrogen species [53] and activation of intracellular proteases and lipases [54], all of which indicate excitotoxicity. This leads to neuronal injury and death [50]. Similar changes have been reported in immature brains as well [55].

In contrast, absence status is felt to be a more benign entity with no neuronal loss demonstrated in animal models [56]. The thalamocortical discharges in absence status are dependent on GABAergic mechanisms, whereas limbic epilepsies are dependent on glutaminergic mechanisms, which may explain the fundamental differences in pathophysiology between the two syndromes.

Although the data on animals are robust, evidence of pathological changes associated with NCSE in humans is largely indirect and anecdotal. In autopsy studies, reduced hippocampal neuronal density was reported among patients who had complex partial NCSE [57], and similar findings have been observed in children as well [58]. Other indirect evidence comes from increased levels of neuron specific enolase, a marker of neuronal injury, in cerebrospinal fluid of patients who had NCSE [59,60]. Moreover, radiological studies demonstrated increased edema acutely [61] and atrophy chronically [62], as well as evidence of neuronal loss on magnetic resonance spectroscopy [63] following NCSE.

Many cases of NCSE are associated with underlying conditions, such as ischemic infarct or infection, it may be challenging to isolate pathology due to NCSE from pathology due to the underlying condition. Similarly, in patients with preexisting epilepsy, there is a question as to what degree of damage is due to NCSE and what is the result of prior seizures. Whether NCSE results in permanent cognitive sequelae is subject to debate in the literature. In animal models of limbic epilepsy, alterations in both memory and behavior have been noted [64,65].

Similar memory and behavioral sequelae were demonstrated in immature rats following a brief episode of status epilepticus [66]. In humans, very few studies have examined the neuropsychological effects of SE. Some showed mild impairment in patients with SE compared with controls [67]. Others have reported mild cognitive deficits immediately following an episode of SE that improved over time [68].

However, one study showed no difference in overall neuropsychological function among patients with epilepsy, with or without NCSE [69]. Although there are no studies specifically examining the neuropsychological outcomes of NCSE, some argue that patients with NCSE may do better than those with GCSE [70,71]. Patients with ASE have not been shown to have any long-lasting neuropsychological effects [67], though this is a subject of debate as well.

7. THE UTILITY OF EEG AND CONTINUOUS EEG MONITORING

As there are no clinical or radiographic findings specific to NCS/NCSE, diagnosis often relies on EEG findings. Thus, the EEG remains the gold standard for making this diagnosis. In critically ill patients, there may be no clinical manifestations of seizure activity at all, and the clinician must have a high degree of suspicion to detect NCSE. Moreover, continuous EEG monitoring, rather than a routine bedside EEG, may be required to detect NCSC. Studies of continuous EEG monitoring in patients in neurological ICUs have shown that electrographic seizures occur in 27–34% of patients with encephalopathy/coma [72]. Furthermore, prolonged monitoring is required to make the diagnosis in most cases of unexplained encephalopathy. Pandian et al. [73] reported twice as many electrographic seizures captured with continuous EEG monitoring as compared with a routine diagnostic EEG, in a cohort of 105 patients. Once the diagnosis is made, the EEG then becomes critical in evaluating the response to treatment.

8. EEG Patterns

In patients who are ambulatory, the most common EEG patterns associated with NCSE are generalized spike-and wave or generalized polyspike-and-wave discharges (in the case of ASE), or rhythmic focal discharges (in the case of CPSE) [74]. In contrast, the EEG patterns in obtunded or comatose patients are more complex and controversial. Electrographic seizures have been defined as generalized spike-and-wave discharges at greater-than or equal-to 3 Hz and clearly evolving discharges of any type that reach a frequency of greater-than or equal-to 4 Hz [75]. However, in comatose patients, rhythmic or periodic patterns often do not clearly fall into "ictal" or "nonictal" categories. These patterns include rhythmic delta activity, generalized triphasic waves, periodic lateralizing epileptiform discharges (PLEDs), generalized periodic epileptiform discharges (GPEDs), bilaterally independent periodic lateralizing epileptiform discharges (BIPLEDs), and stimulus-induced, rhythmic, periodic, or ictal discharges (SIRPIDs) [74,76]. PLEDs have been further divided by some authors into "PLEDs proper" and "PLEDs-plus"; and GPEDs have been divided into periodic short-interval diffuse discharges and periodic long-interval diffuse discharges [77,78]. In this chapter, we discuss some of these patterns further.

8.1. Periodic Lateralizing Epileptiform Discharges

PLEDs have been extensively investigated. Chatrian et al. [79] first described PLEDs as an EEG finding associated with an acute unilateral forebrain lesion. Initially, it was thought that PLEDs signified disconnection between cortical and subcortical structures; however, studies have shown that PLEDs can be associated with lesions of the cortical gray matter, subcortical white matter, subcortical gray matter, or a combination of these [80]. In addition, PLEDs have been reported in patients with no focal lesion at all [81] or with chronic brain lesions [82,83]. Most commonly, PLEDs are seen with an acute structural lesion such as a tumor, infarct, or encephalitis, with or without a superimposed metabolic disturbance [72].

Alcohol withdrawal has been emphasized as an associated factor [74,84]. Although herpes simplex virus is the classic infection associated with PLEDs, a recent series of children with PLEDs reported four cases of influenza-associated encephalopathy and one case of Mycoplasma pneumoniae encephalitis.

Two cases of theophylline toxicity were also reported in this series. Finally, PLEDs can be seen with metabolic problems such as nonketotic hyperglycemia, demonstrating that a broad range of cerebral insults can cause PLEDs [85].

PLEDs generally are self-limited and resolve within days to weeks, although studies have shown that they can be longstanding [83]. PLEDs (Figure 2) consist of periodic spike-and-slow wave or sharp-and-slow wave complexes, typically with a frequency of 1–2 Hz [86]. The complexes can be reflected synchronously in the contralateral hemisphere [74]. The incidence of clinical seizures in the acute setting of PLEDs ranges from 58 to 100%; most commonly these are focal motor seizures or epilepsia partialis continua [86]. Whether PLEDs represents a definitively ictal pattern is debated in the literature. PLEDs have been reported to be "time-locked" with focal motor movements; they have also been reported to be associated with a reversible confusional state [72]. Focal changes in blood flow and glucose metabolism have been documented using SPECT and PET imaging, respectively [87,88]. These findings suggest that PLEDs can sometimes be ictal.

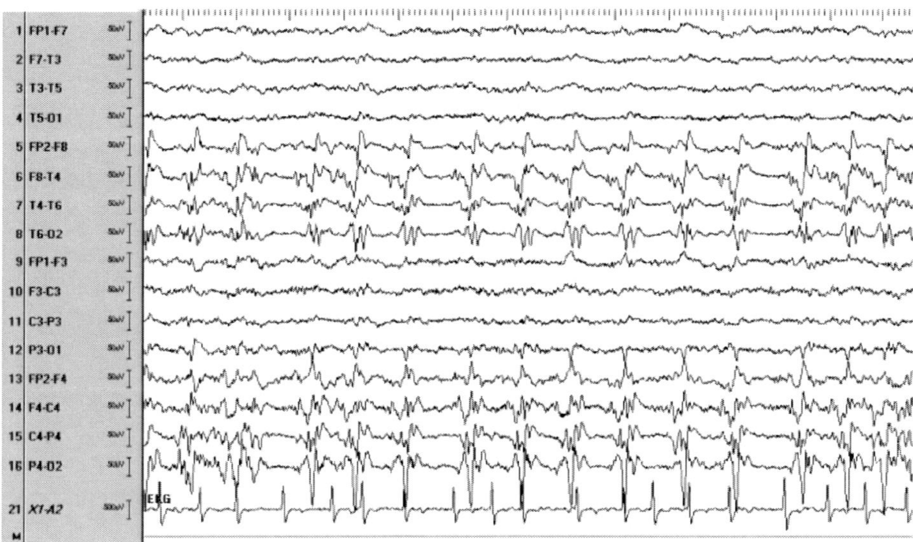

Figure 2. Periodic lateralizing epileptiform discharges (PLEDs) in an 84 year-old woman with a right hemispheric subarachnoid hemorrhage.

However, longstanding PLEDs in ambulatory patients without apparent sequelae have been reported [83], suggesting that that are not ictal. Reiher et al. [78] suggested that PLEDs exist on an ictal–interictal continuum between PLEDs-proper (PLEDs without associated low-amplitude rhythmic discharges), PLEDs-plus (PLEDs with associated low-amplitude rhythmic discharges), and electrographic seizure activity. Clearly, more work is needed in this area. Clinical correlation with the state of the patient is required to make appropriate treatment decisions.

8.2. Bilaterally Independent Periodic Lateralizing Epileptiform Discharges

BIPLEDs (Figure 3) are, by definition, asynchronous discharges and typically differ in morphology, amplitude, and frequency [74]. There are fewer studies addressing the etiology and significance of BIPLEDs compared with PLEDs. De la Paz and Brenner [89] reported that the most frequent causes were anoxic encephalopathy, CNS infection, and chronic epilepsy. Compared with patients with PLEDs, patients with BIPLEDs were more likely to be comatose and had a higher mortality rate [89]. Fushimi et al. [90] reported a case of "benign" chronic BIPLEDs in a patient with bilateral hippocampal infarctions, with mild memory impairment as the only clinical manifestation. BIPLEDs are also highly associated with clinical seizures, 78% of the patients in the series by De la Paz and Brenner [89].

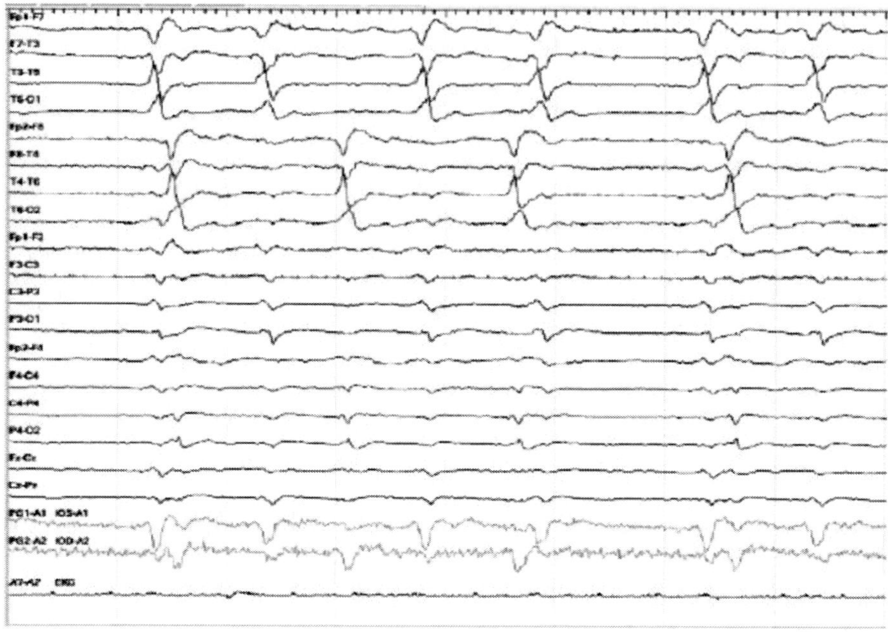

Figure 3. Bilaterally independent, periodic lateralizing epilepileptiform discharges (BiPLEDs) in a in a 74-year-old man with end-stage renal disease and diabetes mellitus who presented with generalized convulsive status epilepticus.

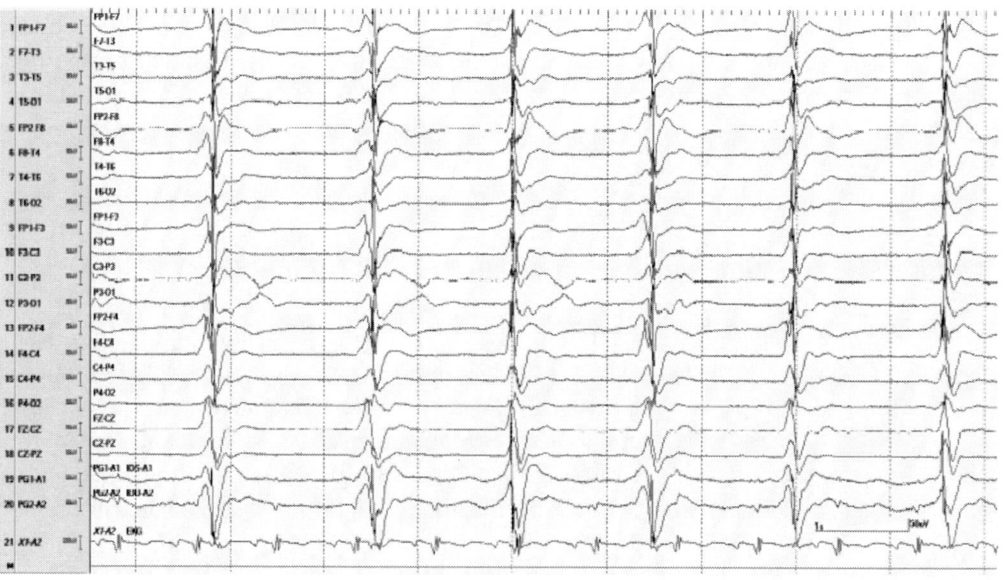

Figure 4. Generalized periodic epileptiform discharges (GPEDs) in a 54 year-old man undergoing hypothermia protocol status post cardiac arrest and anoxic brain injury.

8.3. Generalized Periodic Epileptiform Discharges

GPEDs (Figure 4) are periodic complexes that are bilaterally synchronous, and can have a variety of morphologies. Again, limited data are available, and studies have differed somewhat in their inclusion criteria. Husain et al. [91] included "sharp, slow, and triphasic-like waves," but excluded suppression–burst patterns and continuous triphasic waves, in their series of 25 patients with GPEDs.

Forty percent of the patients had anoxia and a toxic-metabolic encephalopathy, 28% had a toxic-metabolic encephalopathy, and 32% had a primary neurological process (predominantly seizures and stroke). Thirty-two percent of patients met criteria for status epilepticus, defined as electrographic seizure activity, tonic–clonic movements, or a positive response to antiepileptic drug treatment either clinically or electrographically.

In this group, GPED amplitude, duration, and inter-GPED amplitude were significantly higher. These patients also had a lower mortality (50%) compared with patients not in status epilepticus (71%).

Yemisci et al. [92] reported 37 cases of GPEDs; 89.2% of patients had clinical seizures within 48 hours of GPED detection by EEG. Four patients had suppression–burst patterns, 15 had periodic long-interval diffuse discharges (PLIDDs) (interdischarge interval = 4–30 seconds), and 15 had periodic short-interval diffuse discharges (PSIDDs) (interdischarge interval = 0.5–4 seconds).

The most common etiology was metabolic and/or infectious disease (59.5%), followed by subacute sclerosing panencephalitis (SSPE) (29.7%) and Creutzfeldt–Jakob disease (10.8%). Three patients had hypoxic encephalopathy after cardiac arrest. SSPE was more commonly seen in patients with PLIDDs, whereas metabolic/infectious disease and Creutzfeldt–Jakob disease were more common in patients with PSIDDs. One-month mortality was 53.3% for PSIDDs, 20% for PLIDDs, and 100% for suppression–burst patterns.

Classically, three conditions are recognized as being associated with GPEDs: SSPE, Creutzfeldt–Jakob disease, and anoxia [80]. SSPE is typically associated with PLIDDs, whereas Creutzfeldt–Jakob disease is typically associated with PSIDDs (although not in cases of new-variant disease) [80]. In the setting of anoxic injury, GPEDs are universally associated with a poor prognosis [91-94].

8.4. Stimulus-Induced Rhythmic, Periodic, or Ictal Discharges

SIRPIDs are the most recently described periodic EEG pattern [76]. They are defined as "periodic, rhythmic or ictal-appearing discharges... consistently induced by alerting stimuli." Of 150 consecutive, critically ill patients undergoing continuous EEG monitoring, 22% were found to have SIRPIDs. The stimulus-induced pattern was PEDs (including GPEDs, PLEDs, BIPLEDs, and triphasic waves) in 64%; 54% of patients showed evolving patterns that met criteria for "ictal discharges."

Frontal rhythmic delta activity was present in 42%. Fifty-two percent of patients exhibited more than one pattern. Seventy-three percent of patients had an acute brain injury. Fifty-two percent had either clinical or subclinical seizures at some time during their illness, in addition to SIRPIDs. Clinical status epilepticus (but not isolated clinical seizure activity) was more frequent in patients with focal or ictal-appearing SIRPIDs compared with patients without SIRPIDs.

The authors concluded that "further research is necessary to determine the pathophysiologic, prognostic, and therapeutic significance of SIRPIDs" [76].

8.5. Triphasic Waves

Generalized triphasic waves (TWs) (Figure 5) consist of an initial small negative phase, a larger positive phase (usually with the largest amplitude of the three), followed by a final negative phase. The waveforms typically have a duration of 0.25 to 0.5 second. A phase lag, either anterior to posterior or posterior to anterior, can be seen in the longitudinal bipolar montage. TWs can appear in a periodic or quasi-periodic pattern at 0.5- to 1-second intervals [95]. "Typical" TWs have been defined as bilaterally synchronous, symmetric, medium- to high-voltage TWs occurring in rhythmical trains at 1.5–2.5 Hz [96]. However, this is not universally agreed upon, and other authors consider this an unimportant distinction [95].

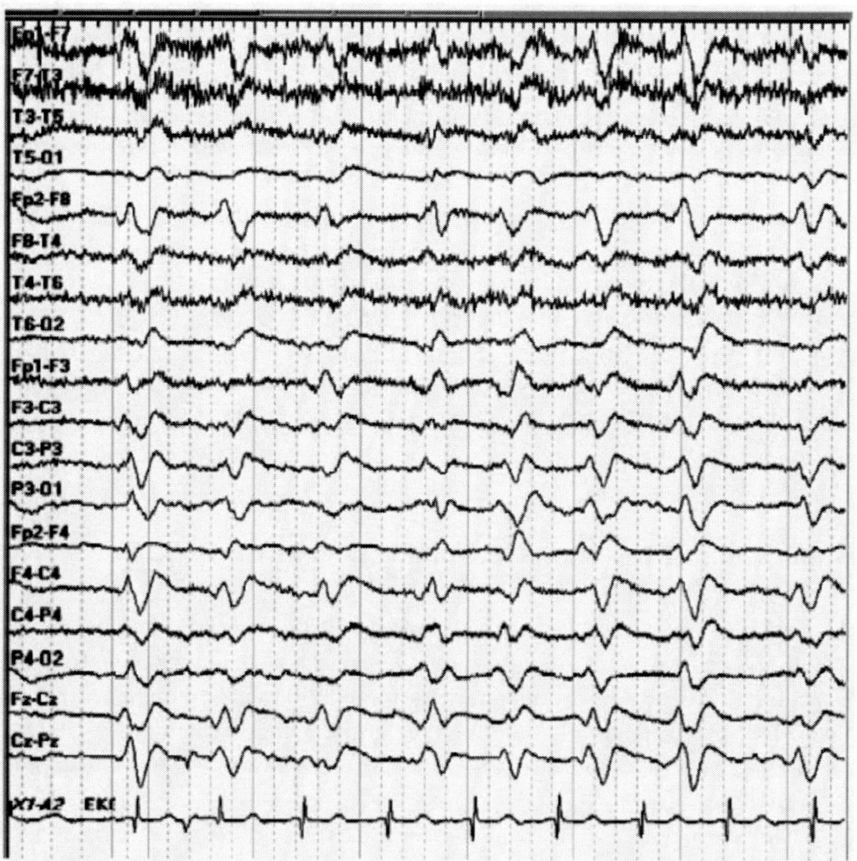

Figure 5. Triphasic waves in a 79-year-old man with renal failure. Observe the prominent second positive phase and the anterior–posterior lag viewed with a longitudinal bipolar montage.

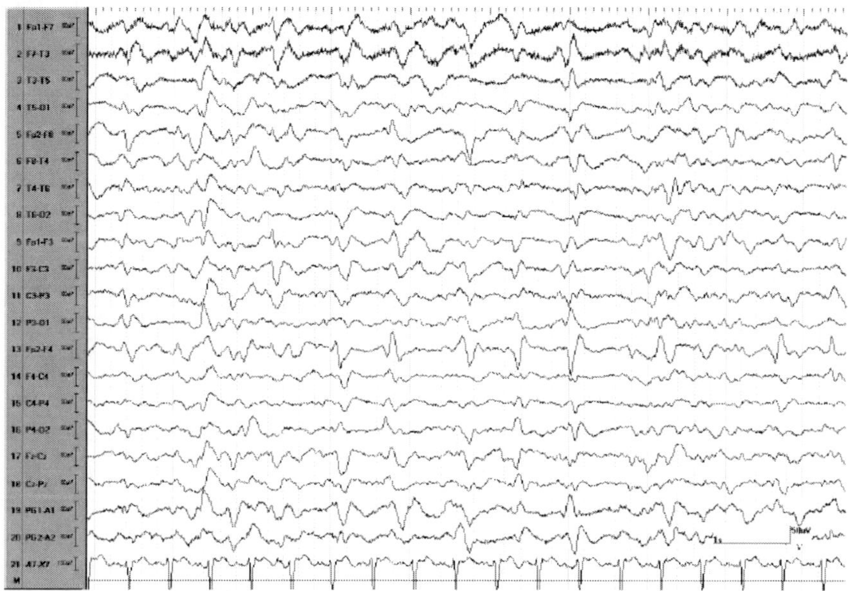

Figure 6. Ambiguous EEG pattern in a 66 year-old female with a ruptured right PCOMM aneurysm and left vertebral aneurysm. Note the bilateral asymmetric triphasic waves and sharply-contoured phase-reversals, though without clear evolution or rhythmicity typically associated with ictal patterns.

Although TWs is the term usually used to imply a pattern of metabolic encephalopathy, this pattern can be indistinguishable from electrographic NCSE. Furthermore, both NCSE and triphasic waves have been shown to clear with intravenous benzodiazepines [74] [80].

It is not clear from the literature when TWs should be considered epileptiform as they may be indistinguishable from GPEDs sometimes. Some authors consider blunted peaks, anteroposterior amplitude gradient, and a time lag as features consistent with TWs, and use these criteria to make the distinction [35]. Others report that focal or bilaterally asymmetric TWs are more likely to be epileptiform [95] [97]. Despite these criteria, many EEG patterns remain ambiguous and difficult to interpret (Figure 6). A recent series reported improvement in mental status and resolution of TWs with antiepileptic treatment in 11 of 15 patients with focal or bilaterally asymmetric TWs [97].

Boulanger et al. reported that TWs associated with metabolic encephalopathies (as opposed to epileptiform discharges in NCSE) tend to have a lower frequency, a dominant phase 2 wave, an anterior–posterior lag, and associated diffuse background slowing.

Interestingly, they also reported that TWs were seen in response to stimulation in 51% of patients; this puts them in the category of SIRPIDs (see above) [98].

However, this was a retrospective study comparing patients who had been diagnosed with NCSE with patients with metabolic encephalopathy. Half of the patients diagnosed with NCSE had anoxic injury, which typically produces EEG patterns that are quite distinct from TWs. This may have biased the findings. However, making the distinction between metabolic periodic discharges and seizure-related periodic discharges is often not possible with EEG alone [80].

In conclusion, there are a number of EEG patterns that are seen in patients with encephalopathy. Some patterns clearly represent NCSE, whereas others are ambiguous.

Moreover, different patterns may be seen within the same patient at different times. Thus, further work is needed to clearly define which patterns represent NCSE and which patterns do not.

9. TREATMENT OF NCSE

There are no systematic prospective trials examining different treatment paradigms and treatment outcomes that encompass all subtypes of NCSE. An existing trial did compare four different treatment arms for convulsive and subtle status epilepticus [99]. Given the risks associated with aggressive treatment, some authors advocate a ''less aggressive'' approach [22].

Others recommend a more aggressive approach in certain situations such as in NCSE with coma [100]. Some forms of NCSE may respond to treatment with first-line agents, and others may be resistant and require a more intensive approach [101].

Thus, optimal treatment of NCSE must account for the specific subtype. Treatment can be further individualized or customized depending on the clinical picture.

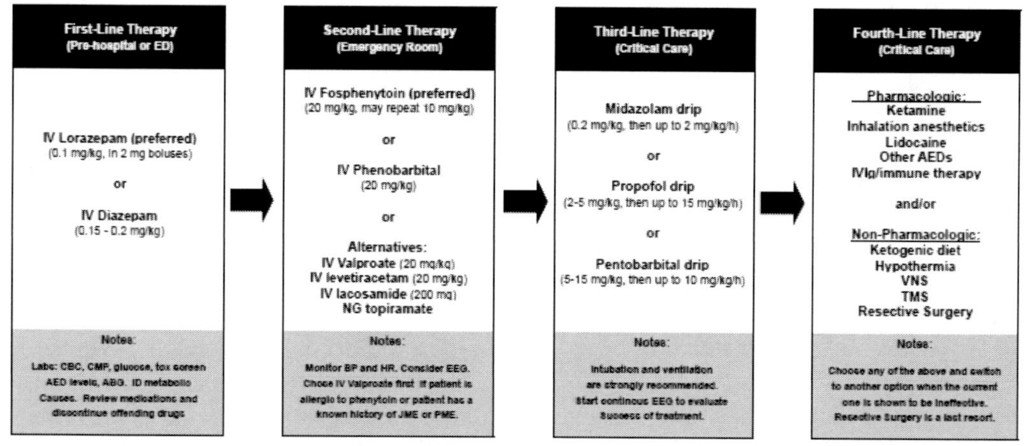

Abbreviations: IV – intravenous; NG – via nasogastric tube; VNS – vagus nerve stimulator; TMS – transcranial magnetic stimulation; ID – identify; AED – antiepileptic drugs; CMP – complete metabolic panel.

Figure 7. Proposed treatment algorithm for aggressive treatment of NCSE [19,50,125,135].

9.1. Aggressive Treatment of NCSE

In patients in whom NCSE developed out of frank convulsive seizures or convulsive status epilepticus, many authors agree that treatment should be initiated as quickly as possible and should be according to accepted therapeutic paradigms for status epilepticus [102]: intravenous benzodiazepines first, followed by intravenous phenytoin, phenobarbital, and then general anesthetics. The outcome in patients with NCSE however, is dependent largely on underlying etiology and timing of treatment. There are ample clinical and basic science studies now to enforce the concept that early treatment intervention is crucial in controlling seizures and improving prognosis.

At this time, commonly employed protocols are based on the treatment of early status epilepticus, focusing on GCSE and refractory SE (Figure 7). Few studies, if any, consider NCSE directly. Furthermore, there is a lack of large controlled studies, and the majority of data regarding second-line drugs come from case series or anecdotal reports. Therefore, treatment for NCSE must be extrapolated from this body of knowledge.

9.1.1. First Line Therapy - Benzodiazepines

The VA Cooperative Study and Pre-Hospital Treatment Status Epilepticus (PHTSE) Study strongly support the position of intravenous lorazepam as first-line therapy, and several other studies suggest that phenytoin or fosphenytoin should be a second-line medication for the treatment GCSE [99,103] (Figure 7).

Lorazepam is the preferred benzodiazepine because of its pharmacokinetics of limited volume distribution and a longer than 12-hour duration of action. Lorazepam is typically given at a dose of 0.1 mg/kg with an infusion rate of 2 mg/min, or as a series of discrete 2 mg boluses. In a large randomized, controlled study comparing treatments, lorazepam was significantly superior to phenytoin in convulsive status. However, phenobarbital was slightly more successful than lorazepam in treating the subgroup of patients with subtle nonconvulsive status, but the difference was not statistically significant [99]. As the duration of status epilepticus increases, however, the effectiveness of benzodiazepines appears to decline. One study showed response rates to lorazepam for patients with subtle status epilepticus were inferior (26%) compared with those for patients in convulsive status (67%) [99].

Diazepam (10–20 mg IV) can be given instead of lorazepam. However, despite its long half-life of 30-60 hours, its high lipid solubility leads to rapid redistribution to peripheral fat stores within 20 to 30 minutes. This limits diazepam's clinical effectiveness and accounts for a high rate of relapse [104]. Diazepam should therefore be followed quickly by second-line AEDs. The commonly reported side effects following administration of benzodiazepines include respiratory suppression, hypotension, and cardiac dysrhythmia.

9.1.2. Second-Line Therapy – Antiepileptic Drugs

If first-line benzodiazepines fail to terminate seizures, anti-epileptic drugs should be initiated (Figure 7). Phenytoin is administered at a loading dose of 18–20 mg/kg in non-glucose-containing solutions at a maximal rate of 50 mg/min. If necessary, an additional 10 mg/kg can be given. Because of phenytoin's cardiovascular complications and injection site reactions, fosphenytoin is preferred to phenytoin in the treatment of SE. Fosphenytoin is a phosphate ester pro-drug of phenytoin that is converted to phenytoin by phosphatases within 8 to 15 minutes following infusion. Fosphenytoin is water-soluble and can be administered faster, at a maximal rate of 150 mg of phenytoin equivalent (PE)/min [50]. Despite this rapid administration, there is no clear evidence that fosphenytoin stops SE faster than phenytoin.

If NCSE continues after benzodiazepines or fosphenytoin, barbiturates are commonly given next. Phenobarbital has been shown in several studies to be effective in treating SE, but its serious adverse effects, including profound respiratory suppression and alteration of consciousness, limit its use. Phenobarbital is usually given at an initial loading dose of 18–20 mg/kg with a maximal infusion rate of 50 mg/min, and an additional 10 mg/kg can be given if needed.

More recently, other alternative anticonvulsants have been employed in NCSE, particularly for those who have compromised cardiovascular function and cannot tolerate the hypotensive effects of other anticonvulsants [105]. These include valproate, topiramate, levetiracetam, and, most recently, lacosamide.

Intravenous valproate appears to be effective for both GCSE and NCSE, including myoclonic, absence, and complex partial status epilepticus [106,107]. In a pilot study by Misra et. al. comparing valproate to phenytoin, no statistical difference in effectiveness was found [24]. Loading doses of 15 to 25 mg/kg have been used for adults, and even higher loading doses in the range 30 to 40 mg/kg were used for children [106]. Despite its effectiveness, one must be cautious as intravenous valproate produces severe persistent encephalopathy in with patients with hyperammonemia or mitochondrial disorders [50,100].

Topiramate in very high doses has also been tried, but is not part of the standard treatment recommendations [108]. Also, because no intravenous formulation is currently available, placement of a nasogastric tube is required for its administration.

Levetiracetam has been used as treatment for status epilepticus, though without conclusive effect [109], and has been implicated in causing nonconvulsive status as well [110]. Potential advantages, however, are lack of interaction with other medications due to renal metabolism and minimal cardiovascular and respiratory side effects. Rapid infusion rates of 4000 mg in 15 minutes, or 2000 mg in 5 minutes have been tolerated [111]. In a series of cases and open studies, around 700 patients with various forms of SE were given levetiracetam. SE was successfully terminated in about 70% [112]. There are no controlled studies, however, evaluating levetiracetam in SE, let alone NCSE.

Lacosamide is a relatively new antiepileptic medication that is available in an intravenous formulation. It has a dual mechanism of action: 1) selective enhancement of sodium channel slow inactivation and 2) modulation of collapsing response mediation protein (CRMP)-2 activity [112]. Several case series show positive results [112]. Patient's were given loading doses of 50-300 mg and maintenance doses of 200-400 mg total daily dose [112]. In a recent study, 10 patients with refractory SE, 8 with focal NCSE and 2 with generalized NCSE, who had failed traditional AEDs and/or drug-induced coma were given lacosamide [113]. NCSE resolved in 7 of 10 patients and partially resolved in another 1 of 10.

9.1.3. Third-Line Therapy– Intravenous General Anesthetics

If standard antiepileptic medication fails to terminate status epilepticus, one may proceed with general anesthetics such as pentobarbital [102,114], thiopental [115], midazolam [116], and propofol [117] (Figure 7). Because these agents cause respiratory depression, patients should be admitted to the ICU and intubated before initiating treatment. Continuous EEG should be employed to evaluate treatment success.

Several factors may be considered when deciding which general anesthetic to start. In a large meta-analysis [118], midazolam, propofol, and pentobarbital were compared in cases of refractory status epilepticus. Treatment failure rates and breakthrough seizures were lower for pentobarbital, and rate of withdrawal seizures was higher for midazolam. The rate of complications such as hypotension requiring pressors was highest for pentobarbital. Pentobarbital is also associated with myocardial depression, ileus, hepatotoxicity, and increased susceptibility to infection. Treatment, with long-term, high-dose propofol, however, puts the patient at risk for "propofol infusion syndrome," characterized by severe metabolic lactic acidosis, rhabdomyolysis, renal failure, hypertriglyceridemia, myocardial depression, bradycardia, and possible death [50]. These drugs are administered at the following doses: pentobarbital 10–20 mg/kg (maintained at an infusion rate of about 1–3 mg/kg/h), propofol 1.0 mg/kg (maintained at 3–10 mg/kg/h), and midazolam 0.2 mg/kg (maintained at 0.1–0.4 mg/kg/h). High-dose thiopental (2–3 mg/ kg followed by maintenance dose of 3–5 mg/kg/h), used in Europe, has also been shown to be effective in refractory cases [115]. There is no agreement as to the depth of coma that should be targeted. Some studies target a suppression-burst pattern, where others target full suppression on EEG [50,111]. Furthermore, there is lack of agreement as to how long the initial induced coma should continue before reducing the dose of anesthetic. In a study by Haltkamp et al., several opinion leaders were surveyed [111]. 22% of responding physicians recommended reducing general anesthetic in the first 24 hours. 72% recommended reducing anesthesia between 24 and 48 hours. 5% recommended between 48 and 72 hours.

Most authors advocate maintaining adequate blood levels of AEDs to assist with seizure control when the dose of anesthetic is ultimately reduced [111]. Typical loading and maintenance doses of anticonvulsants used for status epilepticus are listed in Table 2.

Table 2. Common pharmacologic agents and their dosing in NCSE [111]

Drug	Loading	Infusion	Maintenance dose	Half-life	Adverse effects
Lorazepam	0.1 mg/kg	2 mg/min		8-25 h	Sedation; Respiratory depression
Diazepam	0.15-0.2 mg/kg	5 mg /min		28-54 h	Sedation; Respiratory depression
Phenytoin	18-20 mg/kg	50 mg/min	1.5 mg/kg TID	24 h	Hypotension; Cardiac arrhythmia
Fosfenytoin	18-20 mg/kg	150 mg /min	1.5 mg/kg TID	24 h	Hypotension; Cardiac arrhythmia
Valproic acid	15-30 mg/kg	3-6 mg/kg/min	4-8 mg/kg TID	15 h	Encephalopathy with hyperammonemia or mitochondrial disorder
Levetiracetam	Up to 20 mg/kg (usually 0.5-2 g)	Over 5-15 min	500-1500 mg BID	6-8 h	Mild sedation
Lacosamide	200-300 mg	Over 30 min	100-200 mg BID	13 h	
Phenobarbital	18-20 mg / kg	50-100 mg/min	0.5-1 mg/kg/h	48-120 h	Hypotension; respiratory depression
Midazolam	0.2 mg/kg		0.05-2 mg/kg/h	2 h	Sedation; hypotension; respiratory depression
Propofol	2-5 mg/kg		1-15 mg/kg/hr	2 h	Sedation; hypotension; respiratory depression; infusion syndrome
Pentobarbital	5-15 mg/kg		0.5-10 mg/kg/h	15-60 h	Prolonged sedation; hypotension; respiratory depression; myocardial depression; infections (pneumonia); liver dysfunction; ileus; drug interactions
Thiopental	100-250 mg/kg; 50 mg boluses q2-3 minutes until seizures are controlled		3-5 mg/kg/h	12-36 h	

9.1.4. Late Refractory or Super Refractory SE – Alternative Pharmacologic Therapy

In patients with status epilepticus refractory to the initial generalized anesthetics above, additional treatments have been explored, though the studies have been in the form of small case series or anecdotal reports. Therefore, it is not clear to what degree these therapies are successful in the treatment of NCSE. These have included other general anesthetics, namely ketamine [119], inhalational anesthetics, such as isoflurane[120], lidocaine [24], and magnesium [121] (Table 3).

The rationale for the use of Ketamine stems from the observation that GABA receptors are down-regulated as the duration of SE increases [122], limiting the use of agents with predominantly GABAergic mechanisms of action. Ketamine, an NMDA antagonist, has successfully terminated refractory SE with less hypotension than other anesthetics due to its sympathomimetic properties [122]. Doses up to 7.5 mg/kg/hr have been used. However, outcomes are mixed, and Ketamine is associated with neurotoxicity when used over long periods of time [121].

Inhalational halogenated anesthetic agents have been used in patients who did not respond to intravenous anesthetics. In a case series, isoflurane and desflurane produced EEG suppression-burst and terminated seizure activity in 7 patients with refractory SE [122]. Use of inhalational anesthetics, however, requires specialized equipment, such as gas recovery systems, that are not generally available outside of an operating room [121].

Lidocaine, which modulates sodium channels, has been reportedly administered in boluses up to 5 mg/kg and perfusions up to 6 mg/kg/h [121]. In a retrospective survey of 37 children, 36% of patients with refractory SE responded to lidocaine without major adverse effect [121]. However, serum concentrations greater than 5 mg/L may induce seizures [121].

Magnesium blocks NMDA receptors and has shown mixed results in the treatment of SE [121]. Verapamil may inhibit multi-drug transporters that lower availability of antiepileptic drugs in the brain. Based on several case studies, doses up to 360 mg/day have been shown to be safe [121]. However, the efficacy needs further evaluation.

Some treatments are directed at the underlying cause of SE, and it has become apparent that some refractory SE are immunologically mediated, particularly antibodies against voltage-gated potassium channels and NMDA receptors [123]. In addition, there is increasing evidence that inflammation promotes epileptogenesis, specifically activation of the interleukin-1 receptor/toll-like receptor (IL-1R/TLR) pathway [123]. Therefore, immunological therapy has been employed in cases of cryptogenic, refractory SE, even without clear immunological cause. Several courses of IVIg, high dose steroids, and other immunomodulatory agents, such as rituximab or cyclophosphamide may be employed [125]. Corticosteroids may also provide other non-immunological effects, such as re-closing the blood brain barrier, reversing GABAergic inhibition, and decreasing intracranial pressure [123].

9.1.5. Non-Pharmacologic Treatments

Several non-pharmacologic therapies have been employed when pharmacologic treatments have failed to terminate SE. As with the alternative pharmacologic therapies discussed above, the efficacy of these therapies is undetermined, and most investigations have taken the form of case reports and case series (Table 3).

There has been a resurgence of interest in the Ketogenic diet (KD), and a handful of case reports and case series, with up to 9 subjects, have attempted to study its efficacy in SE. The high ratio of fats to protein and the elimination of carbohydrates induces ketosis and subsequent acidosis [121]. Liquid formulations currently exist that can be given through a nasogastric tube [121,124], allowing the KD to be administered to comatose and critically ill patients. Available studies have looked at patients between 1 and 54 years old with SE due to a variety of etiologies, including Rasmussen encephalitis, head trauma, Sturge-Weber, heterotopias, and others [124]. Response to treatment was seen in 1 to 10 days [124]. In another case series by Nabbout et. al. (Epilepsia 2010;51(10):2033-2037), nine children between the ages of 5 and 8, with fever-induced refractory epileptic encephalopathy (FIRES) who had failed 3-6 antiepileptic drugs, were administered a 4:1 ratio of fat to protein. 7 of 8 children showed rapid improvement. Complications of KD, aside from acidosis, include hypoglycemia, weight loss, and gastroesophageal reflux [124].

Table 3. Alternative therapies for late/super-refractory SE [123]

Pharmacologic	
Ketamine	Up to 7.5 mg/kg/hr. Associated with neurotoxicity when used for a prolonged period [129].
Inhalational anesthetics	Requires specialized equipment.
Lidocaine	Boluses up to 5 mg/kg or perfusions up to 6 mg/kg/h [129]. Serum concentrations greater than 5 mg/L may induce seizures.
Magnesium	Up to 360 mg/day
IVIg / Plasma exchange	To clear antibodies against NMDA receptors or voltage-gated potassium channels. Dosing not established.
Corticosteroids	Reduces inflammation, reverses intracranial pressure and decreases GABAergic inhibition. Dosing not established.

Non-Pharmacologic	
Ketogenic Diet	Administered via NG tube. Response to treatment expected in < 10 days.
Hypothermia	Cool to between 31 and 34 degrees Fahrenheit
Vagus nerve stimulator	Begin stimulation in the OR after implantation and titrate VNS settings rapidly following surgery.
Transcranio-magnetic stimulation	Low frequency stimulation (0.5–1 Hz) at 90-100% of motor threshold. Shown to be useful in simple partial (motor) SE and EPC
Electroconvulsive therapy	Multiple daily sessions over several days.
Resective Surgery	For when a definite, seizure-associated lesion can be identified

Another treatment modality, hypothermia, which is now used regularly for post-cardiac arrest patients, has been investigated in a limited fashion for the purposes of SE, particularly SE that arises as the result of acute brain injury [121]. It is thought to act by reducing energy demands in the brain and diminishing excitatory neurotransmissions [125].

In animal studies, hypothermia was shown to reduce seizure severity, epileptiform discharges, brain edema, and apoptosis [121]. In a series of four adults in refractory SE that were cooled to 31 to 34 degrees Fahrenheit, seizures were controlled in 2 patients and decreased in 1 [125]. The risks of hypothermia include electrolyte disturbances, disseminated intravascular coagulation and other coagulation disorders, infection, cardiac arrhythmias, and paralytic ileus, which is more common with co-administration of barbiturates [121,125].

In patients who have a well-defined seizure focus identified in non-eloquent brain, resective surgery has been utilized [121]. A few case studies have shown that implantation of a vagus nerve stimulator has been effective in a handful of patients [121] when surgical resection is not possible. Transcranial Magnetic stimulation, when administered at low frequency (0.5 – 1 Hz) at 90-100% of motor threshold, was shown to be effective in one patient with simple partial SE [121]. In another case report, investigators preceded the above regimen with an initial high-frequency stimulation up to 100 Hz before starting low frequency stimulations [125].

Lastly, electroconvulsive therapy has been administered to patients with highly resistant refractory status epilepticus. In one study, one to four daily sessions were administered to patients over a few days, which reportedly resulted in lasting control of SE [121].

9.2. Less Aggressive Treatment

Much of the rationale for aggressive treatment stems from studies of GCSE, where prolonged seizures may lead to severe medical conditions—cardiac failure, pulmonary edema, rhabdomyolysis and metabolic acidosis, and metabolic acidosis, to name a few. However, some subtypes of NCSE are felt to be more benign, and treatment of these subtypes may vary from the general principles discussed above.

9.2.1. Absence Status Epilepticus

Absence status epilepticus typically responds very well to benzodiazepines administered intravenously or orally. Lorazepam 2–4 mg might be sufficient; the dose can be repeated, if necessary (maximum of 0.1 mg/ kg) [20]. Resistant cases may respond to intravenous valproate (25–45 mg/ kg) or Phenobarbital (20 mg/kg). An alternative may be rectal diazepam [126].

Some antiepileptic medications, such as phenytoin, carbamazepine, oxcarbazepine, gabapentin, tiagabine, and vigabatrin, may be proconvulsive and trigger absence status [127]. In addition to aforementioned measures, discontinuation of these medications may be necessary to terminate the seizures. Should absence status arise in the context of noncompliance, it is important to reinstitute the prior regimen.

Late-onset "de novo" ASE may be triggered by withdrawal from benzodiazepines, intoxication with alcohol, or initiation of psychotropic drugs that can lower the seizure threshold, possibly in conjunction with other metabolic factors. It is important to treat withdrawal accordingly, that is, by giving benzodiazepines intravenously or orally and stopping any offending drugs [20,21]. If control is not easily achieved, valproate can be successful. However, long-term treatment is not required if provoking factors can be avoided (Table 4).

Treatment of atypical ASE is similar to that of typical absence status.

9.2.2. Simple and Complex Partial Status Epilepticus in Patients with Prior Epilepsy

This is thought to represent a fairly benign entity that typically responds to first- and second line status epilepticus treatment--intravenous benzodiazepines, followed by phenytoin or fosphenytoin, valproate, or, if necessary, phenobarbital, as outlined earlier. To prevent recurrences, antiepileptic treatment should be instituted or the existing regimen adjusted. Recurrence is uncommon though it can be seen in cases that are de novo [128].

New-onset CPSE that occurs after an acute insult is likely within the category of NCSE in comatose patients, and treatment recommendations are less straightforward. Treatment should be determined depending on the seriousness and prognosis of the underlying condition, and the morbidity conferred by the treatment has to be taken into account [129]. The current recommendation is a stepwise escalation of intravenous drugs, starting with lorazepam, followed by phenytoin or fosphenytoin, and valproate or phenobarbital at the doses described earlier [22,129].

9.2.3. NCSE in Coma

NCSE in coma is a diagnosis made by EEG findings suggesting electrical status epilepticus in comatose, severely ill patients. When it is not a consequence of convulsive status epilepticus, many consider it a distinct entity, adding to the confusion regarding diagnosis and treatment of NCSE [22]. The EEG findings can be variable, and unfortunately, the pattern can be ambiguous (see above). This poses a problem for the clinician who does not know whether seizures have preceded the condition and whether it represents an acutely epileptogenic state. Other times, it cannot be established or agreed on whether an EEG pattern represents epileptiform activity.

Several authors suggest aggressive treatment similar to that for subtle status epilepticus, proceeding rapidly to general anesthesia, because response to first-line treatment is poor.

Even if patients are suspected to be in the worst outcome group, according to the neurological insult, a good outcome may be achieved with the most aggressive treatment approach [101]. Some authors question whether treatment should be less aggressive, thinking that the EEG patterns in these patients represent an epiphenomenon of a grave neurological or systemic condition. Although antiepileptic drugs should still be provided, they caution against escalating potentially dangerous treatment, unless there is unequivocal evidence of prior or ongoing epileptic seizures [100]. A study by Litt et al. underscores this notion, documenting that critically ill elderly patients with suspicious EEG patterns were more likely to die after treatment with benzodiazepines than those who did not receive them [14].

9.3. Other Treatment Considerations

Whether patients with epileptic encephalopathies should be treated as having NCSE is controversial. Because the definition of NCSE includes a change in mental status, and patients with epileptic encephalopathy are not cognitively normal, it can be difficult or impossible to determine whether they are in status epilepticus. Although discussion of the pediatric syndromes and their treatment is beyond the scope of this chapter, they exemplify the therapeutic dilemma created by EEG findings in combination with clinical fluctuations in patients with seizures and abnormal baseline cognition [22]. Authors agree that discrete seizures should be treated with long-term antiepileptic regimens [129]. However, because the patients are not considered to be in NCSE, escalation of treatment with rapid loading of phenytoin or phenobarbital or even general anesthesia— to treat the EEG abnormalities—is not recommended [22]. Steroids are used for some syndromes in an attempt to modify the disease process. In patients with continuous spike-and-wave activity in slow-wave sleep, benzodiazepines (clobazam, clonazepam, diazepam) at bedtime have improved cognition and behavior [129].

In summary, most authors agree that treatment should aim at rapidly terminating the clinical and EEG consequences of NCSE. This is usually easily accomplished in cases of ASE or some cases of CPSE. In patients with NCSE evolving out of a convulsive status epilepticus, aggressive treatment is warranted though success is difficult to achieve. Whether aggressive treatment of all comatose patients thought to be in NCSE is helpful or detrimental is a subject of debate. Dedicated clinical trials are required as the treatment itself is associated with high morbidity and mortality.

10. MORTALITY ASSOCIATED WITH NCSE

Data from early studies indicate that status epilepticus is associated with mortality rates as high as 22%, which may be due to the condition itself or the complications associated with the disease and its treatment [8, 130]. Mortality associated with NCSE, however, depends on the type. For example, ASE, strictly defined, is not shown to be associated with increased mortality [131]. Other forms of NCSE, especially CPSE, have been shown to be associated with mortality [68]. Kaplan reported that mortality associated with CPSE is dependent on etiology and level of consciousness [1].

Table 4. Pharmacologic treatment of typical/atypical absence status epilepticus [19]

Recommended	Not Recommended
Start: • Lorazepam 2–4 mg, repeat if needed to a maximum of 0.1 mg/kg Then (choose one or more): • IV valproate (25–45 mg/ kg) • Phenobarbital (20 mg/kg) • Rectal diazepam	• Phenytoin • Carbamazepine • Oxcarbazepine • Gabapentin • Tiagabine • Vigabatrin Note: These AEDs may exacerbate absence seizures

Note: These AEDs may exacerbate absence seizures.

Schneker and Fountain evaluated mortality of NCSE in a prospective fashion and reported a mortality rate of about 18%, with mortality depending on underlying etiology [132]. Moreover, mortality was not a direct consequence of NCSE.

Mortality also depends on the age group. In the pediatric age groups, a mortality rate of 26.3% was reported in a cohort of patients with NCSE, though none died directly as a result of NCSE. In the elderly and those who were critically ill, mortality rates were much higher (56%) [14]. Finally, mortality is influenced by etiology, specifically whether or not patients have preexisting epilepsy. In the study by Schneker and Fountain, 1 of the 53 with preexisting epilepsy died, suggesting low mortality in those with NCSE and preexisting epilepsy [132].

CONCLUSION

Diagnosing and treating NCSE poses many challenges. As mentioned prior, it is a heterogeneous disorder, a repository of varied and potentially disparate physiologic processes united by a common clinical presentation—altered mental status and abnormal rhythmic discharges or patterns on electroencephalogram. The subtypes, themselves, present with varying clinical courses and EEG patterns, in different age groups, and with variable response to treatment.

To identify NCSE in the setting of diminished mental status, one must begin with a high clinical suspicion in order to obtain EEG recording. However, even when an EEG is obtained, distinguishing NCSE from other rhythmic patterns is often not straight forward. The lack of consensus regarding which patterns, or features of patterns, represent ictal patterns and which are more benign may leave the clinician uncertain at best.

There is also disagreement as to how aggressively NCSE should be treated, particularly in critically ill and elderly patients, as treatment paradigms may be associated with serious complications such as multi-organ failure. While animal studies, and some human studies, of generalized convulsive status epilepticus show clear neuronal degradation in a somewhat predictable pattern, there is controversy as to the degree of pathology found in various subtypes of NCSE. Yet, even in subtypes that appear to demonstrate extensive neuronal degradation, it is unclear to what degree there are chronic functional or neuropsychological sequelae. In the face of this uncertainty, the custom has been to treat aggressively.

In the future, to better identify NCSE and optimize treatment, several issues need to be resolved. As ever, the definition of NCSE needs to be solidified with universally accepted criteria. As part of that process, more work must be done to identify the features of the EEG that distinguish ictal patterns requiring treatment from those that are more benign. If the features cannot ultimately be identified by visual inspection, computer analysis of EEG patterns may help to identify distinguishing features. Further studies will have to distinguish the underlying clinical conditions that lead to NCSE, taking age of the patient into account, and evaluate the degree of pathology and neuropsychological consequences in each subtype. Subtypes that involve more serious pathology will thus be approached more aggressively. Researchers, employing prospective multicenter studies, will also have to evaluate treatment modalities for each underlying condition so that therapy may be better "targeted" to the specific subtype. Ultimately, this should improve response to treatment and outcomes in this highly variable disorder.

REFERENCES

[1] Kaplan, P. W. The clinical features, diagnosis, and prognosis of nonconvulsive status epilepticus. *Neurologist* 2005;11:348–61.

[2] Niedermeyer, E., Khalifeh, R. Petit mal status ("spike-wave stupor"): an electro-clinical appraisal. *Epilepsia* 1965;6:250–62.

[3] Treiman, D. M., DeGiorgio, C. M. A., Salisbury, S. M., Wickboldt, C. L. Subtle generalized convulsive status epilepticus. *Epilepsia* 1984;25:653.

[4] Arzimanoglou, A., Guerrini, R., Aicardi, J. *Aicardi's epilepsy in children*. Baltimore: Lippincott Williams and Wilkins; 2004.

[5] Zappoli, R. Two cases of prolonged epileptic twilight state with almost continuous wave-spikes: an electroencephalographic study. *Electroencephalogr. Clin. Neurophysiol.* 1955;7:421–3.

[6] Dan, B., Boyd, S. Nonconvulsive (dialeptic) status epilepticus in children. *Curr. Pediatr. Rev.* 2005;1:7–16.

[7] Niedermeyer, E., Ribeiro, M. Considerations of nonconvulsive status epilepticus. *Clin. Electroencephalogr.* 2000;31:192–5.

[8] DeLorenzo, R. J., Hauser, W. A., Towne, A. R., et al. A prospective, population-based epidemiologic study of status epilepticus in Richmond, Virginia. *Neurology* 1996;46:1029–35.

[9]   Hesdorffer, D. C., Logroscino, G., Cascino, G., et al. Incidence of status epilepticus in Rochester, Minnesota, 1965–1984. *Neurology* 1998;50:735–41.

[10] Coeytaux, A., Jallon, P., Galobardes, B., Morabia, A. Incidence of status epilepticus in French-speaking Switzerland: (EPISTAR). *Neurology* 2000;55:693–7.

[11] Knake, S., Rosenow, F., Vescovi, M., et al. Incidence of status epilepticus in adults in Germany: a prospective, population-based study. *Epilepsia* 2001;42:714–8.

[12] Vignatelli, L., Tonon, C., D'Alessandro, R. Incidence and short-term prognosis of status epilepticus in adults in Bologna, Italy. *Epilepsia* 2003;44:964–8.

[13] Towne, A. R., Waterhouse, E. J., Boggs, J. G., et al. Prevalence of nonconvulsive status epilepticus in comatose patients. *Neurology* 2000;54:340–5.

[14] Litt, B., Wityk, R. J., Hertz, S. H., et al. Nonconvulsive status epilepticus in the critically ill elderly. *Epilepsia* 1998;39:1194–202.

[15] Narayanan, J. T., Murthy, J. M. Nonconvulsive status epilepticus in a neurological intensive care unit: profile in a developing country. *Epilepsia* 2007;48:900–6.

[16] Claassen, J., Myers, S. A., Kowalski, R. G., Emerson, R. G., Hirsch, L. J. Detection of electrographic seizures with continuous EEG monitoring in critically ill patients. *Neurology* 2004;62:1743–8.

[17] Jette, N., Claassen, J., Emerson, R. G., Hirsch, L. J. Frequency and predictors of nonconvulsive seizures during continuous electroencephalographic monitoring in critically ill children. *Arch. Neurol.* 2006;63:1750–5.

[18] Tay, S. K., Hirsch, L. J., Leary, L., Jette, N., Wittman, J., Akman, C. L. Nonconvulsive status epilepticus in children: clinical and EEG characteristics. *Epilepsia* 2006;47:1504–9.

[19] Maganti, R., Gerber, P., Drees, D., Chung, C. Nonconvulsive status epilepticus. *Epilepsy Behav.* 2008;12:572-586.

[20] Thomas, P., Beaumanoir, A., Genton, P., Dolisi, C., Chatel, M. 'De novo' absence status of late onset: report of 11 cases. *Neurology* 1992;42:104–10.

[21] Dunne, J. W., Summers, Q. A., Stewart-Wynne, E. G. Non-convulsive status epilepticus: a prospective study in an adult general hospital. *Q. J. Med.* 1987;62:117–26.

[22] Meierkord, H., Holtkamp, M. Non-convulsive status epilepticus in adults: clinical forms and treatment. *Lancet Neurol.* 2007;6:329–39.

[23] Bauer, G., Trinka, E. Nonconvulsive status epilepticus and coma. *Epilepsia* 2010; 51(2):177-90.

[24] Knake, S., Hamer, H. M., Rosenow, F. Status epilepticus: a critical review. *Epilepsy Behav.* 2009;15(1):10-4.

[25] Mansford, M., Fuller, G. N., Wade, J. P. "Silent diabetes": non-ketotic hyperglycaemia presenting as aphasic status epilepticus. *J. Neurol. Neurosurg. Psychiatry* 1995;59:99–100.

[26] Okura, M., Okada, K., Nagamine, I., et al. Electroencephalographic changes during and after water intoxication. *Jpn. J. Psychiatry Neurol.* 1990;44:729–34.

[27] Eleftheriadis, N., Fourla, E., Eleftheriadis, D., Karlovasitou, A. Status epilepticus as a manifestation of hepatic encephalopathy. *Acta Neurol. Scand.* 2003;107:142–4.

[28] Ficker, D. M., Westmoreland, B. F., Sharbrough, F. W. Epileptiform abnormalities in hepatic encephalopathy. *J. Clin. Neurophysiol.* 1997;14:230–4.

[29] Saurina, A., Vera, M., Pou, M., Cases, A. Nonconvulsive status epilepticus in dialysis patients. *Am. J. Kidney Dis.* 2002;39:440–1.

[30] Chow, K. M., Wang, A. Y., Hui, A. C., Wong, T. Y., Szeto, C. C., Li, P. K. Nonconvulsive status epilepticus in peritoneal dialysis patients. *Am. J. Kidney Dis.* 2001;38:400–5.

[31] Tsuji, M., Tanaka, M., Yamakawa, M., Sagawa, R., Azuma, H. A case of systemic lupus erythematosus with complex partial status epilepticus. *Epileptic Disord.* 2005;7:249–51.

[32] Fernandez-Torre, J. L., Martinez-Martinez, M., Gonzalez-Rato, J., et al. Cephalosporin-induced nonconvulsive status epilepticus: clinical and electroencephalographic features. *Epilepsia* 2005;46:1550–2.

[33] Maganti, R., Jolin, D., Rishi, D., Biswas, A. Nonconvulsive status epilepticus due to cefepime in a patient with normal renal function. *Epilepsy Behav.* 2006;8:312–4.

[34] Koussa, S. F., Chahine, S. L., Samaha, E. I., Riachi, M. E. Generalized status epilepticus possibly induced by gatifloxacin. *Eur. J. Neurol.* 2006;13:671–2.

[35] Kaplan, P. W., Birbeck, G. Lithium-induced confusional states: nonconvulsive status epilepticus or triphasic encephalopathy? *Epilepsia* 2006;47:2071–4.

[36] Yoshino, A., Yoshimasu, H., Tatsuzawa, Y., Asakura, T., Hara, T. Nonconvulsive status epilepticus in two patients with neuroleptic malignant syndrome. *J. Clin. Psychopharmacol.* 1998;18:347–9.

[37] Trinka, E., Unterberger, I., Spiegel, M., et al. De novo aphasic status epilepticus as presenting symptom of multiple sclerosis. *J. Neurol.* 2002;249:782–3.

[38] Velioglu, S. K., Ozmenoglu, M., Boz, C., Alioglu, Z. Status epilepticus after stroke. *Stroke* 2001;32:1169–72.

[39] Labovitz, D. L., Hauser, A., Sacco, R. L. Prevalence and predictors of early seizure and status epilepticus after first stroke. *Neurology* 2001;57:200–6.

[40] Rumbach, L., Sablot, D., Berger, E., Tatu, L., Vuillier, F., Moulin, T. Status epilepticus in stroke: report on a hospital-based stroke cohort. *Neurology* 2000;54:350–4.

[41] Little, A. S., Kerrigan, J. F., McDougall, C. G., et al. Nonconvulsive status epilepticus in patients suffering spontaneous subarachnoid hemorrhage. *J. Neurosurg.* 2007;106:805–11.

[42] Claassen, J., Hirsch, L. J., Frontera, J. A., et al. Prognostic significance of continuous EEG monitoring in patients with poor-grade subarachnoid hemorrhage. *Neurocrit. Care* 2006;4:103–12.

[43] Vespa, P. M., Nuwer, M. R., Nenov, V., et al. Increased incidence and impact of nonconvulsive and convulsive seizures after traumatic brain injury as detected by continuous electroencephalographic monitoring. *J. Neurosurg.* 1999;91:750–60.

[44] Jordan, K. G. Nonconvulsive status epilepticus in acute brain injury. *J. Clin. Neurophysiol.* 1999;16:332–40.

[45] Abend, N. S., Dlugos, D. J. Nonconvulsive status epilepticus in a pediatric intensive care unit. *Pediatr. Neurol.* 2007;37:165–70.

[46] Hussain, N., Appleton, R., Thorburn, K. Aetiology, course and outcome of children admitted to pediatric intensive care with convulsive status epilepticus: a retrospective 5-year review. *Seizure* 2007;16:305–12.

[47] Meldrum, B. S., Brierley, J. B. Neuronal loss and gliosis in the hippocampus following repetitive epileptic seizures induced in adolescent baboons by allylglycine. *Brain Res.* 1972;48:361–5.

[48] Hosford, D. A. Animal models of nonconvulsive status epilepticus. *J. Clin. Neurophysiol.* 1999;16:306–13.

[49] Krsek, P., Mikulecka, A., Druga, R., Kubova, H., Suchomelova, L., Mares, P. Long-term behavioral and morphological consequences of nonconvulsive status epilepticus in rats. *Epilepsy Behav.* 2004;5:180–91.

[50] Rabinstein, A. A. Management of status epilepticus in adults. *Neurol. Clin.* 2010; 28(4):853-62.

[51] Fountain, N. B., Lothman, E. W. Pathophysiology of status epilepticus. *J. Clin. Neurophysiol.* 1995;12:326–42.

[52] Pal, S., Sombati, S., Limbrick, D. D., DeLorenzo, R. D. In vitro status epilepticus causes sustained elevation of intracellular calcium levels in hippocampal neurons. *Brain Res.* 1999;851:20–31.

[53] Cock, H. R. The role of mitochondria and oxidative stress in neuronal damage after brief and prolonged seizures. *Prog. Brain Res.* 2002;135:187–96.

[54] Jope, R. S., Johnson, G. V., Baird, M. S. Seizure-induced protein tyrosine phosphorylation in rat brain regions. *Epilepsia* 1991;32:755–60.

[55] Sankar, R., Shin, D. H., Liu, H., Mazarati, A., Pereira de Vasconcelos, Westerlain, C. G. Patterns of status epilepticus-induced neuronal injury during development and long-term consequences. *J. Neurosci.* 1998;18:8382–93.

[56] Nehlig, A., de Vasconcelos, A. P. The model of pentylenetetrazolinduced status epilepticus in the immature rat: short- and long-term effects. *Epilepsy Res.* 1996;26:93–103.

[57] DeGiorgio, C. M., Gott, P. S., Rabinowicz, A. L., et al. Neuron-specific enolase, a marker of acute neuronal injury, is increased in complex partial status epilepticus. *Epilepsia* 1996;37:606–9.

[58] Tsuchida, T. N., Barkovich, A. J., Bollen, A. W., Hart, A. P., Ferriero, D. M. Childhood status epilepticus and excitotoxic neuronal injury. *Pediatr. Neurol.* 2007;36:253–7.

[59] Rabinowicz, A. L., Correale, J. D., Bracht, K. A., Smith, T. D., DeGiorgio, C. M. Neuron-specific enolase is increased after nonconvulsive status epilepticus. *Epilepsia* 1995;36:475–9.

[60] O'Regan, M. E., Brown, J. K. Serum neuron specific enolase: a marker for neuronal dysfunction in children with continuous EEG epileptiform activity. *Eur. J. Paediatr. Neurol.* 1998;2(4):193–7.

[61] Chu, K., Kan, G. D. W., Kim, J. Y., Chang, K. H., Lee, S. K. Diffusion weighted magnetic resonance imaging in nonconvulsive status epilepticus. *Arch. Neurol.* 2001;58:993–8.

[62] Lansberg, M. G., O'Brien, M. W., Norbash, A. M., Moseley, M. E., Morrell, M., Albers, G. W. MRI abnormalities associated with partial status epilepticus. *Neurology* 1999;52:1021–7.

[63] Lazeyras, F., Blanke, O., Zimine, I., Delavelle, J., Perrig, S. H., Seeck, M. MRI, 1H-MRS, and functional MRI during and after prolonged nonconvulsive seizure activity. *Neurology* 2000;55:1677–82.

[64] Rice, A. C., Floyd, C. L., Lyeth, B. G., Hamm, R. J., DeLorenzo, R. J. Status epilepticus causes long-term NMDA receptor-dependent behavioral changes and cognitive deficits. *Epilepsia* 1998;39:1148–57.

[65] Shorvon, S. Does convulsive status epilepticus (SE) result in cerebral damage or affect the course of epilepsy: the epidemiological and clinical evidence? *Prog. Brain Res.* 2002;135:85–93.

[66] Hoffman, A. F., Zhao, Q., Holmes, G. L. Cognitive impairment following status epilepticus and recurrent seizures during early development: support for the "two-hit hypothesis". *Epilepsy Behav.* 2004;5:873–7.

[67] Dodrill, C. B., Wilensky, A. J. Intellectual impairment as an outcome of status epilepticus. *Neurology* 1990;40(5, Suppl. 2):23–7.

[68] Krumholz, A., Sung, G. Y., Fisher, R. S., Barry, G., Bergey, G. K., Grattan, L. M. Complex partial status epilepticus accompanied by serious morbidity and mortality. *Neurology* 1995;45:1499–504.

[69] Adachi, N., Kanemoto, K., Muramatsu, R., et al. Intellectual prognosis of status epilepticus in adult epilepsy patients: analysis with Wechsler Adult Intelligence Scale— Revised. *Epilepsia* 2005;46:1502–9.

[70] Wasterlain, C. G., Fujikawa, D. G., Penix, L., Sankar, R. Pathophysiological mechanisms of brain damage from status epilepticus. *Epilepsia* 1993;34 (Suppl. 1):S37–53.

[71] Guberman, A., Cantu-Reyna, G., Stuss, D., Broughton, R. Nonconvulsive generalized status epilepticus: clinical features, neuropsychological testing, and long-term follow-up. *Neurology* 1986;36:1284–91.

[72] Jirsch, J., Hirsch, L. J. Nonconvulsive seizures: developing a rational approach to the diagnosis and management in the critically ill population. *Clin. Neurophysiol.* 2007;118:1660–70.

[73] Pandian, J. D., Cascino, G. D., So, E. L., Manno, E., Fulgham, J. R. Digital video-electroencephalographic monitoring in the neurological–neurosurgical intensive care unit: clinical features and outcome. *Arch. Neurol.* 2004;61:1090–4.

[74] Brenner, R. P. EEG in convulsive and nonconvulsive status epilepticus. *J. Clin. Neurophysiol.* 2004;21:319–31.

[75] Hirsch, L. J., Brenner, R. P., Drislane, F. W., et al. for the ACNS Subcommittee on Research Terminology for Continuous EEG Monitoring. Proposed standardized terminology for rhythmic and periodic EEG patterns encountered in critically ill patients. *J. Clin. Neurophysiol.* 2005;22:128–35.

[76] Hirsch, L. J., Claassen, J., Mayer, S. A., Emerson, R. G. Stimulus-induced rhythmic, periodic, or ictal discharges (SIRPIDs): a common EEG phenomenon in the critically ill. *Epilepsia* 2004;45:109–23.

[77] Brenner, R. P., Schaul, N. Periodic EEG patterns: classification, clinical correlation, and pathophysiology. *J. Clin. Neurophysiol.* 1990;7:249–67.

[78] Reiher, J., Rivest, J., Grand'Maison, F., Leduc, C. P. Periodic lateralized epileptiform discharges with transitional rhythmic discharges: association with seizures. *Electroencephalogr. Clin. Neurophysiol.* 1991;78:12–7.

[79] Chatrian, G.-E., Shaw, C. M., Leffman, H. The significance of periodic lateralized epileptiform discharges in EEG: an electrographic, clinical and pathological study. Electroencephalogr *Clin. Neurophysiol.* 1964;17:177–93.

[80] Chong, D. J., Hirsch, L. J. Which EEG patterns warrant treatment in the critically ill? Reviewing the evidence for treatment of periodic epileptiform discharges and related patterns. *J. Clin. Neurophysiol.* 2005;22:79–91.

[81] Garcia-Morales, I., Teresa Garcia, M., Galan-Davila, L., et al. Periodic lateralized epileptiform discharges: etiology, clinical aspects, seizures, and evolution in 130 patients. *J. Clin. Neurophysiol.* 2002;19:172–7.

[82] Gurer, G., Yemisci, M., Saygi, S., Ciger, A. Structural lesions in periodic lateralized epileptiform discharges (PLEDs). *Clin. EEG Neurosci.* 2004;35:88–93.

[83] Westmoreland, B. F., Klass, D. W., Sharbrough, F. W. Chronic periodic lateralized epileptiform discharges. *Arch. Neurol.* 1986;43:494–6.

[84] Chu, N. S. Periodic lateralized epileptiform discharges with preexisting focal brain lesions: role of alcohol withdrawal and anoxic encephalopathy. *Arch. Neurol.* 1980;37:551–4.

[85] Yoshikawa, H., Abe, T. Periodic lateralized epileptiform discharges in children. *J. Child Neurol.* 2003;18:803–5.

[86] Pohlmann-Eden, B., Hoch, D. B., Cochuis, J. L., Chiappa, K. H. Periodic lateralized epileptiform discharges: a critical review. *J. Clin. Neurophysiol.* 1996;13:519–30.

[87] Handforth, A., Cheng, J. T., Mandelkern, M. A., Treiman, D. M. Markedly increased mesiotemporal lobe metabolism in a case with PLEDs: further evidence that PLEDs are a manifestation of partial status epilepticus. *Epilepsia* 1994;35:876–81.

[88] Assal, F., Papazyan, J. P., Slosman, D. O., Jallon, P., Goerres, G. W. SPECT in periodic lateralized epileptiform discharges (PLEDs): a form of partial status epilepticus? *Seizure* 2001;10:260–4.

[89] De la Paz, D., Brenner, R. P. Bilateral periodic lateralized epileptiform discharges: clinical significance. *Arch. Neurol.* 1981;38:713–5.

[90] Fushimi, M., Matsubuchi, N., Sekine, A., Shimizu, T. Benign bilateral independent periodic lateralized epileptiform discharges. *Acta Neurol. Scand.* 2003;108:55–9.

[91] Husain, A. M., Mebust, K. A., Radtke, R. A. Generalized periodic epileptiform discharges: etiologies, relationship to status epilepticus, and prognosis. *J. Clin. Neurophysiol.* 1999;16:51–8.

[92] Yemisci, M., Gurer, G., Saygi, S., Ciger, A. Generalised periodic epileptiform discharges: clinical features, neuroradiological evaluation and prognosis in 37 adult patients. *Seizure* 2003;12:465–72.

[93] Kuroiwa, Y., Celesia, G. G. Clinical significance of periodic EEG patterns. *Arch. Neurol.* 1980;37:15–20.

[94] Jumao-as, A., Brenner, R. P. Myoclonic status epilepticus: a clinical and electroencephalographic study. *Neurology* 1990;40:1199–202.

[95] Fisch, B. J. Electrographic seizure patterns, pseudoperiodic patterns, and pseudoepileptiform patterns. In: *Fisch and Spehlmann's EEG primer: basic principles of digital and analog EEG.* Amsterdam: Elsevier;1999. p. 307–48.

[96] Bauer, G. Coma and brain death. In: Niedermayer, E., Da Silva, F. L., editors. *Electroencephalography: basic principles, clinical applications and related fields.* Baltimore: Lippincott Williams and Wilkins; 2005. p. 471–87.

[97] Kaya, D., Bingol, C. A. Significance of atypical triphasic waves for diagnosing nonconvulsive status epilepticus. *Epilepsy Behav.* 2007;11(4):567–77.

[98] Boulanger, J. M., Deacon, C., Le´cuyer, D., Gosselin, S., Reiher, J. Triphasic waves versus nonconvulsive status epilepticus: EEG distinction. *Can. J. Neurol. Sci.* 2006;33:175–80.

[99] Treiman, D. M., Meyers, P. D., Walton, N. Y., et al. for the Veterans. Affairs Status Epilepticus Cooperative Study Group. A comparison of four treatments for generalized convulsive status epilepticus. *N Engl. J. Med.* 1998;339:792–8.

[100] Walker, M. C. Treatment of nonconvulsive status epilepticus. *Int. Rev. Neurobiol.* 2007;81:287–97.

[101] Treiman, D. M., Walker, M. C. Treatment of seizure emergencies: convulsive and non-convulsive status epilepticus. *Epilepsy Res.* 2006;68 (Suppl. 1):S77–82.

[102] Lowenstein, D. H., Alldredge, B. K. Status epilepticus. *N Engl. J. Med.* 1998;338:970–6.

[103] Lowenstein, D. H., Alldredge, B. K., Allen, F., et al. The prehospital treatment of status epilepticus (PHTSE) study: design and methodology. *Control. Clin. Trials* 2001;22:290–309.

[104] Trieman, D. M. Pharmacokinetics and clinical use of benzodiazepines in the management of status epilepticus. *Epilepsia* 1989;30 (Suppl. 2): S4–S10.

[105] Yu, K. T., Mills, S., Thompson, N., Cunanan, C. Safety and efficacy of intravenous valproate in pediatric status epilepticus and acute repetitive seizures. *Epilepsia* 2003;44:724–6.

[106] Hovinga, C. A., Chicella, M. A., Rose, D. F., Eades, S. K., Dalton, J. T., Phelps, S. J. Use of intravenous valproate in three pediatric patients with convulsive or nonconvulsive status epilepticus. *Ann. Pharmacother.* 1999;33:579–84.

[107] Sheth, R. D., Gidal, B. E. Intravenous valproic acid for myoclonic status epilepticus. *Neurology* 2000;54:1201.

[108] Towne, A. R., Garnett, L. K., Waterhouse, E. J., Morton, L. J., DeLorenzo, R. J. The use of topiramate in refractory status epilepticus. *Neurology* 2003;60:332–4.

[109] Rossetti, A. O., Bromfield, E. B. Levetiracetam in the treatment of status epilepticus in adults: a study of 13 episodes. *Eur. Neurol.* 2005;54:34–8.

[110] Atefy, R., Tettenborn, B. Nonconvulsive status epilepticus on treatment with levetiracetam. *Epilepsy Behav.* 2005;6:613–6.

[111] Seif-Eddeine, H., Treiman, D. M. Problems and controversies in status epilepticus: a review and recommendations. *Expert Rev. Neurother.* 2011;11(12):1747-1758.

[112] Trinke, E. What is the evidence to use new intravenous AEDs in status epilepticus? *Epilepsia.* 2011 Oct.;52 suppl. 8:35-8.

[113] Mnatsakanyan, L., Chung, J. M., Tsimerinov, E. I., Eliashiv, D. S. Intravenous Lacosamide in refractory nonconvulsive status epilepticus. *Seizure.* 2012; 21(3):198-201.

[114] Van Ness, P. C. Pentobarbital and EEG burst suppression in treatment of status epilepticus refractory to benzodiazepines and phenytoin. *Epilepsia* 1990;31:61–7.

[115] Parviainen, I., Uusaro, A., Kalviainen, R., Kaukanen, E., Mervaala, E., Ruokonen, E. High-dose thiopental in the treatment of refractory status epilepticus in intensive care unit. *Neurology* 2002;59:1249–51.

[116] Kumar, A., Bleck, T. P. Intravenous midazolam for the treatment of refractory status epilepticus. *Crit. Care Med.* 1992;20:483–8.

[117] Rossetti, A. O., Reichhart, M. D., Schaller, M. D,. Despland, P. A., Bogousslavsky, J. Propofol treatment of refractory status epilepticus: a study of 31 episodes. *Epilepsia* 2004;45:757–63.

[118] Claassen, J., Hirsch, L. J., Emerson, R. G., Mayer, S. A. Treatment of refractory status epilepticus with pentobarbital, propofol, or midazolam: a systematic review. *Epilepsia* 2002;43:146–53.

[119] Sheth, R. D., Gidal, B. E. Refractory status epilepticus: response to ketamine. *Neurology* 1998;51:1765–6.

[120] Mirsattari, D. M., Sharpe, M. D., Young, G. B. Treatment of refractory status epilepticus with inhalational anesthetic agents isoflurane and desflurane. *Arch. Neurol.* 2004;61:1254–9.

[121] Rossetti, A. O., Lowenstein, D. H. Management of refractory status epilepticus in adults: still more questions than answers. *Lancet Neurol.* 2011; 10(10):922-30.

[122] Smith, M. Anesthetic agents and status epilepticus. *Epilepsia.* 2011 Oct.;52 suppl. 8:42-4

[123] Shorvon, S., Ferlisi, M. The treatment of super-refractory status epilepticus: a critical review of available therapies and a clinical treatment protocol. *Brain.* 2011;134:2802-2818.

[124] Kossof, E. The Fat Is in the Fire: Ketogenic Dient for Refractory Status Epilepticus. *Epilepsy Currents.* 2011 May/June;11(3):88-89

[125] Shorvon, S. The treatment of status epilepticus. *Curr. Opin. Neurol.* 2011 Apr.;24(2):165-70

[126] Collins, M., Marin, H., Rutecki, P., Heller, D. A protocol for status epilepticus in a long-term care facility using rectal diazepam (Diastat). *J. Am. Med. Dir. Assoc.* 2001;2(2):66–70.

[127] Osorio, I., Reed, R. C., Peltzer, J. N. Refractory idiopathic absence status epilepticus: a probable paradoxical effect of phenytoin and carbamazepine. *Epilepsia* 2000;41:887–94.

[128] Cockerell, O. C., Walker, M. C., Sander, J. W., Shorvon, S. D. Complex partial status epilepticus: a recurrent problem. *J. Neurol. Neurosurg. Psychiatry* 1994;57:835–7.

[129] Walker, M. C. Diagnosis and treatment of nonconvulsive status epilepticus. *CNS Drugs* 2001;15:931–9.

[130] Fountain, N. B. Status epilepticus: risk factors and complications. *Epilepsia* 2000;41 (Suppl. 2):s22–30.

[131] Krumholz, A. Epidemiology and evidence for morbidity of nonconvulsive status epilepticus. *J. Clin. Neurophysiol.* 1999;16:314–22.

[132] Shneker, B. F., Fountain, N. B. Assessment of acute morbidity and mortality in nonconvulsive status epilepticus. *Neurology* 2003;61:1066–73.

[133] Cooper, A. D., Britton, J. W., Rabinstein, A. A. Functional and Cognitive Outcome in Prolonged Refractory Status Epilepticus. *Arch. Neurol.* Dec. 2009; 66(12): 1505--9.

[134] Epstein, D., Diu, E., Abeysekera, T., Kam, D., Chan, Y. Review of non-convulsive status epilepticus and an illustrative case history manifesting as delirium. *Australas J. Ageing.* 2009;28(3):110-5.

[135] Chen, J. W. Y., Wasterlain, C. G. Status epilepticus: pathophysiology and management in adults. *Lancet Neurol.* 2006;5:246-56.

Disclosure Statement: Dr. Maganti has been a consultant for Lundbeck and served on speaker's bureau for UCB Pharma and Glaxo-Smith-Kline. Dr. Imerman has no financial conflicts of interest.

In: Encephalitis, Encephalomyelitis and Encephalopathies   ISBN: 978-1-62257-766-8
Editors: Andrew Ruiz and Douglas Fleming   © 2013 Nova Science Publishers, Inc.

Chapter 3

THE IMPLICATIONS OF SENSITIZATION AND KINDLING FOR CHRONIC FATIGUE SYNDROME

Leonard A. Jason[*], *Matthew Sorenson, Meredyth Evans,*
Abigail Brown, Samantha Flores,
Madison Sunnquist and Charles Schafer
DePaul University, Chicago, IL, US

ABSTRACT

Many patients with chronic fatigue syndrome (CFS) have widespread pain which has a large role in patients' activity limitations. Central sensitization has been posited as an explanation of this pain in both Fibromyalgia (FM) and CFS. Repeated or sustained noxious stimulation can lead to central sensitization, which can cause the spinal cord to enter a "hyperexcitable" state. In this article, we will explore the relevance of the central sensitization theory for CFS, as well as link it to the kindling hypothesis that has been previously offered as one explanation for the etiology of CFS. The article also reviews the implications of this theory for both inflammatory markers and central nervous system involvement.

Keywords: Chronic fatigue syndrome, myalgic encephalomyeltits, sensitization, kindling, limbic-hypothalamic-pituitary axis

THE IMPLICATIONS OF SENSITIZATION AND KINDLING FOR CHRONIC FATIGUE SYNDROME

Many patients with chronic fatigue syndrome (CFS) and Myalgic Encephalomyelitis (ME) have widespread pain, and this pain accounts for about 25% of the variability in their

---

[*] Requests for reprints should be sent to Leonard A. Jason, DePaul University, Center for Community Research, 990 W. Fullerton Ave., Chicago, Il. 60614. Funding was provided by NIAID (grant numbers AI 49720 and AI 055735).

activity limitations (Nijs, Van de Velde, & De Meirleir, 2005). As most of the research has used the term CFS, we will use that term in this article. Meeus, Nijs, Huybrechts, and Truijen (2010) found lower pressure pain thresholds for patients with CFS, even at pain-free locations, and psychological factors such as catastrophizing and depression did not account for the findings. Lower pain thresholds for patients with CFS have been found by other investigators (Vecchiet et al., 1996). Central sensitization has been posited as a possible explanation of this pain and lower pain thresholds in CFS (Meeus & Nijs, 2007). In other words, patients with CFS may have a sensitized central nervous system, involving impaired pain inhibition (leading to excessive nociceptive firing in the dorsal horn of the spinal cord). If the pain inhibitory systems are not functioning adequately in patients with CFS, the central nervous system may become hyperexcitable. Central hypersensitivity could explain exaggerated pain due to signals amplified by hyperexcitable neurons. In this article, we will explore the relevance of the central sensitization theory for CFS, as well as link it to the kindling hypothesis that has been previously offered as one explanation for CFS etiology and symptoms (Jason, Sorenson, Porter, & Belkairous, 2011).

THE SENSITIZATION THEORY

Signals for muscle pain travel via nerve fibers to the dorsal horn of the spinal cord, where it prompts the release pro-pain substances (e.g., substance P). Repeated or sustained noxious stimulation can lead to increased neuronal responsiveness or central sensitization (Meeus & Nijs, 2007). In other words, this stimulation can cause the spinal cord to become sensitized, or placed into a "hyperexcitable" state. In support of this theory, Mendell and Wall (1965) have found that, with animals, repetitive C-fiber stimulation can result in progressive increases of electrical discharges from second-order neurons in the spinal cord. Van Wilgen and Keizer (2012) have also proposed that sensitization is a model that may be used for the explanation of the existence of chronic pain. Martinez-Lavin and Solano (2009) speculate that within the dorsal root ganglia, after a trauma or inflammation due to infection, sympathetic neurons sprout and connect to pain sensing neurons, and the dorsal root ganglia become hyperexcitable to painful inputs.

We are beginning to learn the mechanism for this sensitization. Following an injury, the dorsal root ganglion cells are in a state of neuropathic pain, and glia prolong this state of neuronal hypersensitization by releasing substances that act on the immune system (McEwen & Kalia, 2010). Vargas-Alarcon et al. (2012) suggest that for some patients with severe FM, their sodium channels that are located in dorsal root ganglia act as molecular gatekeepers for pain detection. When N-methyl-D-aspartate (NMDA) receptors of neurons are activated, calcium enters into the dorsal horn neurons, leading to the synthesis of nitric oxide (NO) (Bennett, 2000). NO enhances the release of sensory neuropeptides, such as substance P (Luo, & Cizkova, 2000), and this substance increases synaptic excitability. When substance P is released into the neurons, the NMDA receptors become hypersensitive to glutamate, which is the chief excitatory neurotransmitter in the brain (Johnson, 2006). High levels of NMDA receptors on a cell indicate that the cell is hypersensitive to glutamate. As a consequence, spinal neurons are sensitized, and individuals have an increased sensitivity to pain.

THE KINDLING HYPOTHESIS

A related hypothesis involves kindling, in which repeated exposure to an initially sub-threshold stimulus can eventually exceed threshold limits, resulting in persistent hypersensitivity to the stimulus, and ultimately, spontaneous seizure-like activity. Repeated stimulation lowers the threshold for more seizures to occur spontaneously after repetitive sub-threshold stimuli. Chronically repeated, low-intensity stimulation due to an infectious illness may cause kindling, but it may also occur by high-intensity stimulation (e.g., brain trauma). Goddard (1967) found that if rats' brains are electrically or chemically stimulated over a period of weeks at a very low intensity that is known to be sub-threshold for eliciting seizure activity, many of the rats will eventually experience epileptic convulsions. Kindling involves afterdischarge, or neuronal cell populations that continue to fire after the initiating stimulation has ceased (Loescher & Ebert, 1996). Seizure activity can spread to adjacent structures in the brain. Once this system is charged, it can sustain a high level of arousal with little or no external stimulus.

INFECTIONS

Infections have been posited to play a key role in the etiology of CFS. For example, Mycoplasma infections have been reported in patients with CFS and FM (Nasralla, Haier, & Nicolson, 1999), with the M. fermentans species being one of the most prevalent. M. fermentans produces a lipopeptide, which stimulates macrophages (Pall & Satterle, 2001), and macrophages release nitric oxide. It is possible that excessive NO levels can trigger central sensitization. Infection triggers the release of the pro-inflammatory cytokine interleukin-1β (IlB), which can lead to sensitization of peripheral nerve terminals, and these infections can activate spinal cord glia, also leading to the release of NO (Watkins, & Maier, 1999). Elevated NO levels have been found in patients with CFS, and as NO plays an important role in the history of central sensitization, it is possible that central sensitization is at least partially caused by NO. Some investigators have not been able to find increased levels of NO in patients with CFS (Meeus et al., 2010); however, other pro-inflammatory cytokines are produced within the central nervous system in response to infection. Interleukin-six (IL-6), one of the main pro-inflammatory cytokines, is produced by cells within the brain after exposure to viral infections. The production of IL6 may then contribute to the development of seizure activity (Libbey et al., 2011).

Broderick et al. (2010) applied network analysis to cytokines in patients with CFS and healthy controls, and outcomes were consistent with a latent viral infection (i.e., attenuated Th1 and Th17 immune responses, an established Th2 inflammatory milieu, and diminished NK cell responsiveness). Among patients with CFS, the production of pro-inflammatory cytokines (IL-1β and IL-6) is correlated with acute sickness behavior (i.e., fever, malaise, pain, fatigue, and poor concentration). Viruses increase activation of macrophages, which produce a release of interleukin-1beta (IL-1β), a pro-inflammatory cytokine, causing an alteration in the electrical activity of the brain (Maier, Watkins, & Fleshner, 1994). Prolonged exposure to these cytokines may induce a state of chronic activation and kindling (Vollmer-Conna et al., 2004). Pre-existent kindling can also induce the production of pro- and antiinflammaotry cytokines, which could then worsen subthreshold kindling through a process of prolonged activation (Plata-Salamán et al., 2000).

BRAIN DYSFUNCTION

Arnett, Alleva, Korossy-Horwood, and Clark (2011) propose that patients with CFS have relative immunodeficiency that predisposes them to inadequate early control of infections, and ultimately, CFS is due to a long-term inflammatory process on the brain. Kuratsune and Watanabe (2007) believe that brain dysfunction among patients with CFS is caused by reactivation of various herpes viral infections and/or chronic mycoplasma that may cause infection and abnormal production of cytokines. Within seconds of exposure to infection and abnormal production of cytokines, corticotropin-releasing hormone (CRH) is released from nerve terminals to influence hormonal secretion from ACTH in the pituitary and glucocorticoid secretions in the adrenal glands. CRH induces neuronal excitability, which can lead to epileptic output, or seizure activity (Baram & Hatalski, 1998). Fevers and trauma can activate CRH receptors in the hippocampus and amygdala to induce seizures in both children and rats. CRH increases the frequency of spontaneous excitatory postsynaptic currents by 252% (Baram & Hatalski). Infections could cause the sub-threshold kindling effects that eventually increase levels of CRH. Once the kindling has occurred, the CRH may play a less critical role in maintaining the kindling, and after time, CRH levels may become depleted.

Administering the pro-inflammatory cytokine tumor necrosis factor alpha (TNF-α) has been shown to increase seizure activity in animals (Shandra et al., 2002). TNF-α is a cytokine involved in systemic inflammation, and it stimulates the release of CRH, therefore stimulating the HPA axis. Individuals who have higher levels of these pro-inflammatory cytokines may be at greater risk of developing CFS. In support of this proposition, Vollmer-Conna et al. (2008) found that severe illness following an infection was more likely to occur among individuals with high levels of IFN-γ (a pro-inflammatory cytokine) and low levels of IL-10 (an anti-inflammatory cytokine). In addition, elevated levels of pro-inflammatory cytokines can lead to increases in levels of NO, and this nitric oxide can, in turn, react with superoxide to form the powerful oxidant peroxynitrite, resulting in oxidative stress.

In support of immune activation, Natelson et al.'s (2005) research indicated that IL-8 and IL-10 have been found to be significantly elevated in the cerebrospinal fluid of patients with CFS (both of the cytokines are elevated after an acute inflammatory event). Sorenson et al. (2011) also found increased expression of pro-inflammatory cytokine IL-8 in fatigued patients. Another indicator of chronic immune activation is the up-regulated amyloid beta precursor protein (APP) in the cerebrospinal fluid of patients with CFS (Baraniuk et al., 2005), and APP-1 expression is driven by TNF. Baraniuk et al. believe that patients with CFS have a longer rather than shorter version of the gene CNDP1 (carnosine dipeptidase). The longer version of this gene impairs the ability of the brain to protect itself from free radicals. CNDP1 degrades carnosine, which is a free radical scavenger and increases corticosterone levels. Therefore, low carnosine levels could contribute to increased oxidative stress.

Excessive arousal due to sensitization and kindling can lead to an increase in the dendrites of the limbic system, with an increase in excitatory postsynaptic receptors and a decrease in inhibitory presynaptic receptors. Arnsten (2009) has found that dendrites in the prefrontal cortex change after only one week of stress, and dendrites in the amygdala expand in response to chronic stress exposure. This can result in excitatory neurotoxicity, or the death of nerve cells due to very high levels of glutamate (Girdano, Everly, Jr., & Dusek, 1990). de Lange et al. (2005) observed significant reductions in grey matter volume in patients with CFS, and this may be due to inflammation, as grey matter loss in Alzheimer's is due to chronic inflammatory cytokine production in the brain (Clark et al., 2010). Sensitization and kindling may also be what is responsible for the high levels of oxidative stress in patients with CFS due to the dysfunction of ion channels in conjunction with ion transport (Kennedy et al., 2005; Robinson et al., 2009).

In patients with CFS, Baraniuk et al. (2005) believe that the neural circuits running from the spinal cord to the brainstem are not filtering out unnecessary information. The most critical neural circuit, the Papez Circuit, ties together the anterior cingulate, amygdala, and hippocampus, and is associated with heightened awareness (Johnson, 2010). The drug Klonopin often helps patients with CFS because it slows down the overactivity of the brain by increasing production of GABA, a central nervous system inhibitory neurotransmitter. Minor and Hunter (2002) have proposed that prolonged exposure to inescapable stressors will eventually deplete GABA (Minor & Hunter, 2002), thus reducing an important form of inhibition on excitatory glutamate transmission. Doi, Ueda, *Nagatomo,* and Willmore (2009) found that rats with diminished GABA functioning were more likely to develop kindling.

Among patients with CFS, Puri et al. (2011) found reduced grey matter volume in the occipital lobes (right and left occipital poles; left lateral occipital cortex, superior division; and left supracalcrine cortex), the right angular gyrus and the posterior division of the left parahippocampal gyrus, and reduced white matter volume in the left occipital lobe. Areas of the prefrontal cortex and anterior cingulate influence the amygdala (Gupta, 2002), and kindling and sensitzation in these areas could cause continuous sympathetic stimulation which would eventually lead to mental and physical exhaustion as well as glandular depletion. Administration of CRH in rats produces seizures in the amygdala and epileptiform discharges in the hippocampus, but the earliest CRH-induced epileptiform discharges are produced in the amydgala and propagate to the hippocampus (Baram & Hatalski, 1998). A Magnetic Resonance (MR) study examining a pediatric population of patients suffering from chronic EBV infection has shown evidence for the presence of lesions in the hippocampal region (Hausler et al. 2002).

Billiot, Budzynski, and Andrasik (1997) found increased microvolt levels in lower frequencies (5-7 Hz) among patients with CFS, and excess theta waves could be related to cognitive problems (delta waves occurs from 0 to 4 Hz, theta from 4 to 8 Hz, alpha from 8 to 13 Hz, and beta from 13 to 21 Hz). Research using low-resolution electromagnetic brain tomography by Sherlin et al. (2006) has found that twins with CFS, when compared to their healthy co-twins, had higher delta waves in the left uncus and parahippocampal gyrus and higher theta waves in the cingulate gyrus and right superior frontal gyrus. It appears that the slowing of the deeper structures of the limbic system is associated with affect. Flor-Henry, Lind, and Koles (2009) were able to successfully differentiate CFS from controls in 83% of cases using the alpha band during a verbal cognitive condition. Significantly greater source-current activity was found in the left frontal-temporal-parietal regions of the cortex among the patients with CFS.

Using quantified EEG (qEEG) data, Donati, Fagioli, Komaroff, and Duffy (1994) found spike waves for 44% of the patients with CFS compared to only 1.3% of all others. Spikes were most common in the temporal region, which contains the hippocampus. Those in the CFS group also had significantly more sharp waves, more frequent high amplitude alpha, and more frequent bursts of theta waves in the posterior regions. In the patients with CFS, abnormalities were observed that involved high amplitude sharp alpha rhythm (10 Hz) that occurs in the occipital lobes upon closing the eyes. Also, discharges of the type associated with epilepsy were seen in the temporal lobes. These are typically found after head injury and extreme sleep deprivation. Temporal lobes have a predilection for infection by the herpes virus in acute herpes encephalopathy and encephalitis; therefore, the findings may be related to post-viral mild encephalopathy primarily affecting the temporal lobes, which could cause the self-reported memory and attention problems. In a later analysis of these data, Duffy et al. (2009) found that factors derived from the EEG data were able to discriminate with nearly 90% accuracy patients with CFS from healthy controls and from those with major depression.

Patients with CFS and FM have a tendency to sleep lightly (stages 1 and 2), and lack deep sleep (stage 3). Additionally, during sleep there are findings of alpha or awake-like brain waves. Kishi et al. (2010) found that a sleep disruption specific to CFS was a significantly enhanced probability of transition from REM sleep to waking. They also found that those with CFS and FM had greater probabilities of transitioning from waking, REM sleep and Stage 1 to Stage 2, and those from slow-wave sleep to Stage 1. Using a multiple sleep latency test, in which patients are given the opportunity to fall asleep during five 20-minute nap periods, Spitzer and Broadman (2010) found that 80% of FM and CFS patients fell asleep in under eight minutes, an indication of excessive daytime sleepiness. In addition, an immunological marker DQB1*0602 that is present in about half of people with narcolepsy, was present in 43% of patients, five times higher than in healthy people. People with narcolepsy sleep poorly at night and have excessive daytime sleepiness. Spitzer and Broadman believe that patients with CFS and FM have a lesion in the ventral-lateral preoptic nucleus of the hypothalamus, which is critical to initiating and maintaining sleep.

Previous research has found a genetic link to some seizures (Haug et al., 2003; Berkovic, Howell, Hay, & Hopper, 1998). For example, Haug et al. found three heterozygous mutations in ten genes causing distinct forms of idiopathic epilepsy. The three mutations caused the following: loss of function of CIC-2 channels, decreased transmembrane chloride gradient needed for inhibition of GABA, and changes in voltage gating which may cause membrane depolarization and neuronal hyperexcitability, the latter of which is exhibited in patients with CFS. These genetic mutations may be applicable to the kindling found in patients with CFS patients.

An intriguing set of experiments by Hilty and colleagues (2010, 2011, 2011) found that nerve impulses from the muscle inhibit the primary motoric area during energy-demanding exercise, but after narcotization of the spinal cord, the corresponding fatigue-related inhibition processes become significantly weaker. The brain regions that exhibit an increase in activity shortly before the interruption of a tiring, energy-demanding activity are the thalamus and the insular cortex, and the inhibitory influences on motoric activity are actually mediated via the insular cortex. Communication between the insular cortex and the primary motoric area became more intensive as the fatigue progressed. These findings further indicate that the brain plays a major role in muscle fatigue. Napadow, Kim, Clauw, and Harris (2012) found that intrinsic brain connectivity may be used as an objective marker that tracks changes in spontaneous chronic pain in FM.

CEREBRAL BLOOD FLOW (CBF)

Costa, Tannock, and Brostoff (1995) have found that patients with FM exhibit significantly lower rCBF levels during rest in the thalamus and the caudate nucleus. These dysregulations may contribute to the abnormal pain modulation (Willis, 1997), as the thalamus also plays an important role in pain modulation (Saade, Kafrouni, Saab, Atweh, & Jabbur, 1999). It is posible that pain experiences of patients with CFS may be related to low resting state levels of functional activity in the brain stem. Low brain stem rCBF levels may contribute to abnormal function of the locus ceruleus, which controls descending anti-nociceptive pathways from the brain to the spinal dorsal horn. Neary et al. (2008) tested whether patients with CFS have reduced oxygen delivery to the brain during an exercise challenge. They found that, in addition to significant exercise intolerance, patients evidenced reduced prefrontal oxygenation in comparison to controls, suggesting altered cerebral oxygenation and blood volume in the brain.

Below, we examine the evidence for low cerebral blood flow in patients with CFS. Using SPECT scanning, Costa, Tannock, and Brostoff (1995) and Schwartz et al. (1994) found regional deficits of perfusion in the cerebral hemispheres and brainstems of patients with CFS. Deficits in CFS cerebral flow and perfusion have also been found using near-infrared spectroscopy (Tanaka, Matsushima, Tamai, & Kajimoto, 2002), Xenon gas diffusion computerized tomography (Yoshiuchi, Farkas, & Natelson, 2006), and magnetic resonance arterial spin labeling (Biswal, Kunwar, & Natelson, 2011). In a neuroimaging study, Shungu et al. (2012) found increased ventricular lactate and decreased cortical glutathione, as well as lower regional cerebral blood flow in the left anterior cingulate cortex and the right lingual gyrus in patients with Chronic Fatigue Syndrome. However, work by Fischler et al. (1996) and MacHale et al. (2000) could not confirm any deficits in CFS cerebral perfusion. SPECT, CT, and MRI-based methods are limited as they cannot be used during tilt table tests.

In an effort to discover more consistent findings, others have examined cerebral impairments during orthostatic challenges. For example, Ocon et al. (2009) studied a subset of subjects with Postural Orthostatic Tachycardia Syndrome (POTS) who, after being placed upright during tilt-table testing, had decreased cerebral blood flow. Additionally, Low et al. (1999) found decreased cerebrovascular regulation in subjects with POTS. However, Schondorf et al. (2005) found that cerebral autoregulation was preserved in subjects with POTS, and Razumovsky et al. (2003) did not find any CFS versus control differences in cerebral blood flow velocity.

These discrepant findings regarding cerebral blood flow may be due to the differing ways of measuring the response of cerebral blood flow velocity to arterial pressure. For example, Panerai et al. (2005) have found that the critical closing pressure (CCP) and resistance area product (RAP) provide a more consistent two-parameter interpretation of cerebral blood flow responses induced by mental activation tasks than cerebrovascular resistance alone, which has been used in most prior Orthostatic Intolerance (OI) studies. Pilot data from Julian Stewart's laboratory (personal communication, May 17, 2011) has found that increasing orthostatic stress impairs neurocognitive abilities in CFS/POTS, but these impairments are not related to cerebral blood flow using cerebrovascular resistance alone. However, when using CCP and RAP, cerebral blood flow was related to neurocognitive performance: those who did poorly on N-back testing (a cognitive test) had little change in cerebral blood flow, while those who performed best had the largest increments in cerebral blood flow throughout testing. These findings are of importance as studies have found that cognitive activation should increase cerebral blood flow (Sabri et al., 2003). Tilt-table testing accentuated the relation between brain blood flow and cognitive success, and using the CCP and RAP approach allowed for improved separation of cognitive performance based on cerebral blood flow-related parameters.

Hollingsworth, Hodgson, MacGowan, Blamire, and Newton (2011) found the ME and CFS group had substantially reduced left ventricular mass (reduced by 23%), end-diastolic volume (30%), stroke volume (29%) and cardiac output (25%). These results suggest that, compared to controls, patients have significant impairments in stroke volume and cardiac output.

NEUROENDORCRINE SYSTEMS

Stress can trigger mast cells, which are heavily populated in the thalamus (located next to the sleep/wake center in the hypothalamus), to release the stimulant histamine. Excessive mast cells and their release of stimulants could be one of the reasons that sleep is interrupted in patients with CFS and FM. Mast cells act as an immunologic defense against external pathogens, and there are 5 to 14 fold increases of these cells in the top layer of the skin in 100% of FM patients (Blanco et al., 2010). Kindling and sensitization may impact mast cells and the release of histamine in the thalamus, resulting in disrupted sleep patterns among patients with CFS.

There is also evidence for the existence of a persistent hyperserotonergic state in patients with CFS, and this refers to synaptic serotonin concentrations. This state may be related to the inducible form of nitric oxide synthase that is produced during inflammation. As mentioned earlier, high nitric oxide concentrations can activate the NMDA receptor, which antagonizes the serotonin receptor signal transduction pathway. Arnett et al. (2011) proposed that, as the pathways of NMDA and serotonin are antagonistic, this hyperserotonergic state may be an attempt to overcome the chronic inhibition of serotonergic pathways due to increased activation of the NMDA pathways.

Vassallo et al. (2001) found evidence of elevated activity of presynaptic serotonin neurons, which could be an area affected by kindling. The serotonin hypothesis links fatigue to increases in serotonin synthesis and elevations of activities of serotonergic neurons. Patients with CFS have an abnormally high level of brain serotonin, and this may contribute to the persistent central fatigue (e.g., Bakheit et al., 1992). One pilot study found that medications that block serotonin (5-HT3) receptors were followed by at least a 35% improvement in about one-third of patients with CFS (Spath, Welzel, & Farber, 2000). Still, there may be subtypes of CFS patients that in fact show decreases in serotonin levels. One study found decreased brain serotonin levels in patients with CFS (Badawy et al., 2005). Yamamoto et al. (2004), using PET, found that the density of 5-HTT (the serotonin transporter involved in the reuptake of serotonin from the synaptic cleft immediately after its release) of the rostral subdivision of the anterior cingulate cortex was significantly reduced in patients with CFS. These findings suggest that an alteration in the serotonergic neurons in the anterior cingulate cortex, specifically a depletion of serotonin, may play a role in the pathophysiology of CFS. There are at least seven receptor subtypes (5-HT1A, 5-HT1B, 5-HT1C, 5-HT1D, 5-HT2, 5-HT3, 5-HT4) in the brain, and direct-acting agonists and antagonists can have selective affinity for specific receptor subtypes (Fuller, 1991). Cleare, Messa, Rabiner, and Grasby (2005), for example, found widespread reduction in 5-HT1A receptor binding potential, and this reduction was particularly marked in the hippocampus bilaterally, where a 23% reduction was observed.

Among patients with CFS, Cleare et al. (1995) have found hypocortisolism along with increased serotonin neurotransmitter function. Hypofunction of the HPA axis could contribute to CFS by failing to modulate the immune system. However, Arnett et al. (2011) suggest that it is more likely that an immune dysfunction progresses to CFS rather than a hypoactive HPA axis dysfunction predisposing someone to CFS. Supportive evidence for this is that the length of the illness is positively correlated with HPA axis dysfunction, and efforts to treat CFS with corticosteroids have not been effective. It is also of interest that glucocorticoids have a more immunosuppressant effect on men than women (Rohleder et al., 2001), and this functional difference in immune systems may result in a higher pro-inflammatory response to infection in females. Accordingly, about 75% of patients with CFS are female.

Histone deacetylases (HDACs) are a group of enzymes that inhibit the process of DNA unwinding (Yuan et al., 2009). Among an elderly sample with CFS, Jason, Sorenson et al. (2011) recently found increased histone deacetylases activity and lower total antioxidant power in the context of decreased plasma cortisol and increased plasma dehydroepiandrosterone, concomitant with decreased expression of the encoding gene for the glucocorticoid receptor. Therefore, it is possible that increased HDAC activity may in turn contribute to a chronic pro-inflammatory state that may result in the expression of fatigue, through the inhibition of gene expression.

Differences have also been found in the expression of glucocorticoid receptor (GR) (NR3C1) in individuals with CFS when compared to controls (Smith, White, Aslakson, Vollmer-Conna, & Rajeevan, 2006). Those with CFS may have decreased sensitivity to the effects of cortisol due to a down-regulation of GR (Kavelaars et al., 2000). In a pediatric CFS sample, Jason et al. (2010) found hypocortisolism and the down-regulated expression of NR3C1 (the encoding gene for the glucocorticoid receptor expression GR), NFKB1, and NFKB2. It is possible that epigenetic alterations in expression of NR3C1 leads to an inflammatory immunologic profile, which further suppresses cortisol levels through a process of feedback through bidirectional pathways. The reduced expression of the gene for the glucocorticoid receptor expression provides evidence for dysfunction of the HPA axis in those with CFS.

Chronic cortisol deficiency can cause an overproduction of pro-inflammatory cytokine interleukin-6 (IL-6), which has been associated with symptoms of CFS (Arnold et al., 2002). Lower cortisol (Pall, 2007), as well as an overactive sympathetic nervous system, could be responsible for the findings of ejection fraction decreases (the fraction of blood pumped out of the ventricles per heartbeat) and lower cardiac output among patients with CFS (Peckerman, Chemitiganti, et al., 2003).

TREATMENT IMPLICATIONS

Post-exertional malaise is a key symptom of CFS, as exercise lowers the pain threshold for patients with CFS (Whiteside, Hansen, & Chaudhuri, 2004); therefore, avoiding physical activity is likely a consequence rather than the cause of central sensitization. In healthy individuals, sustained exercise with gradual exertion increases lymphocytes and NK cells (Adams et al., 2011) and an anti-inflammatory response, and there are no adverse effects, as the pro- and anti-inflammatory effects are balanced. In individuals with underlying inflammatory states, exercise has a pro-inflammatory effect (Cooper, 2006). Arnett et al. (2011) hypothesize that exercise is pro-inflammatory for those with high circulating cytokine concentrations, whereas the same exercise may be anti-inflammatory for those with less severe persistent peripheral inflammation. These findings suggest that non-pharmacologic interventions that attempt to increase exercise and activity may have negative effects for many patients with high circulating cytokine concentrations, who are already exhausted due to limited energy levels and stamina.

Recently, Jason, Benton, Torres-Harding, and Muldowney (2009) found that patients who exerted more energy than they had available did not improve, whereas those patients who were able to stay within their energy boundaries made significant improvements over time. These findings suggest that when an individual with CFS avoids overexertion, maintaining an optimal level of activity over time, it may be associated with some improvements in physical functioning and fatigue. This study suggests that being overextended and going beyond energy reserves can be an impediment to improving functionality and fatigue levels. Kindling is an explanation for what may occur when patients with CFS overexert themselves and deplete energy reserves. The kindling hypothesis suggests that once this system is charged, either by high-intensity stimulation or by chronically repeated low-intensity stimulation, activities that involve going beyond energy reserves may enhance an already high level of arousal. In a sense, patients with CFS may have this type of cortical excitability that may be due to kindling, and then when they go beyond their energy reserves, the kindling produces high arousal that has implications for the hypothalamus, the autonomic nervous system, and the immune system.

Jason, Torres-Harding, Brown, et al. (2008) combined the four treatment groups into two groups, improvers and non-improvers, based on a measure of physical functioning (as measured by the SF-36, with higher scores indicating better functioning). About half of the participants in each group were improvers and the other half were non-improvers. For these two groups, there were no significant baseline differences in physical functioning. However, at follow-up, physical functioning scores for improvers increased from 43.9 to 66, whereas non-improvers' scores declined from 50.4 to 42.2. What was most remarkable between these two groups was that improvers at baseline had decreased T and B cells and elevated NK percentage numbers, whereas non-improvers at baseline had an elevated humoral immune response (in other words, a dominance of the Type 2 over the Type 1 immune response). Those with the most severe immune baseline characteristics tended to be non-improvers. As this illness is associated with a shift toward a Type 2 immune response, those with this pattern at baseline tended not to improve over the course of the trial. We also categorized patients into abnormal versus normal baseline cortisol levels. We categorized the readings as abnormal if cortisol over five testings during one day continued to rise, was flat, or was abnormally low over time (Jason Torres-Harding, Maher, et al., 2007). We found that patients with normal cortisol at baseline had the most improvement over time for activity levels, fatigue severity, depression, anxiety, and immune system markers. Patients with normal baseline cortisol evidenced improvements on a number of immunologic and self-report measures, whereas patients most impaired on hypothalamic-pituitary-adrenal (HPA) functioning at baseline may be least able to improve when provided non-pharmacologic interventions.

Lerner, Beqa, Fitzgerald, Gill, Gill, and Edington (2010) had treatment success with patients with CFS who had EBV, HCMV, and HHV6 in single or multiple infections. They found that 79 of 106 (74.5%) patients experienced significant improvements in functioning after herpes virus subset-directed antiviral treatment (Lerner et al., 2010). Those with other co-occurring disorders (e.g., Lyme disease) had less favorable outcomes. Other evicence for the persistence of infectious agents was found by Embers et al. (2012), who infected Rhesus macaques with B. burgdorferi and then provided them with aggressive antibiotic therapy. These investigators found that B. burgdorferi can withstand antibiotic treatment, administered post-dissemination, in a primate host, suggesting the same may occur in humans.

Tzartos et al. (2012) provide additional information that in active multiple sclerosis lesion, latent Epstein-Barr virus infection can trigger interferon-alpha production. In other words, while the virus was not actively replicating, it was releasing small RNA molecules in the brain, causing inflammation, damaging nerve cells in the brain, and causing symptoms. This is of particular interest as Capuron et al. (2007) found that interferon-α was associated with increases in glucose metabolism in the basal ganglia and cerebellum, and decreases in the dorsal prefrontal cortex glucose metabolism, and this may be contributing to fatigue in medically ill patients. In another study, Fluge et al. (2011) found that administration of rituximab (Rituxan), which depletes B cells, led to moderate reductions in fatigue in 67% of ME and CFS patients, in contrast to 13% in the placebo control group. However, in most patients, improvements faded within eight to 44 weeks.

Working with patients with FM, Diers et al. (2012) examined changes in pain-evoked brain activation following behavioral extinction training. Findings showed a relation between successful behavioral treatment and higher activation bilaterally in the posterior insula and in the contralateral primary somatosensory cortex.

Light et al. (2009) maintain that exercise could send a continuous signal of muscle sensory fatigue to the central sympathetic nervous system, causing dysregulation of sympathetic nervous system reflexes, and ultimately producing the recognition of enhanced fatigue. Light et al. found that, after exercise, patients with CFS demonstrated increases in mRNA for gene receptors that can detect muscle produced metabolites, genes that are essential for sympathetic nervous system processes, and immune function genes that reliably exceeded responses of control subjects. The researchers concluded that patients with CFS may have an enhanced sensory signal for fatigue that is increased after exercise. In a more recent study, Light et al. (2011) found that the FM group differed from controls at baseline, and had significantly higher mRNA for sensory receptors 2PX4 and TPRIV1, and for the cytokine IL-10, yet the CFS group did not differ at baseline from controls on any receptor values. However, after moderate exercise, two subtypes of changes occurred within the CFS group. In 71% of the CFS group, large gene expression occurred for multiple systems, including sensory receptors (2PX4, 2PX5, TPRIV1), adrenergic receptors (sympathetic nervous system) (Alpha 2a, Beta-1, Beta-2, COMT), and cytokine receptors (IL-10).

However, for 29% of the CFS group, decreases after exercise were only found in the Alpha 2a mRNA, indicating that for this group, there was only adrenergic sympathetic nervous system dysregulation (71% of these patients had orthostatic intolerance, but only 18% had this symptom in the larger CFS subgroup). Because Alpha 2a normally causes a decrease in sympathetic outflow, the decrease in transcription of Alpha 2a in this subgroup may be a response to an abnormally low level of sympathetic outflow, and result in decreased cardiac output and global vasodilation. Sensitization could lead to excessive arousal that leads to an increase in excitatory postsynaptic receptors and a decrease in inhibitory presynaptic receptors.

There are reports of the Lights (cited above) having some success using propranolol, a beta blocker that blocks activity of both epinephrine and norepinephrine and reduces excitation of the sympathetic nervous system. During exercise, this medication reduces the heart rate and the contracting forces of the heart muscle. The researchers use low doses of propranolol (1/5 to 1/10 the dose prescribed for blood pressure control) to block the sensory receptors, reducing the total signal to the sympathetic nervous system (Johnson, 2011).

Nijs, Meeus et al. (2011) suggest that acetaminophen, serotonin-reuptake inhibitor drugs, selective and balanced serototin and norepinephrine-reuptake inhibitor drugs, the serotonin precursor tryptophan, opioids, N-methyl-d-aspartate (NMDA)-receptor antagonists, calcium-channel alpha(2)delta (a2δ) ligands, transcranial magnetic stimulation, transcutaneous electric nerve stimulation (TENS), manual therapy and stress management could theoretically be used to desensitize the central nervous system in patients.

DISCUSSION

Long-term sensory receptor activation may lead to sensitization of spinal cord and brain systems that transmit fatigue signals, causing long-term fatigue enhancement within the central nervous system (Cook et al., 2007). In addition, vascular smooth muscle adrenergic receptors desensitize due to the constant release of catecholamines (Kaufman & Hayes, 2002). Therefore, this dysregulation could lead to bouts of increased metabolites that would further activate sensory receptors.

Neurotropic viral infections could be responsible for the appearance of lesions in the brain and the presence of focal epileptiform seizure activity. It is possible that kindling could play a major role in the promotion of these seizures. Reactivation of various herpes viral infections and/or chronic mycoplasma infection causes abnormal production of cytokines, which can lead to increases in levels of CRH. CRH elevates the frequency of spontaneous excitatory postsynaptic currents by 252% (Baram & Hatalski, 1998). Consequently, CRH receptors in the amygdala may induce seizures (Baram & Hatalski, 1998), and stressors may even cause dendrites in the amygdala to expand (Arnsten, 2009). The earliest CRH induced epileptiform discharges in rats are produced in the amygdala and propagate to the hippocampus (Baram & Hatalski, 1998). In some cases, cortical lesions caused by herpes viridae infections fade before MR documentation can take place. Lesions may then reappear under specific conditions of environmental stimuli, a process that fits well with the relapsing and remitting nature of CFS. Within the brain, areas of the prefrontal cortex and anterior cingulate influence the amygdala (Gupta, 2002), and kindling in these areas could cause continuous sympathetic nervous stimulation that would eventually lead to glandular depletion.

Gupta (2002), borrowing on the work of LeDoux (1998), has suggested that an infection or chemical or physiological stressor can act to create a cell assembly within the unconscious amygdala, which can create sympathetic stimulation through the hypothalamus and other brain pathways involving the flight or fight response. The amygdala first determines whether a stimuli poses a threat, and if so, the amygdala initiates autonomic and endocrine responses to help the organism survive. Areas of the prefrontal cortex and anterior cingulate are involved in attention to dangerous or negative stimuli, which ultimately influence the amygdala. In long-term potentiation, synaptic strength does increase between co-firing neurons after brief but repetitive stimulation, and this has many similarities to kindling. LeDoux (1998) refers to these cell assemblies as being particularly resistant to extinction; so, for some patients, this hard-wiring may only be regulated rather than extinguished. Gupta (2002) believes that activation of the amygdala causes continuous sympathetic stimulation that is a predominantly unconscious process over which patients have little control, but it eventually leads to mental and physical exhaustion as well as glandular depletion.

Wyller, Eriksen, and Malterud (2009) proposed compatible theories, stating that sustained arousal is the primary mechanism of CFS, and they also reviewed findings on how arousal responses can be modified by sensitization. Wyller et al. suggest clonodine may effectively reduce this arousal. Morriss, Robson, and Deakin (2002) have found that low doses of clonidine act pre-synaptically at alpha-2 adrenoceptors to inhibit noradrenaline function, and using this drug with patients with ME/CFS enhances growth hormone and cortisol release, and increases speed in the initial stage of a planning task.

Glass et al. (2004) found that healthy individuals with certain biological patterns (i.e., lower cortisol, more heart rate variability, and NK attenuated response to stress) developed somatic symptoms when asked to stop exercising for a week. These biological patterns may be some of the other predisposing neuroendocrine and immunologic irregularities of some individuals who are at increased risk for sensitization and kindling, and ultimately, developing CFS.

In summary, central sensitization has been posited as an explanation of pain in CFS. Resarch suggests that repeated or sustained noxious stimulation can lead to central sensitization, which can cause the spinal cord to enter a "hyperexcitable" state. This central sensitization theory has many commonalities with the kindling hypothesis, which has also been offered as one explanation for the etiology of CFS. These theories help explain many complex CNS and neuroendorcrine findings within the CFS area, and have important treatment implications. New ways of imaging the brain, revealing pervasive 3D grid structures (Wedeen et al., 2012), should help aid investigators in the future in both the diagnosis and treatment of these types of brain disorders.

ACKNOWLEDGEMENT

The authors thank Tara Lauriat, Elisa Grant-Holler, and Sandra Virtue for their helpful comments.

REFERENCES

Adams, G.R., Zaldivar, F.P., Nance, D.M., & Cooper, D.M. (2011). Exercise and leukocyte interchange among central circulation, lung, spleen, and muscle. *Brain, Behavior, and Immunity,* 14, 14.

Arnett, S.V., Alleva, L.M., Korossy-Horwood, R., & Clark, I.A. (2011). Chronic fatigue syndrome- A neuroimmunological model. *Medical Hypotheses,* doi: 10.1016/j.mehy.2011.03.030.

Arnold, M. C., Papanicolaou, D. A., O'Grady, J. A., Lotsikas, A., Dale, J. K., Straus, S., et al. (2002). Using an interleukin-6 challenge to evaluate neuropsychological performance in chronic fatigue syndrome. *Psychological Medicine,* 32, 1075–1089.

Arnsten, A. F. T. (2009). Stress signalling pathways that impair preforntal cortex structure and function. *Nature Reviews Neuroscience,* 10, 410-422.

Badawy, A. B., Morgan, C. J., Llewelyn, M. B., Selwyn R. J. Albuquerque, S. R. J., & Farmer, A. (2005). Heterogeneity of serum tryptophan concentration and availability to the brain in patients with the chronic fatigue syndrome. *Journal of Psychopharmacology,* 19, 385-391.

Bakheit, A M., Behan, P.O., Dinan, T.G., & O'Keane, V.,(1992). Possible upregulation of hypothalantic 5- hydroxytryptamine receptors in patients with postviral fatigue syndrome. *British Medical Journal,* 304, 1010-12.

Baram, T. Z., & Hatalski, C. G. (1998). Neuropeptide-mediated excitability: A key triggering mechanism for seizure generation in the developing brain. *Trends in Neuroscience,* 21, 471-476.

Baraniuk, J. N., Casado, B., Maibach, H., Clauw, D. J., Pannell, L. K., & Hess, S. S. (2005). A Chronic fatigue syndrome-related proeome in human cerebrospinal fluid. *BMC Neurology,* 1, 5:22. PMCID: PMC1326206

Bennett, G.J. (2000) Update on the neurophysiology of pain transmission and modulation: focus on the NMDA-receptor. *Journal of Pain Symptom Management,* 19, S2–S6.

Berkovic, S. F., Howell, R. A., Hay, D. A., & Hopper, J. L. (1998). Epilepsies in twins: genetics of the major epilepsy syndromes. *Annals of Neurology,* 43, 435-445.

Billiot, K. M., Budzynski, T. H., & Andrasik, F. (1997). EEG patterns and chronic fatigue syndrome. *Journal of Neurotherapy,* 2(2), 20-30 (available at *http://www.snr-jnt.org/JournalNT/JNT(2-2)4.html).*

Biswal, B., Kunwar,P. and Natelson,B.H. (2011) Cerebral blood flow is reduced in chronic fatigue syndrome as assessed by arterial spin labeling. *Journal of the Neurologic Sciences,* 301, 9-11.

Blanco, I., Béritze, N., Argüelles, M., Cárcaba, V., Fernández, F., Janciauskiene, S., Oikonomopoulou, K., de Serres, F. J., Fernández-Bustillo, E., & Hollenberg, M. D. (2010). Abnormal overexpression of mastocytes in skin biopsies of fibromyalgia patients. *Clinical Rheumatology.* (Epub ahead of print).

Broderick, G., Fuite, J., Kreitz, A., Vernon, S.D., Klimas, N., & Fletcher, M. A. (2010). A formal analysis of cytokine networks in Chronic Fatigue Syndrome. *Brain, Behavior, and Immunity.* 2010 May 4. [Epub ahead of print]

Capuron, L, Pagnoni, G., Demetrashvili, M.F., Lawson, D.H., Fornwalt, F.B., Woolwine, B., Berns, G.S., Nemeroff, C.B., & Miller, A.H. Basal ganglia hypermetabolism and symptoms of fatigue during Interferon-α therapy. (2007), *Neuropsychopharmacology, 32,* 2384-2392.

Clark, I.A., Alleva, L.M., Vissel, B. (2010). The roles of TNF in brain dysfunction and disease. *Pharmacology & Therapeutics, 128,* 519-548.

Cleare, A. J., Bearn, J., Allain, T., McGregor, A., Wessely, S., Murray, R. M., et al. (1995). Contrasting neuroendocrine responses in depression and chronic fatigue syndrome. *Journal of Affective Disorders,* 34, 283-289.

Cleare, A. J., Messa, C., Rabiner, E. A, & Grasby, P. M. (2005). Brain 5-HT1A receptor binding in chronic fatigue syndrome measured using positron emission tomography and [11C]WAY-100635. *Biological Psychiatry,* 57(3), 239-246.

Cook, D. B., O'Connor, P. J., Lange, G., & Steffener, J. (2007). Functional neuroimaging correlates of mental fatigue induced by cognition among chronic fatigue syndrome patients and controls. *NeuroImage,* 36(1), 108-122.

Cooper, D.M., Radom-Aizik, S., Schwindt, C., & Zaldivar, Jr. F. (2006). Dangerous exercise: Lessons learned from dysregulated inflammatory response to physical activity. *Journal of Applied Physiology,* 103, 700-709.

Costa, D.C., Tannock, C., & Brostoff, J. (1995) Brainstem perfusion is impaired in chronic fatigue syndrome. *QJM: An International Journal of Medicine,* 88, 767–773

de Lange, F. P., Kalkman, J. S., Bleijenberg, G., Hagoort, P., van der Meer J. W. M., & Toni, I. (2005). Gray matter volume reduction in the chronic fatigue syndrome. *NeuroImage,* 26, 777-781.

Diers, M., Yilmaz, P., Rance, M., Thieme, K., Gracely, R.H., Rolko, C., Schley, M.T., Kiessling, U., Wang, H. & Flor. H.(2012). Treatment-related changes in brain activation in patients with fibromyalgia syndrome. *Experimental Brain Researc.* 2012 Mar 17. [Epub ahead of print]

Doi, T., Ueda, Y., Nagatomo, K., & Willmore, L. J. (2009). Role of Glutamate and GABA Transporters in development of Pentylenetetrazol-Kindling. *Neurochemistry Research,* 34(7), 1324-1331. DOI 10.1007/s11064-009-9912-0.

Donati, F., Fagioli, L., Komaroff, A. L., & Duffy, F. H. (1994, Oct.). *Quantified EEG findings in patients with chronic fatigue syndrome.* Paper presented at the American Association for Chronic Fatigue Syndrome, Ft. Lauderdale, Florida.

Duffy, F. H., McAnulty, G. B., McCreary, M., Albert, M. S., Cucharal, G., Shatzberg, A. F., et al. (2009, March). *Electroencephalographic data distinguish patients with CFS from healthy and depressed controls.* Paper presented at the 9th International Association of CFS/ME, Reno, NV.

Embers, M. E., Barthold, S. W., Borda, J. T., Bowers, L., Doyle, L., Hodzic, E., Jacobs, M. B., Hasenkampf, N. R., Martin, D. S., Narasimhan, S., Phillippi-Falkenstein, K. M., Purcell, J. E., Ratterree, M. S., & Philipp, M. T. (2012). Persistence of Borrelia burgdorferi in Rhesus macaques following antibiotic treatment of disseminated infection. *PLoS ONE,* 7(1), 1-12. doi: 10.1371/journal.pone.0029914

Fischler, B., D'Haenen, H., Cluydts, R. et al. (1996) Comparison of 99m Tc HMPAO SPECT scan between chronic fatigue syndrome, major depression and healthy controls: an exploratory study of clinical correlates of regional cerebral blood flow. *Neuropsychobiology* 34, 175-183.

Flor-Henry, P., Lind, J.C., & Koles, Z.J. (2009). EEG source analysis of chronic fatigue syndrome. *Psychiatric Research.* PMID: 20006474.

Fluge, Ø., Bruland, O., Risa, K., Storstein, A., Kristoffersen, E.K., et al. (2011) Benefit from B-Lymphocyte Depletion Using the Anti-CD20 Antibody Rituximab in Chronic Fatigue Syndrome. A Double-Blind and Placebo-Controlled Study. *PLoS ONE* 6(10): e26358. doi:10.1371/journal.pone.0026358

Fuller, R.W. (1991). Role of serotonin in therapy of depression and related disorders. *Journal of Clinical Psychiatry,* 52 Suppl:52-7.

Girdano, D. A., Everly, Jr., G. S., & Dusek, D. E. (1990). *Controlling stress and tension.* Englewood Cliffs, N.J.: Prentice Hall.

Glass, J. M., Lyden, A. K., Petzke, F., Stein, P., Whalen, G., Ambrose, K., et al. (2004). The effect of brief exercise cessation on pain, fatigue, and mood symptom development in healthy, fit individuals. Journal of Psychosomatic Research, *57, 391-398.*

Goddard, G. V. (1967). Development of epileptic seizures through brain stimulation at low intensity. *Nature, 214,* 1020-1021.

Gupta, A. (2002). Unconscious amygdalar fear conditioning in a subset of chronic fatigue syndrome patients. *Medical Hypotheses,* 59, 727-735.

Haug, K., W., Warnstedt, M., Alekov, A.K., Sander, T., Ramirez, A., Poser, B., Maljevic, S., Hebeisen, S., Kubisch, C., Rebstock, J., Horvath, S., Hallmann, K., Dullinger, J.S., Rau, B., Haverkamp, F., Beyenburg, S., Schulz, H., Janz, D., Geise, B., Muller-Newen, G., Propping, P., Elger, C.E., Fahlke, C., Lerche, H., & Heils, A., (2003). Mutations in clcn2 encoding a voltage-gated chloride channel are associated with idiopathic generalized epilepsies.*Nature Genetics,* 33. doi: 10.1038/ng1121

Hausler, M., Ramaekers, V. T., Doenges, M., Schweizer, K., Ritter, K. & Schaade, L. (2002). Neurological complications of acute and persistent Epstein-Barr Virus infection in paediatric patients. *Journal of Medical Virology,* 68, 253-263.

Hilty, L., Jäncke, L., Luechinger, R., Boutellier, U., & Lutz, K. (2010). Limitation of Physical Performance in a Muscle Fatiguing Handgrip Exercise Is Mediated by Thalamo-Insular Activity. *Human Brain Mapping,* 32: 2151–2160.

Hilty, L., Langer, N., Pascual-Marqui, R., Boutellier, U., & Lutz, K. (2011). Fatigue-induced increase in intracortical communication between mid /anterior insular and motor cortex during cycling exercise. *European Journal of Neuroscience,* 34: 2035–2042.

Hilty, L., Lutz, K., Maurer, K., Rodenkirch, T., Spengler, C. M., Boutellier, U., Jäncke, L. & Amann, M. (2011). Spinal opioid receptor-sensitive muscle afferents contribute to the fatigue-induced increase in intracortical inhibition in healthy humans. *Experimental Physiology,* 96*:* 505–517.

Hollingsworth, K. G., Hodgson, T., MacGowan, G. A., Blamire, A. M. & Newton, J. L. (2011), Impaired cardiac function in chronic fatigue syndrome measured using magnetic resonance cardiac tagging. *Journal of Internal Medicine.* doi: 10.1111/j.1365-2796.2011.02429.x

Jason, L.A., Benton, M., Torres-Harding, S., & Muldowney, K. (2009). The impact of energy modulation on physical functioning and fatigue severity among patients with ME/CFS. *Patient Education and Counseling, 77, 237-241.* PMCID: PMC2767446

Jason, L.A., Sorenson, M., Porter, N., & Belkairous, N. (2011). An etiological model for Myalgic Encephalomyelitis/chronic fatigue syndrome. *Neuroscience & Medicine, 2, 14-27.* doi:10.4236/nm.2011.21003 Retrieved from *http://www.scirp.org/journal/nml*

Jason, L.A., Sorenson, M., Porter, N., Brown, M., Lerch, A., Mikovits, J., Roberts, L. J., Sebally, K., Alkazemi, D., & Kubow, S. (2011*). Increased HDAC is associated with hypocortisolism in older adults.* Manuscript submitted for publication.

Jason, L.A., Sorenson, M., Porter, N., Brown, M., Lerch, A., Van der Eb, C., & Mikovits J. (2010). Possible genetic dysregulation in pediatric CFS. *Psychology,* 1, 247-251.

Jason, L.A., Torres-Harding, S., Brown, M., Sorenson, M., Donalek, J., Corradi, K., Maher, K., & Fletcher, M.A. (2008). Predictors of change following participation in non-pharmacologic interventions for CFS. *Tropical Medicine and Health,* 36, 23-32. Retrieved from *http://www.jstage.jst.go.jp/article/tmh/36/1/23/_pdf*

Jason, L.A., Torres-Harding, S., Maher, K., Reynolds, N., Brown, M., Sorenson, M., Donalek, J., Corradi, K., Fletcher, M.A., & Lu, T. (2007). Baseline cortisol levels predict treatment outcomes in chronic fatigue syndrome non-pharmacologic clinical trial. *Journal of Chronic Fatigue Syndrome,* 14, 39-59. doi: 10.1080/10573320802092039

Johnson, C. (2006) Fibromyalgia: A brain disorder? Retrieved on 6/24/2011 at: *http://aboutmecfs.org.violet.arvixe.com/Rsrch/FibromyalgiaICNS.aspx*

Johnson, C. (2011). Light on ME/CFS I: Bad Reception: A Key to ME Uncovered? The Light Gene Expression Studies. Phoenix Rising website. Retrieved on Jan. 22, 2012 from *http://phoenixrising.me/archives/5790*

Johnson, C. (2010). Proteins on the Brain: Spinal Tapping for ME/CFS. Phoenix Rising website. Retrieved on April 9, 2010 from *http://www.aboutmecfs.org/News/Brain Proteome Mar10.aspx.*

Kaufman, M. P., & Hayes, S. G. (2002).The exercise pressor reflex. *Clinical Autonomic Research,* 12, 429-439.

Kavelaars, A., Kuis, W., Knook, L., Sinnema, G., & Heijnen, C. J. (2000). Disturbed neuroendocrine-immune interactions in chronic fatigue syndrome. *Journal of Clinical Endocrinology and Metabolism,* 85, 692-696.

Kennedy, G., Spence, V. A., McLaren, M., Hill, A., Underwood, C. & Belch, J. (2005). Oxidative stress levels are raised in chronic fatigue syndrome and are associated with clinical symptoms. *Free Radical Biology & Medicine,* 39, 584-589.

Kishi, A., Natelson, B.H., Togo, F., Struzik, Z.R., Rapoport, D.M., & Yamamoto, Y. (2010). Sleep stage transitions in chronic fatigue syndrome patients with or without fibromyalgia. *Proceedings of the International Conference of the IEEE Engineering in Medicine and Biology Society,* 1,5391-4.

Kuratsune, H. & Watanabe, Y. (2007). Chronic fatigue syndrome. In Y. Watanabe, B. Evengard, B. H. Natelson, L. A. Jason, & H. Kuratsune (Eds.). *Fatigue Science for Human Health.* (pp.67-88). Tokyo: Springer.

LeDoux, J. (1998). *The emotional brain. The mysterious underpinnings of emotional life.* New York: Simon & Schuster.

Lerner AM, Beqaj S, Fitzgerald JT Gill K, Gill C, & Edington D. (2010). Subset-directed antiviral treatment of 142 herpesvirus patients with chronic fatigue syndrome. *Virus Adaptation and Treatment.* 2010. 2:1-11.

Libbey, J.E., Kennett, N.J., Wilcox, K.S., White, H.S., & Fujinami, R.S. (2011). Interleukin-6, Produced by Resident Cells of the Central Nervous System and Infiltrating Cells, Contributes to the Development of Seizures following Viral Infection. *Journal of Virology,* 85(14):6913-6922.

Light, A. R., Bateman, L., Jo, D., Hughen, R.W., VanHaitsma, T.A., White, A. T., & Light, K. C. (2011). Gene expression alternations at baseline and following moderate exercise in patients with chronic fatigue syndrome and Fibromyalgia Syndrome. *Journal of Internal Medicine, 271*, 64-81.

Light, A. R., White, A. T., Hughen, R. W., & Light, K. C. (2009). Moderate exercise increases expression for sensory, adrenergic, and immune genes in chronic fatigue syndrome patients but not in normal subjects. *The Journal of Pain,* 10(10), 1099-1112. doi:10.1016/j.pain.2009.06.003

Loescher, W., & Ebert, U. (1996) The role of the Piriform Cortex in kindling. *Progress in Neurobiology, 50,* 427-482.

Low, P.A., Novak, V., Spies,J.M., Novak,P. & Petty,G.W. (1999) Cerebrovascular regulation in the postural orthostatic tachycardia syndrome (POTS). *Am J Med.Sci.* 317, 124-133.

Luo, Z.D., Cizkova, D. (2000) The role of nitric oxide in nociception. *Current Review of Pain, 4,* 459–466.

MacHale,S.M., Lawrie,S.M., Cavanagh,J.T. et al. (2000) Cerebral perfusion in chronic fatigue syndrome and depression. *Br.J Psychiatry* 176, 550-556.

Maier, S. F., Watkins, L. R., & Fleshner, M. (1994). Psychoneuroimmunology. The interface between behavior, brain, and immunity. *American Psychologist,* 49, 1004-1017.

Martinez-Lavin, M., & Solano, C. (2009). Dorsal root ganglia, sodium channels, and fibromyalgia sympathetic pain. *Medical Hypothesis,* 72, 64-66.

McEwen, B.S., & Kalia, M. (2010). The role of corticosteroids and stress in chronic pain conditions. *Metabolism,* 59 Suppl 1:S9-15.

Meeus, M., & Nijs, J. (2007). Central sensitization: a biopsychosocial explanation for chronic widespread pain in patients with fibromyalgia and chronic fatigue syndrome. *Clinical Rheumatology,* 26(4), 465–473.

Meeus, M., Nijs, J., Huybrechts, S., & Truijen, S. (2010). Evidence for generalized hyperalgesia in chronic fatigue syndrome: a case control study *Clinical Rheumatology* (2010) 29:393–398.

Mendell LM, Wall PD (1965) Responses of single dorsal cord cells to peripheral cutaneous unmyelinated fibres. *Nature,* 206, 97–99.

Minor, T. R. & Hunter, A. M. (2002). Stressor controllability and learned helplessness research in the United States: Sensitization and fatigue processes. *Integrative Physiological & Behavioral Science,* 37, 44-58.

Morriss, R.K., Robson, M.J., & Deakin, J.F.W. (2002). Neuropsychological performance and noradrenaline function in chronic fatigue syndrome under conditions of high arousal. *Psychopharmacology,* 163, 166-173.

Napadow, V., Kim, J., Clauw, D. J., & Harris, R. E. (31 January, 2012). Decreased intrinsic brain connectivity is associated with reduced clinical pain in fibromyalgia. *Arthritis & Rheumatism.* doi: 10.1002/art.34412

Nasralla, M., Haier, J., & Nicolson, G.L. (1999) Multiple mycoplasmal infections detected in blood of patients with chronic fatigue syndrome and/or fibromyalgia syndrome. *European Journal of ClinicalMicrobiology & Infectious Diseases,* 18, 859–865.

Natelson, B.H., Weaver, S.A., Tseng, C.L., & Ottenweller, J.E. (2005). Spinal fluid abnormalities in patients with chronic fatigue syndrome. *Clinical and Diagnostic Laboratory Immunology, 12,* 52-55.

Neary, J.P., Roberts, A.D.W., Leavins, N., Harrison, M.F., Croll, J.C., & Sexsmith,J.R. (2008). Prefrontal cortex oxygenation during incremental exercise in chronic fatigue syndrome. *Clinical Physiology and Functional Imaging*, doi: 10.1111/j.1475-097X.2008.00822.x

Nijs, J., Meeus, M., Van Oosterwijck, J., Roussel, N., De Kooning, M., Ickmans, K., & Matic, M. (2011). Treatment of central sensitization in patients with 'unexplained' chronic pain: what options do we have? *Expert Opinion Pharmacotherapy*, 12(7), 1087-98.

Nijs, J., Van de Velde, B., & De Meirleir, K. (2005). Does nitric oxide trigger central sensitisation? *Medical Hypotheses*, 64, 558–562.

Ocon, A.J., Medow, M.S., Taneja,I., Clarke,D. and Stewart,J.M. (2009) Decreased upright cerebral blood flow and cerebral autoregulation in normocapnic postural tachycardia syndrome. *Am.J.Physiol Heart Circ.Physiol* 297, H664-H673.

Pall, M. (2007). Explaining "unexplained illnesses": Disease paradigm for chronic fatigue syndrome, Multiple Chemical Sensitivity, *Fibromyalgia, Posttraumatic Stress Disorder, Gulf War Syndrome and others*. Bighamton, N.Y.: Haworth Press.

Pall, M.L., & Satterle, J.D. (2001). Elevated nitric oxide/peroxynitrite mechanism for the common etiology of multiple chemical sensitivity, chronic fatigue syndrome, and posttraumatic stress disorder. *Annals New York Academy Sciences*, 933, 323–329.

Panerai, R. B., Moody, M., Eames, P. J., & Potter, J. F. (2005). Cerebral blood velocity during mental activation: Interpretation with different models of the passive pressure-velocity relationship. *Journal of Applied Physiology*, 99, 2352-2362.

Peckerman, A., Chemitiganti, R., Zhao, C., Dahl, K., Natelson, B. H., Zuckler, L., et al. (2003). Left ventricular function in chronic fatigue syndrome (CFS): Data from nuclear ventriculography studies of responses to exercise and portural stress. *FASEB*, 17(F Suppl: Part 2), A853.

Plata-Salamán, C.R., Ilyin, S.E., Turrin, N.P., Gayle, D., Flynn, M.C., Romanovitch, A.E., Kelly,M.E., Bureau, Y., Anisman, H., & McIntyre, D.C. (2000). Kindling modulates the IL-1beta system, TNF-alpha, TGF-beta1, and neuropeptide mRNAs in specific brain regions. *Molecular Brain Research*, 75(2, 248-258.

Puri, B.K., Jakeman, P.M., Agour, M., Gunatilake, K.D.R., Fernando, K.A.C.,Gurusinghe, A.I., Treasaden, I. H., Waldman, A.D., & Gishen, P. (2001). Regional grey and White matter volumetric changes in myalgic encephalomyelitis (chronic fatigue syndrome): a Voxel based morphometry 3-T MRI study. *British Journal of Radiology*, doi:10.1259/bjr/93889091

Razumovsky, A.Y., DeBusk,K., Calkins,H. et al. (2003) Cerebral and systemic hemodynamics changes during upright tilt in chronic fatigue syndrome. *J Neuroimaging* 13, 57-67.

Robinson, M., Gray, S. R., Watson, M. S., Kennedy, G., Hill, A., Belch, J. J., et al. (2009). Plasma IL-6, its soluble receptors and F-isoprostanes at rest and during exercise in chronic fatigue syndrome. *Scandinavian Journal of Medicine & Science in Sports*, 13, 1-9. doi: 10.1111/j.1600-0838.2009.00895.x

Rohleder, N., Schommer, N.C., Hellhammer, D.H., Engel, R., & Kirschbaum, C. (2001). Sex differences in glucocorticoid sensitivity of proinflammatory cytokine production after psychosocial stress. *Psychosomatic Medicine*, 63, 966-972.

Saade, N.E., Kafrouni, A.I., Saab, C.Y., Atweh, S.F., & Jabbur, S.J. (1999). Chronic thalamotomy increases pain-related behavior in rats. *Pain, 83,* 401–409.

Sabri, O., Owega, A., Schreckenberger, M., Sturz, L., Fimm, B., Kunert, P., Meyer, P.T., Sander, D., & Klingelhofer, J. (2003). A truly simultaneous combination of functional Transcranial Doppler Sonography and H2 15O PET adds fundamental new information on differences in cognitive activation between Schizophrenics and healthy control subjects *The Journal of Nuclear Medicine, 44*, 671-681.

Schondorf, R., Benoit, J. & Stein,R. (2005) Cerebral autoregulation is preserved in postural tachycardia syndrome. *J.Appl.Physiol* 99, 828-835.

Schwartz, R.B., Komaroff, A.L., Garada, B.M. et al. (1994) SPECT imaging of the brain: comparison of findings in patients with chronic fatigue syndrome, AIDS dementia complex, and major unipolar depression. *AJR Am J Roentgenol.* 162, 943-951.

Shandra, A. A., Godlevsky, L. S., Vastyanov, R. S., Oleinik, A. A., Konovalenko, V. L., Rapoport, E. N., et al. (2002). The role of TNF-alpha in amygdala kindled rats. *Neuroscience Research*, 42, 147-153.

Sherlin, L., Budzynski, T., Kogan-Budzynski, H., Congedo, M., Fischer, M. E., & Buchwald, D. (2006). Low-resolution brain tomography (LORETA) of monozygotic twins disconcordant for chronic fatigue syndrome. *NeuroImage,* 34(4), 1438–1442.

Shungu, D. C., Weiduschat, N., Murrough, J. W., Mao, X., Pillemer, S., Dyke, J. P., Medow, M. S., Natelson, B. H., Stewart, J. M., & Mather, S. J. (2012). Increased ventricular lactate in chronic fatigue syndrome. III. Relationships to cortical glutathione in clinical symptoms implicate oxidative stress in disorder pathophysiology. *NMR in Biomedicine.* doi: 10.1002/nbm.2772

Smith, A. K., White, P. D., Aslakson, E., Vollmer-Conna, U., & Rajeevan, M. S. (2006). Polymorphisms in genes regulating the HPA axis associated with empirically delineated classes of unexplained chronic fatigue. *Pharmacogenomics*, 7, 387-394.

Sorenson, M., Porter, N., Jason, L.A., Lerch, A. & Matthews, H. (2011*). IL-8 increased in patients with CFS.* Manuscript submitted for publication.

Spath, M. Welzel D, & Farber L. (2000). Treatment of chronic fatigue syndrome with 5-HT3 receptor antagonists -- preliminary results. *Scandinavian Journal of Rheumatology. Supplement*, 113, 72-77.

Spitzer, A.R., & Broadman, M. (2010). Treatment of the narcoleptiform sleep disorder in chronic fatigue syndrome and fibromyalgia with sodium oxybate. *Pain Practice,* 10, 54-9.

Tanaka, H., Matsushima,R., Tamai,H. & Kajimoto,Y. (2002) Impaired postural cerebral hemodynamics in young patients with chronic fatigue with and without orthostatic intolerance. *J Pediatr.* 140, 412-417.

Tzartos, J. S., Khan, G., Vossenkamper, A., Cruz-Sadaba, M., Lonardi, S., Sefia, E., Meager, A., Elia, A., Middeldorp, J. M., Clemens, M., Farrell, P. J., Giovannoni, G., & Meier, U. C. (3 January, 2012). Association of innate immune activation with latent Epstein-Barr virus in active MS lesions. *Neurology* 78(*1*), 15-23. doi: 10.1212/WNL. 0b013e31823ed057\

Van Wilgen, P., & Keizer, D. (March 2012). The sensitization model to explain how chronic pain exists without tissue damage. *Pain Management Nursing* 13(1), 60-65. doi: 10.1014/j.pmn.2012.03.001

Vargas-Alarcon, G., Alvarez-Leon, E., Fragoso, J. M., Vargas, A., Martinez, A., Vallejo, M., & Martinez-Lavin, M. (2012). A SCN9A gene-encoded dorsal root ganglia sodium channel polymorphism associated with severe fibromyalgia. *BMC Musculoskeletal Disorders*, 13 (23). doi: 10.1186/1471-2474-13-23

Vassallo, C. M., Feldman, E., Peto, T., Castell, L., Sharpley, A. L., & Cowen, P. J. (2001). Decreased tryptophan availability but normal post-synaptic 5-HT receptor sensitivity in chronic fatigue syndrome. *Psychological Medicine*, 31, 585-591.

Vecchiet, L., Montanari, G., Pizzigallo, E., Iezzi, S., de Bigontina, P., Dragani, L., Vecchiet, J., & Giamberardino, M.A. (1996) Sensory characterization of somatic parietal tissues in humans with chronic fatigue syndrome. *Neuroscience Letters* 208, 117–120.

Vollmer-Conna, U., Fazou, C., Cameron, B., Li, H., Brennan, C., Luck, L., et al. (2004). Production of pro-inflammatory cytokines correlates with symptoms of acute sickness behaviour in humans. *Psychological Medicine*, 34, 1-9.

Vollmer-Conna U., Piraino B. F., Cameron, B., Davenport, T., Hickie I, Wakefield, D., et al. (2008). Cytokine polymorphisms have a synergistic effect on severity of the acute sickness response to infection. *Clinical Infectious Diseases*, 47, 1418-25.

Watkins, L.R., & Maier, S.F. (1999) Implications of immune-to-brain communication for sickness and pain. *Proceedings of the National Academy of Sciences*, 96, 7710–7713.

Wedeen, V.J., Rosene, D.L., Wang, R., Dai, G., Mortazavi, F., Hagmann, P., Kaas, J.H., Tseng, W.Y.(2012). The geometric structure of the brain fiber pathways. *Science*, 335(6076), 1628-34.

Whiteside, A., Hansen, S., & Chaudhuri A. (2004). Exercise lowers pain threshold in chronic fatigue syndrome. *Pain*, 109, 497–499.

Willis, W.D. Jr. (1997) Nociceptive functions of thalamic neurons. In: M. Steriade, E.G. Jones, D.A. McCormick (Eds.). *Thalamus: experimental and clinical aspects*. (pp. 373–424). Elsevier Science: Oxford.

Wyller, V. B., Eriksen, H. R., & Malterud, K. (2009). Can sustained arousal explain the chronic fatigue syndrome. *Behavioral and Brain Functions*, 5:10. doi:10.1187/1744-9081-5-10.

Yamamoto, S., Ouchi, Y., Onoe, H., Yoshikawa, E., Tsukada, H., Takahashi, H., et al. (2004). Reduction of serotonin transporters of patients with chronic fatigue syndrome. *Brain Imaging*, 15, 2571-2574.

Yoshiuchi, K., Farkas, J. and Natelson, B.H. (2006) Patients with chronic fatigue syndrome have reduced absolute cortical blood flow. *Clinical Physiology and Functional Imaging*, 26, 83-86.

Yuan, Z., Rezai-Zadeh, N., Zhang, X., & Seto, E. (2009). Histone Deacetylase Activity Assay. In S. Chellappan (ed.), *Chromatin Protocols* (2nd ed.), pp. 279-293. Springer.

In: Encephalitis, Encephalomyelitis and Encephalopathies   ISBN: 978-1-62257-766-8
Editors: Andrew Ruiz and Douglas Fleming   © 2013 Nova Science Publishers, Inc.

Chapter 4

TREATMENT OF THE TICK-BORNE ENCEPHALITIS: PAST, PRESENT AND FUTURE

Olga V. Morozova

Institute of Chemical Biology and Fundamental Medicine of Siberian
Branch of the Russian Academy of Sciences, Novosibirsk, Russia
Ivanovsky Virology Institute of the Ministry of Health, Moscow, Russia

ABSTRACT

Comparative analysis of successful treatment based on induction of innate immunity, currently available drugs and up-to-date development of new principles to control virus infections may help to solve public health problems. Main criteria for anti-viral medicines should include not only selective inactivation of virus-specific proteins and/or nucleic acids but also minimal possible influence on host cellular biopolymers, prolonged action to avoid multiple frequent administrations as well as should take into consideration both innate resistance and immunity status of host organism. Despite long-term numerous efforts to develop specific and effective anti-viral medications beginning from the time of virus discovery there is no curative therapy for many viral infections including tick-borne encephalitis (TBE) till now. TBE is the most important flavivirus infection of the central nervous system (CNS) in Eurasia. The etiological agent, the TBE virus (TBEV) is transmitted to man by tick bytes. Geographic natural habitat of the TBEV appeared to be discontinuous and extended throughout southern part of Eurasian forest belt from Pacific to Atlantic ocean mainly within distribution areas of the virus vectors – ixodid ticks. In European endemic regions supportive treatment includes paracetamol, aspirin and other nonsteroidal anti-inflammatory drugs. In severe cases, some clinicians administer corticosteroids, although their use has not been validated. For patients with severe CNS symptoms intubation and ventilation are required to prevent coma or neuromuscular paralysis. In Russia TBE cure is based on the virus-specific immunoglobulin from donor blood sera, analogs of inteferons (viferon, reaferon-EC-lipint (human recombinant interferon α-1 and α-2b), interferon induction (by using larifan, neovir, tiloron, amixin, cycloferon, remantadin, ridosin, cameron, iodantipirin, enerion, mannitol, nootropil, pentoxifillin and others), as well as ribonuclease A from bovine pancreas. However, high molecular weight proteins such as immunoglobulins and RNases are not known to be able to penetrate into both host cells and enveloped viruses. Additionally for treatment of serious encephalitic manifestations artificial lung ventilation, panangin and glucose solutions can be used. In China oriental phytotherapy includes more than 10 elixirs with vitamins, microelements, as well as antiviral, antimicrobial, immunomodulation and anti-inflammatory effects, most of them are permitted to use in Russia. Numerous attempts to inhibit the TBEV reproduction by nucleoside analog ribavirin currently widely used for treatment of infections caused by plus-strand RNA-containing hepatitis C virus and poliovirus were not successful. Both aldehyde-containing and 4-N-exo-base-substituted photoreactive analogs of NTP, NDP and NMP could bind with RNA replicase subunits – the TBEV large nonstructural proteins NS3 and NS5 *in vitro* but their interaction did not completely inhibit the TBEV reproduction in infected cells.

New approach based on low molecular weight artificial ribonucleases - derivatives of aminoacids, short peptides, peptidomimetics and diazabicyclooctane (DABCO) has been suggested. Some of artificial RNases can serve as models of catalytic sites of natural RNases resulting in simple peptides or peptide-like molecules whereas others are based on the acceleration of RNA spontaneous hydrolysis due to the distortion of RNA secondary structure in the presence of polycationic molecules. In spite of complete cleavage of both viral and cellular RNA in the presence of the artificial RNases *in vitro* the degradation of the TBEV genome within extracellular virions and inside infected cells was not exhaustive. Further study should be aimed at development of specific affinity reagents with enhanced penetration into enveloped viruses or into infected cells.

1. TBE Etiology and Epidemiology

Encephalitis is an acute inflammation of the brain. Symptoms include headache, fever, confusion, drowsiness, and fatigue. More severe clinical manifestations cause seizures or convulsions, tremors, hallucinations and memory problems. Viral encephalitis may be resulted from acute infection or long-term neurological/neuropsychiatric sequelae of a latent or persistent infection.

Potentially fatal neurological infection in Europe and Asia is the tick-borne encephalitis (TBE) caused by the TBE virus (TBEV) (Gritsun et al., 2003). TBE clinical manifestations vary from inapparent, fever forms to severe encephalitis with lethal outcomes. The TBE had been firstly described in 1936-1940 by Russian physicians A.G. Panov, A.N. Shapoval, M.B. Krol and I.S. Glasunov. The causative agent – the TBEV had been isolated in 1937 by Soviet virologists L.A. Zilber, E.N. Levkovich, A.K. Shubladze, V.P. Chumakov, V.D. Solovyev and A.D. Sheboldaeva.

TBE outbreaks have been registered in northern China and Japan in the east, through Russia to more than 30 European countries including France, northern Italy and Norway in the west with the highest morbidity rates in Russia, Austria, Czech Republic, Slovenia and the Baltics (Latvia, Lithuania and Estonia) (Gritsun *et al.*, 2003; Mansfield *et al.*, 2009). In France, Italy, Greece, Norway and Denmark, TBE is of minor importance. In the United Kingdom, Ireland, Belgium, the Netherlands, Luxembourg, Spain and Portugal, TBE is not indigenous and no TBE cases have been reported as yet. The TBEV persists in endemic regions or so-called natural foci, where it circulates among vertebrate hosts (mainly small rodents and insectivorous) and the arthropod hosts and vectors (ixodid ticks). Years of observations of the distribution of TBE incidences suggest that such natural foci are very stable. Formation, development and stability of the TBE natural foci are determined by the coincidence of several ecological factors including temperature, relative humidity of air, soil humidity, vegetation properties of a biotope, population density and dynamics of ixodid ticks and their hosts, susceptibility of reservoir hosts to the TBEV, proportion of immune hosts and the virus prevalence among both ticks and vertebrate hosts (Tick-Borne Encephalitis (TBE) and its Immunoprophylaxis, 1996 and references therein). Reservoir host species abundance, multiple horizontal and vertical transmission cycles and adaptation of the TBEV to its different hosts cause long-term resistance of the parasitic system in endemic regions.

The majority of TBE cases occur through a tick bite with a few of them through consuming infected unpasteurized milk and dairy products (Dumpis et al., 1999). Alternative rare way is direct neural infection of an olfactory tract under laboratory conditions. The number of TBE cases is increasing worldwide with spread of the virus to previously non-endemic countries in Europe (France) and Asia (China, Mongolia, Japan and South Korea). In endemic regions TBEV transmission has been found to occur in one of about 200 tick bites. Moreover, tick bites are not often noticed and in the case histories references to tick bites are mentioned in 10-85% (Tick-Borne Encephalitis (TBE) and its Immunoprophylaxis, 1996). One of the striking epidemiological features of TBE has been periodic variation in the occurrence and severity of TBEV infections in different endemic regions from Far Eastern Russia to Europe. Peak values last 1-2 years and trough values continue during 6-7 years separated by intervals of gradual transition over 1-5 years (Bakhvalova *et al.*, 2011 and references therein). Maximal TBE morbidity rate had been registered in 1956 (5,163 cases) and 1964 (5,205 incidences). Then until 1974 TBE prevalence gradually declined to 1,119 cases. During 1976-1989 an average annual morbidity level in Europe and Russia was 2,755 and between 1990 and 2007 - an average of 8,755 reported cases of TBE per year (Mansfield et al., 2009). In 1999 11,356 cases of TBE in Eurasia (www.tbe-info.com) (and among them 9,955 – in Russia alone) render the highest sickness level in all endemic regions. However, these underestimations of TBE rate are based on ELISA-confirmed hospitalized cases of severe encephalitis or meningoencephalitis only and comprise nearly 20-30% of real TBEV infection prevalence among populations in endemic regions. Detailed epidemiological statistics from 1990 onwards can be obtained from the website of the International Scientific Working Group on TBE [http://www.isw-tbe.info].

Following infection with closely related tick-borne flaviviruses including the TBEV, louping ill virus (LIV) circulating in the United Kingdom, Spanish sheep encephalomyelitis virus (SSEV), Greek goat encephalomyelitis virus (GGEV), Turkish sheep encephalomyelitis virus (TSEV), Omsk hemorrhagic fever virus (OHFV) (Gritsun *et al.*, 2003) the viruses are known to first replicate at the site of inoculation and then in the lymph nodes that drain the inoculation site (Mansfield *et al.*, 2009 and references therein). Thus, the TBEV has been found in the Langerhans cells of the skin before reaching the regional lymphatic nodules via the lymphatic system. Virus replication in the draining lymph nodes is followed by development of plasma viraemia. Short primary viraemia gives place secondary viraemia at the end of incubation period during reproduction of the TBEV in organs and its penetration into CNS. During the last viraemic phase, many extra-neural tissues are infected and the release of the virus from these tissues enables the viraemia to continue for several days. Haematogenic spread allows different organs to be infected, especially those of the reticulo-endothelial system (spleen, liver and bone marrow), and the virus to pass through the blood–brain barrier and to invade CNS, where viral replication causes inflammation, lysis and cellular dysfunction (Dumpis *et al.*, 1999). Neuroinvasion of the TBEV in humans has been well reported, although the mechanisms by which an acute febrile infection develops into a severe, possibly fatal CNS disease are not clearly understood. Blood-brain barrier breakdown is not necessary for the TBEV receptor-mediated entry into the brain as shown by means of penetration of sodium fluorescein into brain of laboratory mice after intraperitoneal infection with the TBEV (Růžek *et al.*, 2011). The permeability of the blood-brain barrier increases at TBE later stages when high viral loads are detected in the brain. The increased permeability of the hematoencephalic barrier is associated with dramatic upregulation of proinflammatory cytokine/chemokine mRNA expression in the brain and does not depend on T-cell immunity (Růžek *et al.*, 2011). Direct intracerebral TBEV infection causes encephalitis with possible death or recovery of laboratory animals depending on the TBEV infection doses. Rare injuries of lower limbs do not correspond to tick bite locations mainly in these sites that suggest the virus tropism to neurons of neck segments and their analogs in the bulbar departments of the medulla oblongata (Mansfield *et al.*, 2009 and references therein). Meningeal and meningoencephalitic forms of TBE are known to occur after haematogenic spread of the virus whereas polyomyelitic and polyradiculoneuritic symptoms - after lymphogenic way.

TBEV reproduction in CNS is accompanied by the inflammation of the brain blood vessels and arachnoid membranes. Although the Far Eastern subtype of TBEV causes a monophasic course of illness, infection with a Western European (Dumpis *et al.*, 1999) and Siberian subtype usually produces a biphasic course of illness (Gritsun *et al.*, 2003). The incubation period is generally 7–14 days and during a typical biphasic infection, symptoms during the initial short febrile period can include fatigue, headache and pain in the neck, shoulders and lower back, accompanied by high fever and vomiting (Gritsun *et al.*, 2003). This is often followed by an asymptomatic period lasting 2–10 days and if the disease progresses to neurological involvement, this leads to the second phase, characterized by acute CNS symptoms with a high fever. CNS infection can manifest in the meninges (where inflammation causes meningitis), the brain parenchyma (to cause encephalitis), the spinal cord (myelitis), the nerve roots (radiculitis) or indeed any combination of these. Acute TBE is characterized by encephalitic symptoms in 45–56% of patients. Symptoms range from mild meningitis to severe meningoencephalomyelitis, which is characterized by muscular weakness (paresis) which develops 5–10 days after remission of the fever. Severely affected patients may demonstrate altered consciousness and a poliomyelitis-like syndrome that may lead to long-term disability (Dumpis *et al.*, 1999; Gritsun *et al.*, 2003). Besides common febrile, meningeal and meningoencephalitic forms TBE may be associated with poliomyelitic and polyradiculoneuritic clinical manifestations (Gritsun *et al.*, 2003). After prodromal period paralytic disorder develops, paresis of the neck, shoulder and upper limbs intensifies and the muscles begin to atrophy. A chronic form of TBE has been observed in patients infected mainly with the Siberian subtype of the TBEV in different endemic regions of the former USSR (reviewed by Gritsun *et al.*, 2003). There are two forms of chronic TBE, the first being long-term sequelae of any of the acute forms of TBE, where the development of neurological symptoms may take years postinfection. Clinical symptoms include Kozshevnikov's epilepsy, progressive neuritis of the shoulder plexus, lateral and dispersed sclerosis, a Parkinson's-like disease and progressive muscle atrophy. Often the physical deterioration is accompanied by mental deterioration and even death. A second chronic form of TBE is associated with hyperkinesias and epileptoid syndrome. Hyperkinesia occurs frequently and may arise during the acute phase. One should differ slow infection after long incubation period from latent and persistent forms of TBE.

Proportions of the TBE different forms periodically vary in different endemic regions. The TBEV is divided into 3 subtypes: Far Eastern, Siberian and European (Ecker *et al.*, 1999). Despite their names all 3 subtypes co-circulate throughout most of the TBEV endemic areas. The TBEV different genetic subtypes can cause various manifestations ranging from asymptomatic infection to meningoencephalitis. The Far Eastern subtype is associated with the highest mortality rate 20-60% (Gritsun *et al.*, 2003) whereas Siberian and European subtypes - with death rates of 6-8% and 1-2%, respectively but the Siberian subtype causes the greatest risk of chronic infection. In Russia about 80% of TBE cases result in a fever without neurological sequelae, 7–8% paralytic forms and chronic TBE in about 4–5% (Zlobin and Gorin, 1996). Although the incidence of TBE in Far Eastern Russia is lower than in Siberia, fatality and disability rates are higher, in some regions reaching 60%. In European countries such as Austria the fatality rate was 1% when vaccination was not readily available and now fatal infections are rarely recorded in Austria where immunization has been actively encouraged.

Although magnetic resonance imaging (MRI) is usually normal, abnormalities have been shown, including pronounced bilateral lesions in the thalamus, cerebral peduncles and the left caudate nucleus (Mansfield *et al.*, 2009 and references therein).

2. FLAVIVIRUS INNATE RESISTANCE

TBE clinical manifestations and their treatment success are known to depend on genetic properties of both patient and the TBEV (Brinton and Perelygin, 2003). Resistance to flavivirus infections was first discovered in the 1920s in mice and was subsequently shown to be controlled by the resistant allele of a single dominant autosomal gene. The resistant allele has been found to segregate in wild mammals populations in many different parts of the world. However, the majority of current laboratory mouse strains have a homozygous susceptible phenotype. Resistance is flavivirus specific and extends to both mosquito- and tick-borne flaviviruses. Resistant animals are infected productively by flaviviruses but produce lower virus titers, especially in their brains, as compared to susceptible mice. An intact immune response is required to clear flaviviruses from resistant mice. The resistant phenotype is expressed constitutively and does not require interferon induction. The *Flv* gene was discovered using positional cloning approach and identified as gene *Oas1b* encoding 2'-5'-oligoadenylate synthetase (2'-5'-OAS). A C820T transition in the 4th exon of the gene introduced a premature stop-codon and was found in all susceptible mouse strains. Therefore, susceptible mice produce a truncated OAS1b protein (Brinton and Perelygin, 2003 and references therein).

There are 4 human genes, 3 of them are encoding 2'-5'-OAS – OAS1, OAS2 and OAS3 and located as cluster of q24 site of human chromosome 12, and 4th gene of OAS-like protein localized in other site of the same chromosome 12. The genes are interferon-induced and play important roles of innate cellular protection against the TBEV infection. The 2'-5'-OASs are activated by double-stranded RNA including replicative forms of viral origin, are needed ATP as substrate and catalyze the reaction of AMP polymerization resulting in 2'-5'-oligoadenylate production. The 2'-5'-oligoadenylates interact with latent endoribonuclease L thus causing its dimerization and activation. After the induction RNase L hydrolyzes both cellular and viral RNA thus inhibiting the virus reproduction. Currently available data suggest a possible association between five 2'-5'-OAS gene single nucleotide polymorphisms (SNPs) and the TBE outcome in Russian population (Barkhash *et al.*, 2010). Recently, the CD209 gene promoter region mutation was shown to be associated with predisposition to severe forms of TBE in Russian population (Barkhash *et al.*, 2012).

Based on the available data the TBEV treatment scheme should consider innate resistance, cytokine status, T- and B-cell immune response of patients as well as the TBEV viral loads and genetic type.

3. CYTOKINES AND TBE

Currently available data on the role of cytokines and chemokines in the TBEV-induced pathogenesis are rather limited. In sera and CSF of patients with TBE elevated levels of inflammation cytokines such as tumour necrosis factor α (TNF-α), interleukin (IL) 1α and IL-6 were detected. During the first week of disease, the levels of those 3 cytokines gradually declined and an inhibitor of cytokine production Il-10 amount increased (Kindberg *et al.*, 2008, Shelly *et al.*, 2009). One should note immunosupression of Th1 key cytokine gene expression of interferon gamma and interleukin (Il) 12 in 2 days after infection of mice with the TBEV-containing tick suspensions with subsequent recovery of original levels of the gene expression (data not shown, in press). However, simultaneous activation of Th2 cytokines Il4 and Il10 gene expression without any delay with maximum in 4 days and subsequent decline up to 16 days after infection were observed. The immunomodulation could be caused by immunosupressors from chitin or tick saliva (Morozova *et al.*, in press).

Interferon was found to play an important role in the control of replication of tick-borne flaviviruses including the TBEV (Shelly *et al.*, 2009). Dendritic cells are the main producers of interferon and are first to be infected with the TBEV. However, the TBEV NS5 protein has been recently shown to act as interferon antagonist inhibiting the expression of antiviral genes (Werme *et al.*, 2008; Mansfield *et al.*, 2009 and references therein). Deletion in the CCR5 chemokine receptor gene is a genetic marker associated with severe forms of TBE (Kindberg *et al.*, 2008). Early interferon response is modulated not only by the TBEV but also by the tick vector and tick salivary proteins (Robertson *et al.*, 2009).

In response to the TBEV infection, type I interferons induce several genes of unknown functions. Tripartite motif (TRIM) protein, TRIM79α, is an interferon-stimulated gene product that specifically restricts TBEV replication by degradation of the RNA-dependent RNA polymerase subunit - NS5 protein in cellular lysosomes. The TBEV specificity of TRIM79α reveals a remarkable ability of the innate immunity to differentiate between closely related flaviviruses (Taylor *et al.*, 2011).

4. TBE AS AN IMMUNOPATHOLOGICAL DISEASE

With an evident tropism to lymphoid tissue the TBEV significantly affects the immune system (Holub *et al.*, 2002). Both 2-fold increase in concentrations of B cells and decrease in the relative and absolute number of T-lymphocytes in the peripheral blood were found.

During 6 weeks after infection the TBEV-specific antibodies levels have been observed to increase in both sera and cerebrospinal fluid (CSF): maximal IgM levels were revealed at the early disease stage and later on up to 6 weeks, whereas peak IgG – in late convalescent sera (around 6 weeks). However, IgM antibodies can persist for a few months after infection typically accompanied by the chronic virus infection, whereas IgG – for a lifetime. In CSF, mononuclear cells are predominantly composed of CD4+ T lymphocytes and less numerous CD8+ T lymphocytes, with limited natural killer cells and B-lymphocytes (Mansfield et al., 2009).

TBE is an immunopathological disease, where the inflammatory CD8+ T cell-mediated reactions contribute to neuronal damage and could lead to a fatal outcome (Růžek *et al.*, 2009). Key role of CD8(+) T-cells in the immunopathology of TBE had been demonstrated by prolonged survival of SCID or CD8(-/-) mice, following infection, when compared with immunocompetent mice or mice with adoptively transferred CD8(+) T-cells (Růžek *et al.*, 2009).

Thus, the impaired immune response might be an important factor in the pathogenesis of flaviviruses and should be taken into consideration for personalized medicine.

5. CONVENTIONAL TREATMENT OF TBE

Despite long-term attempts to develop anti-viral medications no specific treatment for TBE is known so far and therapy is usually symptomatic. Reliably tested specific antiviral agents are few in number and are used with limited success in treatment of viral infection, with the exception of herpes simplex encephalitis. Since man-to-man transmission of the virus has never been reported, there is no need to isolate patients with TBE. Treatment of the TBE is performed according to general principles which do not depend on previous vaccination or specific immunoglobulin administration. During acute period of the TBE rest cure and rational nutrition with necessary vitamins B and C (300-1000 mg each day) are recommended.

In European endemic regions strict bed rest for at least 10 days is imperative and supportive treatment includes paracetamol, aspirin and other nonsteroidal anti-inflammatory drugs. In severe cases, some clinicians administer corticosteroids, although their use has not been validated (Mansfield *et al.*, 2009). Corticosteroids (mainly, methylprednisolone) are used to reduce brain swelling and inflammation. The corticosteroids apparently lead to a rapid temperature decrease and an improvement of subjective symptoms but at the same time seem to prolong hospitalization as compared to patients received only symptomatic treatment (Tick-Borne Encephalitis (TBE) and its Immunoprophylaxis, 1996 and references therein). Therefore, glucocorticosteroids are prescribed for treatment of serious forms of TBE only. Sedatives may be needed for irritability or restlessness. In many Austrian hospitals, patients with TBE are referred to intensive care units for continuous surveillance as a precaution. Only when the temperature is down to normal, neurological symptoms have subsided, and normal CSF values were obtained the patient is permitted to leave bed briefly but to avoid complications predominantly bed rest is recommended for additional 2 weeks. Maintenance of the water and electrolyte balances, sufficient caloric and vitamin intake as well as administration of analgesics and antipyretics constitute main directions of clinical management. Physiotherapy of paralyzed limbs is essential to prevent muscular atrophy (Tick-Borne Encephalitis (TBE) and its Immunoprophylaxis, 1996 and references therein).

In Russia, conventional treatment includes the TBEV-specific polyclonal antibodies from vaccinated donors blood sera and an induction of innate immunity by using analogs of interferons (viferon, reaferon-EC-lipint (human recombinant interferon α-1 and α-2b), interferon induction (by using larifan, neovir, tiloron, amixin, cycloferon, remantadin, ridosin, cameron, iodantipirin, enerion, mannitol, nootropil, pentoxifillin and others), as well as ribonuclease A from a bovine pancreas.

The TBEV-specific antibodies are believed to neutralize the extracellular TBEV in the blood thus preventing further infection development. During last years immunoglobulin is purified from blood plasma of donors living in the TBE endemic regions. Different schemes of early administration of the TBEV-specific immunoglobulin depend on the TBE forms. For treatment of fever form of the TBE 0.1 ml/kg of body weight once a day during 3-5 days but not less than 21 ml of immunoglobulin is used. For meningeal infection immunoglobulin is injected twice a day with intervals between injections 10-12 hours for 5 days but not less 70 ml. For encephalitic and other severe complications the specific immunoglobulin is recommended 2-3 times a day with intervals 8-12 hours during at least 5-6 days and 80-130 ml in average. Usually temperature decrease and pain relief are observed in 12-24 hours after γ-globulin intramuscular injections.

However, phenomenon of antibody-dependent enhancement of flavivirus infectivity in the presence of poly- and monoclonal antibodies against flavivirus glycoproteins E and M is also well known (Peiris and Porterfield, 1979; Phillpotts *et al.*, 1985). The antibody-dependent enhancement results in average life time reduction and even death of immunized laboratory animals after infection (Peiris and Porterfield, 1979; Phillpotts *et al.*, 1985). Immune complexes of whole extracellular virions with flavivirus-specific antibodies can penetrate into monocytes through Fc-receptors thus causing more productive secondary infections or primary infection of previously immunized animals (Thomas, 1993). The infection of monocytes with flaviviruses in complexes with immunoglobulins is accompanied by growth of both cytokine levels and lymphocyte quantities thus resulting in cascade enhancement of flavivirus infectivity. Antibody-dependent enhancement is epitope-specific and is not induced with any monoclonal antibodies against glycoprotein E (Phillpotts *et al.*, 1985). Alternative possible mechanism of the antibody-dependent enhancement is associated with RNA replication activation after binding of the antibodies with glycoprotein E shielding the TBEV RNA (Morozova *et al.*, 1990). Therefore, manufacturers do not recommend to inject the TBEV-specific immunoglobulin after 96 hours after tick bite.

One should note that in Western European TBE endemic regions the virus-specific immunoglobulin is not recommended for treatment in spite of its production. In nearly all patients IgM and IgG antibodies can be detected at the time of their hospitalization. Moreover, the TBEV-specific antibody titers may reach maximal values during the first blood test. So, the administration of additional IgG concentrates is hardly possible to result in immune defence (Tick-Borne Encephalitis (TBE) and its Immunoprophylaxis, 1996 and references therein). But a risk of donor blood contamination with viruses or other infectious agents cannot be absolutely excluded and is one of the evident reasons of restrictions of the TBEV-specific immunoglobulin use. Other cause is the absence of convincing evidence of possible penetration of high molecular weight immunoglobulins from donor blood or even recombinant antibodies into the TBEV-infected cells and through blood-brain barriers.

Binding of flavivirus extracellular virions with specific antibodies can cause antibody-dependent enhancement (Peiris and Porterfield, 1979; Phillpotts *et al.*, 1985). Allogenic recombinant antibodies usually induce specific immune response and are removed from blood of laboratory animals.

For severe TBE treatment ribonuclease A from bovine pancreas is also used in Russia only. The protein of molecular weight 13,7-14,7 kDa is supposed to penetrate through the blood-brain barrier and to inhibit the TBEV reproduction in CNS. However, experimental evidences and reports about reliable clinical trials are not available now. Therefore, the treatment of TBE patients with RNase obtained from bovine pancreas has not been generally accepted (Tick-Borne Encephalitis (TBE) and its Immunoprophylaxis, 1996 and references therein).

Despite that RNase A is recommended for intramuscular injection in isotonic solutions of NaCl diluted immediately before use. Total amount should be 180 mg per a day (30 mg for each injection with intervals between them 4 hours). The treatment continues for 4-5 days and usually coincides with normalization of body temperature. Serious allergic complications including anaphylactic shock and sudden death could be due to injections of allogenic proteins – bovine RNases and sometimes equine TBEV-specific immunoglobulins. Therefore, doses and schemes of the TBE treatment are carefully defined and restricted to the most dangerous cases.

Recent improvement of the TBE treatment is based on intramuscular, intravenous, endolumbal and endolymphatic introduction of analogs of interferons (viferon, reaferon, reaferon-EC-lipint (human recombinant interferon α-1 and α-2b leikinferon and others) as well as interferon inductors (larifan, neovir, tiloron, amixin, cycloferon, remantadin, ridosin, cameron, iodantipirin, enerion, mannitol, nootropil, pentoxifillin and others). However, one should take into account that the $(1-3)*10^6$ ME of interferons are known to possess immunodepressive properties and cell resistance to a virus infection does not directly correlate with interferon titers. Therefore, relatively low doses of interferon analogs or interferon inductors (larifan (double-stranded RNA of phage 2), amixin, camedon and others) cause better immunomodulation and protection from the TBEV infection.

Detoxication of organisms is carried out by peroral and parenteral liquid introduction allowing to keep the water and electrolyte balances. Anticonvulsive, neuroleptic and cardiovascular drugs are used in exceptionally hard cases. Central paralysis are treated with antispasmodic medications (midocalm, melliktin, baclofen, liorezal and others) and drugs aimed at improvement of the blood microcirculation in vessels and especially blood supply of damaged brain (sermion, trental, kavinton, stugeron, nicotinic acid with glucose intravenously). Muscle relaxants include seduxen, skutamil C and sibazon. Hyperkinetic syndrome is treated with nootropil and piracetam, during acute period or myoclonic paroxysm sodium and litium oxibutirat are used intravenously.

Additionally, artificial lung ventilation, panangin and glucose solutions can be used for complicated encephalitis treatment. Therefore, improvements in specific treatment confirmed by randomized controlled trials are highly desirable.

6. NUCLEOSIDE AND NUCLEOTIDE ANALOGS

Numerous attempts to inhibit the TBEV reproduction by the nucleoside derivative ribavirin currently widely used for treatment of infections caused by plus-strand RNA-containing poliovirus and hepatitis C virus were not successful. Ribavirin could inactivate neither extracellular virions nor intracellular TBEV at different concentrations and under various experimental conditions such as purification and crystallization as well as schemes of the TBEV treatment before, simultaneously and after infection of permissive cell lines or laboratory suckling mice (data not shown). Addition of interferons did not change the absence of anti-TBEV effect of the ribavirin.

Both aldehyde-containing and 4-N-exo-base-substituted photoreactive analogs of NTP, NDP and NMP nucleotides could bind with RNA replicase subunits – the TBEV large nonstructural proteins NS3 and NS5 *in vitro* but their interaction did not completely inhibit the TBEV reproduction in infected cells.

Affinity labelling using aldehyde-containing reactive analogs of purine nucleotide involves the covalent modification of the replicase subunints with analogs of initiating NTP and subsequent elongation with radioactive second NTP. Analogues of the initiating substrates that bind outside the active center or attach to other proteins cannot be elongated thus providing a highly specific introduction of the radioactive label (Morozova *et al.*, 1990, 1991). The affinity reagents contained aldehyde groups capable of forming Schiff bases with primary amines near the substrate-binding active center of RNA polymerases (ε-amino group of Lys residues or the α-amino group of the N-terminal amino acid of the protein). Schiff bases must be reduced with $NaBH_4$ to increase the stability of the linkage between the reagent and protein.

$$E\text{-}NH_2 + OHC\text{-}Rp_nX \longrightarrow E\text{-}N\text{-}CH\text{-} Rp_nX$$

$$\xrightarrow{NaBH_4} E\text{-}NH\text{-}CH_2\text{-} Rp_nX$$

$$\xrightarrow{pp^*pY} E\text{-}NH\text{-}CH_2\text{-} Rp_nX^*pY,$$

where $E\text{-}NH_2$ is the enzyme, for example RNA-dependent RNA polymerase of the TBEV, $OHC\text{-}Rp_nX$ is the affinity reagent (R is the reactive residue and X is the nucleoside base), n is 1, 2 or 3, and pp^*pY is the radioactive second NTP corresponding to the viral RNA growing chain nucleotide sequence.

At the early stage of the TBEV replication up to 8 hours after infection of permissive porcine embryo kidney (PS) cells the TBEV genomic plus-strand RNA can serve as the template for complementary minus-strand RNA synthesis in replicative intermediate or replicative form (RF). Later on RF is used for plus-strand RNA accumulation.

The synthesis, purification and analysis of an o-formylphenyl ester of ATP, p-formyl-o-oxymethylphenyl esters of GMP, GDP, GTP, 4-[N-methyl-N-2-(guanylyl-5'-diphosphoryl)ethylamino]benzaldehyde, o-formylphenyl ester of GMP, a formylmethylamide derivative of GMP and 4-[N-methyl-N-2(guanylyl-5'-monophosphoryl)ethylamino]-benzaldehyde were performed as previously described (Morozova 1990, 1991 and references therein). Affinity labelling of the TBEV replicative complex in 8 hours postinfection resulted in a single band of molecular weight approximately 100 kDa. The radioactive product was not degraded upon treatment with DNases or RNases but was in the presence of proteinase or pronase thus proving it to be a protein. Competitive inhibition of the affinity labelling was observed after addition of unmodified NTP into cell-free replication system.

Covalent attachment of the reagent via Schiff base formation was confirmed because without $NaBH_4$ reduction the labeled protein was not detected. No modification was revealed for control uninfected cells thus suggesting virus-specific product of affinity labelling. According to the TBEV molecular organization the only protein of molecular weight ~ 100 kDa is the largest nonstructural protein NS5. Western blotting with monoclonal antibodies against the TBEV NS5 protein proved the coincidence of affinity labelled product and the viral NS5 protein mobility. Analogous procedures with corresponding controls for the TBEV-infected cells at the late stage postinfection (24-48 hours) and immunoblotting with monoclonal antibodies against the TBEV NS3 protein revealed the only affinity labelled NS3 protein. Taken together, selective modification of the TBEV large nonstructural proteins NS5 and NS3 took place at the early and late stage postinfection, respectively. The NS5 protein may play a role in the initiation of minus-strand RNA replication at the early stage of infection whereas NS3 protein can function in the initiation of plus-strand RNA replication from double-stranded RF.

In order to modify elongation subunints of the TBEV replicative complex affinity modification with photoreactive base-substituted NTP analogs has been developed. Base-substituted photoreactive analogs of NTPs containing arylazydo groups attached by linkers have appropriate photochemical properties to permit cross-linking by UV-light 300-360 nm far from cross-linking of nucleic acids and proteins and can serve as elongation substrates used by many RNA polymerases. Base-substituted CTP analogs: exo-N-[2-(2-nitro-5-azidobenzoylamino)-ethyl]-cytidine-5'-triphosphate; exo-N-[2-(4-azidotetrafluoro benzoylamino)-ethyl]-cytidine-5'-triphosphate; exo-N-{2-[O-(4-azidotetrafluoro benzylidene aminooxy)-methylcarbamoyl]-ethyl}-cytidine-5'-triphosphate; exo-N-[(4-azidotetrafluoro benzylideneaminooxy)-butyloxy]-cytidine-5'-triphosphate and exo-N-[(4-azidotetrafluoro benzylidene hydrazinocarbonyl)butylcarbamoyl]-cytidine-5'-triphosphate (Figure 1) were used for affinity binding with the TBEV replicase proteins (Morozova *et al.*, 1998 and references therein). Affinity binding included: 1) incorporation of analogs into growing viral RNA chain due to replicase activity; 2) covalent photocross-linking of newly synthesized RNA to proteins through photoreactive arylazido groups. To reveal the TBEV modified proteins labelling of RNA-protein complex with [α-^{32}P]NTP with subsequent RNase treatment to hydrolyze unprotected oligoribonucleotide and SDS-PAAG electrophoresis and Western blotting with monoclonal antibodies were used. Host cell RNA synthesis and consequently affinity labelling were inhibited by means of preliminary incubation with actinomycin D. DNase I, RNase A and proteinase K treatment confirmed that labelled product were proteins and RNA. Affinity labelling was not detected in the absence of the photoreactice CTP analogs or without UV irradiation.

Optimal concentration for all the analogs was 1 μM coincided with known intracellular concentrations of NTP. Addition of CTP competitively inhibited affinity labeling that disappeared in the presence of 1 mM CTP. Western immunoblotting with monoclonal antibodies and radioimmunoprecipitation with Sepharose CL-4B with immobilized monoclonal antibodies proved that labelled proteins of molecular weight 100 and 69 kDa were the TBEV large nonstructural proteins NS5 and NS3, respectively.

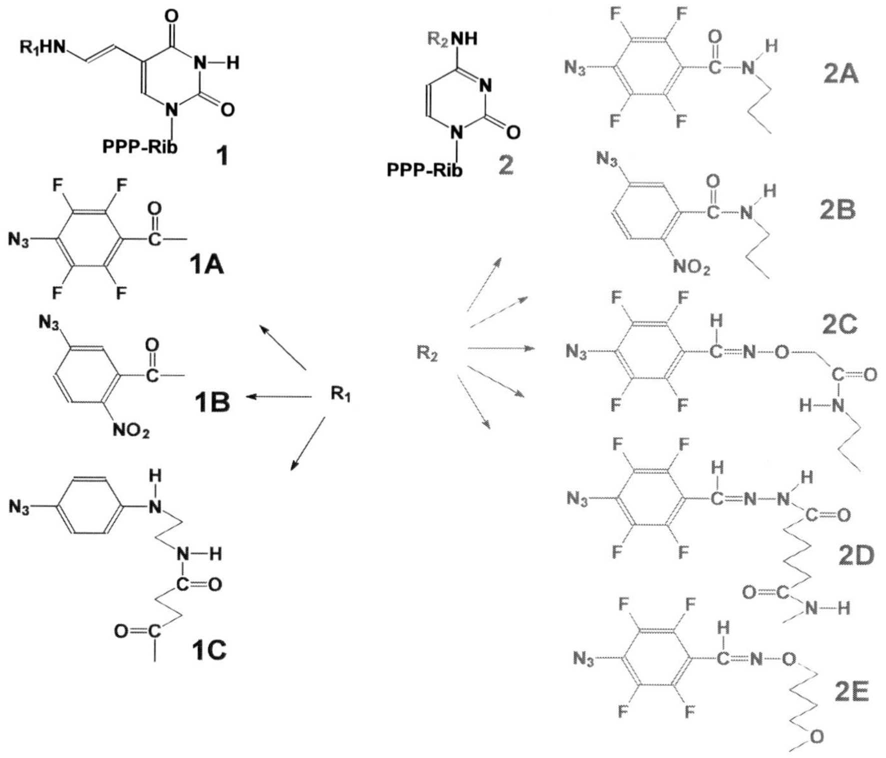

Figure 1. Nucleotide photoreactive analogs used for affinity modification of the TBEV replicase proteins.

The photoreactive NTP analogs could covalently bind with the TBEV replicase subunits at different postinfection stages.

Photoaffinity modification of the viral proteins *in vivo* is complicated by problems of nucleotide analogues delivery and irradiation. Less than 30% photoreactive nucleotide analogues can penetrate into living eukaryotic cells. Among the photoreactive analogs of CTP the only exo-N-[(4-azidotetrafluorobenzylideneaminooxy)-butyloxy]-cytidine-5'-triphosphate was toxic for eukaryotic cells at concentrations 0,1-1 mM (Morozova and Safronov, 2001).

7. ARTIFICIAL RNASES

Multiple RNase activities have been reported from several body fluids of mammals (Ramaswamy *et al.*, 1993 and references therein). Usually RNases observed in the body fluids range in their molecular weight from 12.3-13.7 kDa for human urine RNases to 45 kDa for RNase from human serum. However, the human serum RNase of 45 kDa was shown to aggregate resulting in molecular weight up to 150 kDa. RNases have been recognized to constitute a superfamily, in which several diverse proteins such as angiogenin and eosinophil cationic protein are shown to share sequence homology with ribonucleases (Ramaswamy *et al.*, 1993 and references therein). Many other proteins including immunoglobulins, albumins and lactoferrin possess ribonuclease activity in addition to other various functions (Nevinsky and Buneva, 2010 and references therein). In addition, a neurotoxin isolated from the granules of an eosinophil named eosinophil-derived neurotoxin was shown to have ribonuclease activity and has a sequence identical to human nonsecretory ribonuclease (Ramaswamy *et al.*, 1993 and references therein). RNase-like domain was found even in DNA-directed RNA polymerase II and might work in proofreading, as in RNA-directed RNA polymerase of influenza virus (Shirai and Go, 1991).

The ubiquitous presence of RNases in body fluids has made it difficult to assign a precise role for these enzymes. However, for RNase activity in milk, a protective role in retroviral infection has been envisaged. RNA-containing orthomyxoviruses seem to be sensitive to the elevated levels of RNases in blood (Smirnov *et al.*, 1981). Therefore, design, synthesis and analysis of artificial RNases of low molecular weight with possibly enhanced penetration into extracellular virions of single-stranded RNA-containing viruses and into virus-infected cells are promising directions of anti-viral drug development.

Unlike natural eukaryotic and bacterial RNases the known artificial ribonucleases include unspecific low molecular weight compounds and sequence-specific antisense oligonucleotide derivatives. First class includes complexes of transition metals (Cu^{2+}, Zn^{2+}, Ln^{3+}, Eu^{3+}) with organic ligands, biogenic amines, some peptides, and other low molecular weight organic compounds. Site-directed specific artificial ribonucleases are based on antisense oligonucleotides and ribozymes (Fouace *et al.*, 2004 and references therein). For rational design of low molecular weight artificial ribonucleases 2 approaches has been suggested (for review Koroleva *et al.*, 2007). One of them is based on structural and functional modeling of catalytic sites of natural RNases and DNases resulting in simple peptides or peptide-like molecules. Other way to construct artificial ribonucleases is based on the acceleration of its spontaneous hydrolysis due to the distortion of RNA secondary structure in the presence of polycationic molecules. The length of the rigid linker group of such polycationic aRNases is comparable with the distance between adjacent phosphate groups of RNA. The interaction of these cationic molecules with RNA leads to the optimization of the geometry of the complex, which facilitates the RNA hydrolysis via an "in line" mechanism. Such approach results in compounds, where two residues of quaternized 1,4-diazabicyclo[2.2.2]octane with alkyl substituents of different lengths linked by different linkers (Gulevich *et al.*, 2011).Part of studied artificial RNases of different structures with unspecific nuclease activity is shown in Figure 2.

To estimate and compare nuclease activity of the novel compounds the TBEV-specific RNA quantities has been measured by means of reverse transcription with subsequent real time PCR (($RT)^2$-PCR) with primers and fluorescent hydrolysis probe specific to the TBEV NS1 gene. Cleavage near the middle of the viral single-stranded genomic RNA is believed to result in its virulence decrease. According to previous estimations lengths of products of RNA cleavage with artificial RNases were less than 100 nucleotides so the TBEV NS1 specific PCR fragment length of 156 bp seemed to be convenient. The studied aRNases were not shown to inhibit reverse transcription and PCR as shown by PCR with the TBEV cDNA in the presence or absence of the compounds. Ribonuclease activity of the synthesized compounds was compared *in vitro* by cleavage of the total cellular and the TBEV-specific RNA from infected cells with subsequent detection by using ($RT)^2$-PCR (Figure 3). Complete cleavage of the TBEV RNA was revealed for peptidomimetic 1, peptides 6-7 and for derivatives of diazabicyclo-[2.2.2]-octane 8-12.

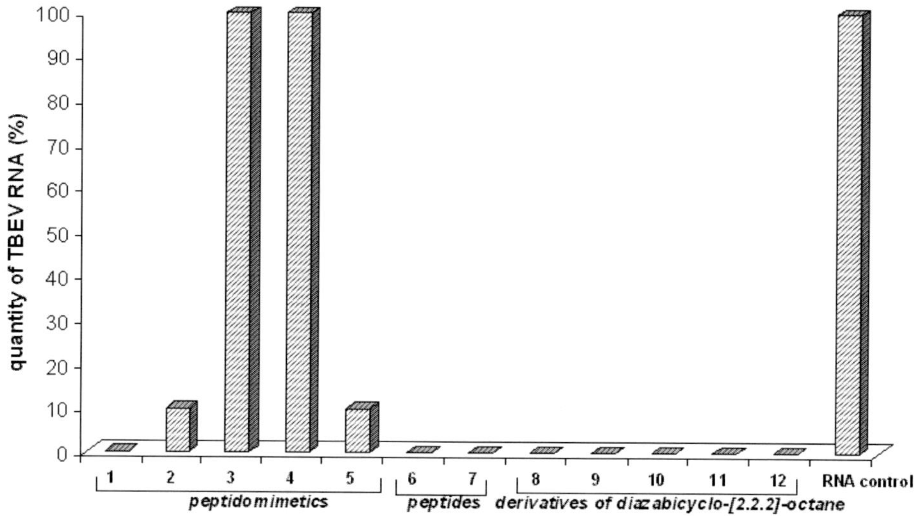

Figure 2. Artificial ribonucleases of different types: peptidomimetics (1-5), peptides (6, 7), and polycationic molecules (8-12).

Figure 3. Comparison of RNA cleavage in the presence of 1mM artificial RNases 1-12 *in vitro* after 2 hours incubation with the TBEV RNA in H₂O.

Among peptidomimetics complete RNA cleavage was observed only for compound 1 containing lysine residues (Figure 3). One should note that cleavage of the viral RNA was accompanied by complete degradation of total RNA isolated from the infected cells as shown by electrophoresis in SDS-agarose gels as previously described (Gulevich *et al.*, 2011).

Functional stability of artificial RNases was studied *in vitro* after storage of fresh stock solution at 4°C for 7 days, freezing at -70°C or heating at 100°C for 5 min. All the analyzed compounds appeared to keep their ribonuclease activity after storage at 4°C. After incubation at 100°C for 5 min the only compound **7** was shown to become inactive despite complete cleavage of total RNA in the presence of the same peptide before heating that suggest possible hydrolysis of ester bond under the extremal conditions resulting in hydrophobic alkyl group loss. Freezing of aRNases at -70°C resulted in complete ribonuclease activity loss for compounds 2 и 7 and partial – for artificial RNases 10 perhaps caused by possible aggregation of hydrophobic molecules in water solutions during cooling. Taken together, the data proved remarkable stability of the artificial RNases similar to majority of known natural RNases with the only exception of the peptide 7.

Complete cleavage of total RNA isolated from the infected cells *in vitro* could suggest toxic properties of artificial RNases. Comparison of cytotoxicity was performed by addition of artificial RNases in subsequent 2-fold dilutions into culture media of monolayer tissue cultures of the pig embryo kidney (PS) cells, green monkey kidney Vero cells, Madine Dabin canine kidney (MDCK) cells and mouse fibroblasts L929 with subsequent microscopic observations for 7 days and final MTT. Part of available data is shown in Table.

In spite of complete cleavage of both viral and cellular RNA in the presence of artificial RNases *in vitro* the degradation of the virus genomes within extracellular virions and inside infected cells was not exhaustive (Figure 4).

Table. Cytotoxicity of artificial RNases expressed in concentrations of test compounds that causes degradation of 50% monolayer cells (CC$_{50}$)

Compound	PS	Vero	MDCK	L929
1	2 mM	4 mM	0,2 mM	-
2	4 mM	1 mM	0,25 mM	0,5 mM
3	1 mM	5 mM	0,02 mM	0,3 mM
5	0,05 mM	1 mM	0,25 mM	0,5 mM
6	5 mM	10 mM	0,4 mM	1 mM
7	5 mM	5 mM	0,2 mM	1 mM
8	0,01 mM	0,1 mM	0,01 mM	0,001 mM
9	-	-	0,06 mM	0,02 mM
10	0,05 mM	0,1 mM	0,005 mM	0,5 mM

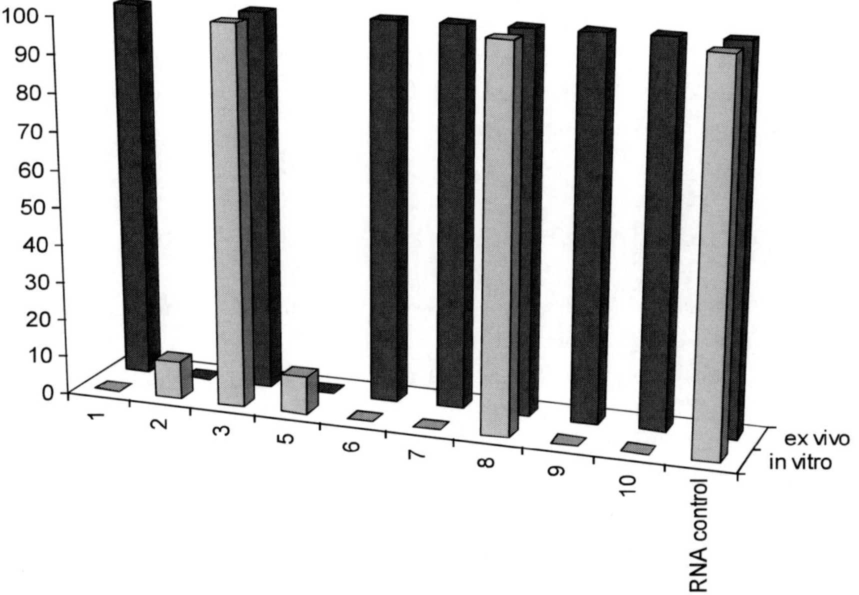

Figure 4. Comparison of RNA cleavage activity of artificial RNases after incubation *in vitro* and *ex vivo*.

Despite RNA degradation within extracellular virions in the presence of the artificial RNases 2 and 5 the TBEV antigen E was not affected as shown by ELISA with monoclonal antibodies using the TBEV antigen detection system of "Vector-Best" (Novosibirsk. Russia). ELISA titers varied in the range 1:128-1:256 and did not significantly change after treatment with 1 mM solutions of aRNases for 2 hours or overnight. However, the TBEV infectivity slightly reduced from 7-8 lgTCID$_{50}$ to 5-6 lgTCID$_{50}$ after long treatment of extracellular virions in the presence of 10 mM peptidometitics and peptides.

Direct comparison of the TBEV-neutralizing antibodies from infected or vaccinated mouse sera and the artificial RNases using the ELISA, (RT)^2-PCR and the TBEV titering based on cytopathic effect formation revealed evident advantage of the first (data not shown, in press).

8. TARGET-SPECIFIC VIRUS INACTIVATION

Inhibition of virus reproduction in infected cells could be achieved by treatment with derivatives of oligonucleotides complementary to viral genomes (Cohen, 1989). Oligonucleotide transport into cells is known to be more efficient in comparison with NTP analogues due to specific receptor for nucleic acids on the surface of eukaryotic cells (Yakubov et al., 1989). But antisense oligonucleotides can bring additional target specificity including both viral and cellular RNA. Unfortunately, oligodeoxyribonucleotides get destroyed with cellular enzymes within several hours after administration (Yakubov et al., 1989 and references therein) and oligoribonucleotides without special protection substituents even faster. Moreover, high concentrations of antisense oligonucleotides comparable with the viral loads during TBEV infection are toxic for permissive tissue cultures (data not shown). Specific delivery of modified nucleotides in infected cells by using immunoliposomes with monoclonal antibodies against virus-specific proteins might locally inhibit virus reproduction (Jensen et al., 1995 and references therein).

9. VIRUS INACTIVATION IN CLINICAL TRIALS

Among currently available anti-viral drugs are nucleoside analogues 3'-azido-2',3'-dideoxythymidine (AZT), 2',3'-dideoxyinisine (ddI) and 2',3'-dideoxycytidine (ddC) which terminate intracellular synthesis of any nucleic acids including virus-specific RNA after phosphorylation.

Ribavirin is another anti-viral nucleoside antimetabolite drugs. When metabolized that prodrug resembles purine RNA nucleotides thus interfering with RNA synthesis. The primary observed serious adverse side effect of ribavirin is hemolytic anemia, which may worsen preexisting conditions and disease outcome. Ribavirin is active against a number of DNA and RNA viruses including flaviviruses (especially yellow fever virus, West Nile virus and dengue virus as well as hepatitis C virus), influenza viruses and many viruses of hemorrhagic fevers. In Europe and the U.S. the oral (capsule or tablet) form of ribavirin is used in the treatment of hepatitis C, in combination with pegylated interferons. Ribavirin was shown to potentiate the antiviral effect of acyclovir (Pancheva, 1991). Ribavirin present generic status is expected to slow research into new uses. Evidently, that unspecific action of the clinically used nucleoside analogs and toxicity for host cells limit their effectiveness.

Besides that nonnucleoside inhibitors of viral enzymes such as dipyridodiazepinone (nevirapine) and thiobenzimidazolones – noncompetitive inhibitors of HIV-1 reverse transcriptase as well as telaprevir and boceprevir - inhibitors of hepatitis C protease. Two last new protease inhibitors were approved by FDA in 2011 for treatment of hepatitis C only in combination with two previously approved agents, pegylated interferon and ribavirin. Combination of multiple antivirals in a single treatment is known to provide greater benefit than use of any one antiviral drug alone. To our knowledge the experimental flavivirus protease inhibitors action against the TBEV remains unclear.

Different methods of virus removal or inactivation in blood including washing, filtration, absorbtion, inactivation with heat or diol epoxides, ozone, halogenated oxidizing agents, extracorporal photochemotherapy or transcutaneous photodynamic therapy by means of illumination of small animals with red light without skin photosensitivity (described in details earlier in review of Morozova and Safronov, 2001) are not in the TBE therapy progress because of the TBEV accumulation in organs at the first fever stage and in brain later but not in patient blood. Really, viraemia period is unpredictable short that hamper the TBEV antigen or RNA detection in the blood.

Further study should be aimed at development of specific affinity reagents with enhanced penetration into enveloped viruses or into infected cells. Main criteria for anti-virals should include not only selective degradarion of virus-specific proteins and/or nucleic acids but also minimal possible influence on host cellular biopolymers, prolonged action to avoid multiple frequent administrations as well as probable interaction with host innate immunity.

REFERENCES

Bakhvalova V.N., Panov V.V., Morozova O.V. (2011) Tick-borne encephalitis virus quasispecies rearrangements in ticks and mammals. // Chapter in the book "*Flavivirus encephalitis*". /Daniel Růžek (Ed.), ISBN: 978-953-307-669-0, "InTech". – 2011. – 213-234 pp.

Barkhash A.V., Perelygin A.A., Babenko V.N., Myasnikova N.G., Pilipenko P.I., Romaschenko A.G., Voevoda M.I., Brinton M.A. (2010) Variability in the 2'-5'-oligoadenylate synthetase gene cluster is associated with human predisposition to tick-borne encephalitis virus-induced disease. *J. Infect. Dis.* V. 202(12), pp. 1813-1818.

Barkhash A.V., Perelygin A.A., Babenko V.N., Brinton M.A., Voevoda M.I. (2012) Single nucleotide polymorphism in the promoter region of the CD209 gene is associated with human predisposition to severe forms of tick-borne encephalitis. *Antiviral Res.* V. 93(1), pp. 64-68.

Brinton M.A. and Perelygin A.A. (2003) Genetic resistance to flaviviruses. *Advances in Virus Research*, 2003, Elsevier Inc., Vol. 60, pp. 43-85.

Dumpis U., Crook D., Oksi J. (1999) Tick-borne encephalitis. *Clin. Infect. Dis.* 28, pp. 882–890.

Fouace S., Gaudin C., Picard S., Corvaisier S., Renault J., Carboni B., Felden B. (2004) Polyamine derivatives as selective RNaseA mimics. *Nucleic Acids Res.* V. 32(1), pp. 151-157.

Gritsun T.S., Lashkevich V.A., Goul E.A. (2003) Tick-borne encephalitis. *Antiviral Res.* V. 57, pp. 129–146.

Gulevich A.V., Koroleva L.S., Morozova O.V., Bakhvalova V.N., Silnikov V.N., Nenajdenko V.G. (2011) Multicomponent synthesis of artificial nucleases and their RNase and DNase activity. *Beilstein J. Org. Chem.*, V. 7, pp. 1135-1140.

Holub M., Klučková Z., Beran O., Aster V., Lobovská A. (2002) Lymphocyte subset numbers in cerebrospinal fluid: comparison of tick-borne encephalitis and neuroborreliosis. *Acta Neurol. Scand.* V. 106, pp. 302–308.

Jensen K.B., Atkinson B.L., Willis M.C., Koch T.H., Gold L. (1995) Using in vitro selection to direct the covalent attachment of human immunodeficiency virus type 1 Rev protein to high-affinity RNA ligands. *Proc. Natl. Acad. Sci. U S A,* V. 92(26), pp. 12220-12224.

Kindberg E., Mickiene A., Ax C., Akerlind B., Vene S., Lindquist L., et al. (2008) A deletion in the chemokine receptor 5 (CCR5) gene is associated with tick-borne encephalitis. *J. Infect. Dis.*, V. 197, pp. 266-269.

Koroleva L.S., Serpokrylova I.Y., Vlassov V.V., Silnikov V.N. (2007) Design and synthesis of metal-free artificial ribonucleases. *Protein Pept. Lett.*, V. 14(2), pp. 151-163.

Mansfield K.L., Johnson N., Phipps L.P., Stephenson J.R., Fooks A.R. and Solomon T. (2009) Tick-borne encephalitis virus – a review of an emerging zoonosis. *Journal of General Virology* (2009), 90, pp. 1781–1794.

Morozova O.V., Mustaev A.A., Belyavskaya N.A., Zaychikov E.F., Kvetkova E.A., Wolf Yu.I. and Pletnev A.G. (1990) Mapping of the region of the tick-borne encephalitis virus replicase adjacent to initiating substrate binding center. *FEBS Letters,* V. 277(1-2), pp. 75-77.

Morozova O.V., Belyavskaya N.A., Zaychikov E.F., Kvetkova E.A., Mustaev A.A., Pletnev A.G. (1991) Identification of RNA replicase subunits responsible for initiation of RNA synthesis of tick-borne encephalitis virus by affinity labelling. *Biomedical Science*, V. 2, pp. 183-186.

Morozova O.V., Safronov I.V., Bahvalova V.N., Dobrikov M.I. (1998) Affinity labelling of the tick-borne encephalitis virus RNA replicase proteins by 4-N-exo-base-sustituted photoreactive CTP analogs. *Bioorganic and Medicinal Chemistry Letters*, V. 8, pp. 787-792.

Morozova O.V. and Safronov I.V. (2001) Viral protein functions study by affinity modification. *Mini Rev. Med. Chem.* V. 1(3), pp. 283-291.

Nevinsky G.A., Buneva V.N. (2010) Natural catalytic antibodies in norm, autoimmune, viral and bacterial diseases. *Scientific World Journal.* V. 10, pp. 1203-1233.

Pancheva S.N. (1991) Potentiating effect of ribavirin on the anti-herpes activity of acyclovir. *Antiviral Res.* V. 16 (2), pp. 151–161.

Peiris J.S.M. and Porterfield J.S. (1979) Antibody-mediated enhancement of flavivirus replication in macrophage cell lines. *Nature* (London), V. 282, pp. 509-511.

Phillpotts R.J., Stephenson J.R., Porterfield J.S. (1985) Antibody-dependent enhancement of tick-borne encephalitis virus infectivity. - *Journal of General Virology,* V. 66(8), pp. 1831-1837.

Ramaswamy H., Swamy Ch.V.B., Das M.R. (1993) Purification and characterization of a high molecular weight ribonuclease from human milk. *The Journal of Biological Chemistry*, V. 268 (6), pp. 4181-4187.

Robertson S.J., Mitzel D.N., Taylor R.T., Best S.M., Bloom M.E. (2009) Tick-borne flaviviruses: dissecting host immune responses and virus countermeasures. *Immunol. Res.*, V. 43(1-3), pp. 172-186.

Růžek D., Salát J., Palus M., Gritsun T.S., Gould E.A., Dyková I., Skallová A., Jelínek J., Kopecký J., Grubhoffer L. (2009) *CD8+ T-cells mediate immunopathology in tick-borne encephalitis.* V. 384(1), pp. 1-6.

Růžek D., Salát J., Singh S.K., Kopecký J. (2011) Breakdown of the blood-brain barrier during tick-borne encephalitis in mice is not dependent on CD8+ T-cells. *PLoS One*, V. 6(5), p. e20472.

Robertson S.J., Mitzel D.N., Taylor R.T., Best S.M., Bloom M.E. (2009) Tick-borne flaviviruses: dissecting host immune responses and virus countermeasures. *Immunol. Res.*, V. 43, pp. 172–186.

Shirai T., Go M. (1991) RNase-like domain in DNA-directed RNA polymerase II. *Proc. Natl. Acad. Sci. U S A.* V. 88(20), pp. 9056-9060.

Smirnov Iu.A., Kolodkina V.P., Kaverin N.V. (1981) Action of hydrolytic enzymes on influenza virus A ribonucleoprotein. *Vopr. Virusol.* V. 4, pp.477-481 (In Russian).

Taylor R.T., Lubick K.J., Robertson S.J., Broughton J.P., Bloom M.E., Bresnahan W.A., Best S.M. (2011) TRIM79α, an interferon-stimulated gene product, restricts tick-borne encephalitis virus replication by degrading the viral RNA polymerase. *Cell Host Microbe.* V. 10(3), pp. 185-196.

Thomas D.B. (1993) *Viruses and the cellular immune response.* New York, Basel, Hong Kong.

Tick-Borne Encephalitis (TBE) and its Immunoprophylaxis. *Immuno AG,* Vienna, Austria, 1996.

Tick-borne encephalitis. Microgen, www.microgen.ru, Moscow, 2010.

Werme K., Wigerius M., Johansson M. (2008) Tick-borne encephalitis virus NS5 associates with membrane protein scribble and impairs interferon-stimulated JAK-STAT signalling. *Cell Microbiol.* V. 10(3), pp. 696-712.

Yakubov L.A., Deeva E.A., Zarytova V.F., Vlassov V.V. (1989) Mechanism of oligonucleotide uptake by cells: involvement of specific receptors? - *Proc. Natl. Acad. Sci. USA*, V.86, pp. 6454-6458.

Zlobin V.I., Gorin O.Z. (1996) Tick-Borne Encephalitis: Etiology, Epidemiology and Prophylactics in Siberia. Nauka, Novosibirsk, 177 pp.

In: Encephalitis, Encephalomyelitis and Encephalopathies   ISBN: 978-1-62257-766-8
Editors: Andrew Ruiz and Douglas Fleming   © 2013 Nova Science Publishers, Inc.

Chapter 5

THE IMMUNOLOGY OF ENCEPHALOMYELITIS: A REVIEW OF PATHOGENETIC MECHANISMS AND CLINICAL DRUG TRIALS

Haruhiko Suzuki

Department of Immunology,
Nagoya University Graduate School of Medicine, Showa-ku, Nagoya, Japan

ABSTRACT

The immune system is closely associated with the pathogenesis of encephalomyelitis and influences susceptibility to the disease. However, the pathogenetic mechanisms underlying encephalomyelitis are still unclear. Consequently, an effective therapy for this intractable disease is not yet available. Encephalomyelitis in humans most commonly manifests in the form of multiple sclerosis (MS). Experimental autoimmune encephalomyelitis (EAE) is a widely used animal model for human MS, although the relevance of the animal model to the human disease has been questioned by many neurologists.

In this chapter, I focus on the immunologic mechanisms underlying the development of encephalomyelitis. In the first half of this chapter, I review the effector immune responses that induce encephalomyelitis and cause deterioration. This section covers both basic studies on the EAE animal model and clinical studies on MS patients. Oligopeptide fragments of myelin basic protein (MBP) and myelin oligodendrocyte glycoprotein (MOG) have been identified as antigens for T cell activation, and immunization of mice with these peptides induces encephalomyelitis. These observations confirm the involvement of T cells in the pathogenesis of this disease. Therefore, I primarily focus on T cell involvement, although many different types of cells are involved in the development of encephalomyelitis. In the second half of this chapter, I review the regulatory immune responses that are involved in the prevention or improvement of encephalomyelitis. Mature T cells that express the $\alpha\beta$-type T cell receptor (TCR) are classified as either CD4$^+$ or CD8$^+$. Regulatory T cells are thought to be part of both the CD4$^+$ and CD8$^+$ populations, although research on regulatory T cells during the last decade increasingly suggests that regulatory T cells are a part of the CD4$^+$ T cell population. In this section, I describe both CD4$^+$ and CD8$^+$ regulatory T cells as new potential tools for overcoming not only encephalomyelitis but also other diseases caused by autoimmune reactions.

INTRODUCTION

Encephalomyelitis is a general term for inflammation of the central nervous system (CNS), i.e. the brain and spinal cord. The inflammation may be caused by numerous factors, including infection by pathogenic microorganisms, physical injury, vascular stroke, or autoimmune attack. In the first half of the 20th century, the focus of medical researchers studying encephalomyelitis was infection by pathogenic microorganisms or viruses, including malaria [1] and measles [2], as well as other bacterial and viral infections. Thus, while encephalomyelitis can be used for a wide variety of diseases, in this chapter, I concentrate on encephalomyelitis caused by immune activities, most of which are considered self-reactive responses, i.e. autoimmune reactions.

HISTORY OF RESEARCH ON IMMUNE-RELATED ENCEPHALOMYELITIS

In the early part of the 20th century, encephalomyelitis of an unknown cause was occasionally observed during convalescence from viral infections such as smallpox, vaccinia, and measles, as well as during or following vaccination against rabies. To resolve the etiology of this form of encephalomyelitis, a number of investigators sought to reproduce encephalomyelitis in experimental animal models. In the 1930s, Rivers and colleagues succeeded in inducing encephalomyelitis in monkeys by injecting emulsions or extracts of rabbit brain [3, 4]. In this case, however, monkeys were immunized with xenogeneic rabbit tissue, thus providing little insight into the mechanisms of spontaneous encephalomyelitis. Induction of encephalomyelitis by immunizing animals with tissue from the same species was first reported by Morgan in the mid 20th century [5, 6]. She injected the CNS tissue from monkeys, emulsified with adjuvants, into other monkeys and succeeded in inducing encephalomyelitis. The involvement of an immune reaction in the development of encephalomyelitis was thus demonstrated by this work. After this successful induction of encephalomyelitis in monkeys, researchers attempted to reproduce the disease in numerous other animals, including guinea pigs [7], rats [8], rabbits [9], and mice [10].

The term *EAE* was first used by Waksman and Adams in 1955, as an abbreviation for experimental allergic encephalomyelitis [9]. In the following 2 decades, more than 50 articles describing EAE were published, although the etiology remained largely unknown. While an adaptive immune reaction was strongly implicated in the development of encephalomyelitis, the antigen(s) targeted by the lymphocytes remained unknown. Consequently, researchers avoided using the term *autoimmune* in their description of EAE, most likely as they considered that the identification of a self-antigen was required to postulate an autoimmune mechanism. At this time, molecular and cellular biology techniques had not developed sufficiently to identify the cells, antigens, or effector molecules involved in the pathogenesis of encephalomyelitis.

Bernard and Carnegie first coined the term *experimental autoimmune encephalomyelitis* in 1975, while maintaining the same acronym (EAE) [11]. At that time, they likely had no idea of the antigen recognized by the T-cell receptor (TCR), although they already knew that EAE could be induced by injecting native (homogenized) or synthetic myelin basic protein (MBP) mixed with Freund's complete adjuvant (FCA) [12, 13]. Because the structures of peptide antigen-complexed MHC class I and class II proteins would not be solved for another 13 years [14-17], they likely did not know how the peptide functioned as an antigen. At the same time, however, they must have been confident that the protein used for immunization of mice worked as an antigen to use the term *autoimmune* (a reasonable concept at the time because MBP was known to be a self-protein). As allergies are caused by foreign antigen(s), it is reasonable to use the term *autoimmune* for EAE because MBP is a self-protein that triggers the immune reaction targeting the CNS. Consequently, the acronym EAE is primary used to represent experimental autoimmune encephalomyelitis. Furthermore, myelin oligodendrocyte glycoprotein (MOG) and proteolipid protein (PLP), which are commonly used for the induction of EAE, are also self-proteins [18-23].

Similar to the discovery of the pivotal role of the autoimmune response, the relationship of EAE in animal models to multiple sclerosis (MS) in human patients also has a fascinating history. As is always the case of animal models of human disease, EAE was developed to represent human MS. However, many neurologists, especially those working in the clinical field, continue to doubt the validity of EAE as a model of MS, and consider it of limited use. These neurologists focus on the differences in neurological symptoms between animals with EAE and MS patients. From the establishment of the various EAE models to the recent advances in our understanding of the mechanisms of autoimmunity, the study of autoimmune encephalomyelitis has primarily advanced because of the effort of immunologists. However, future progress in the study of immune-related encephalomyelitis will definitely depend on the cooperation of immunologists and neurologists.

IMMUNE REACTIONS UNDERLYING ENCEPHALOMYELITIS

Many different methods have been used to induce EAE in mice and other rodents. Induction methods for EAE in non-human primates have also been established. Even if we restrict our focus to EAE in mice, there are numerous variables significantly affecting the outcome. For example, if the environment of the mice is changed, the experimental result may change consequently. Therefore, even if an experiment is performed in exactly the same manner as that described in a published paper, it would not be surprising if the same result is not obtained, especially in the case of *in vivo* experiments. Described below are a number of variables that may affect experimental outcome, and which should be taken into consideration in the design of experiments:

Animals

Strain. As EAE is thought to be a typical Th1 (+ Th17)-type response, C57BL/6 mice are more susceptible to EAE induction than BALB/c mice, which are resistant to EAE. SJL mice, which are susceptible to EAE, have often been used [11, 24, 25]. In rats, there are EAE susceptible and resistant strains as well [26, 27].

Age. There is a report that susceptibility to EAE is reduced in old BALB/c (an EAE-resistant strain) and old SJL (an EAE-susceptible strain) mice [28]. Reduced susceptibility to EAE was also observed in old rats [29].

Gender. Female mice are usually used for experiments on autoimmune diseases. There is a report that male SJL mice do not relapse after EAE induction by PLP immunization [30].

Antigen

Proteins. MBP, MOG and PLP are commonly used proteins for the induction of EAE.

Peptides. The use of proteins has gradually been replaced by the use of peptides, 9–23 amino acids in length, derived from the above-mentioned proteins that fit in the groove of class II MHC molecules.

Dose of peptide antigen. Potentially a very important factor, although there is no standard yet.

Adjuvant

Complete Freund's adjuvant (CFA). CFA containing typical numbers of killed mycobacteria is occasionally used, but the use of higher amounts of killed mycobacteria is a common strategy used to increase the efficiency of EAE induction.

Immunization

Mixing. Mixing of antigen solution and CFA is a critical step in the induction of EAE. Formation of a good emulsion by thorough mixing must be assured.

Site of injection. Hypodermic injection to the tail base is usually recommended, but injection at other sites is also possible.

Dose. Adequate amount of emulsified sample should confer an optimal result.

Injection protocol. Usual method is a single injection, but can be modified based on other factors.

The factors described above influence the outcome of EAE induction. Therefore, the optimal combination of factors must be determined by preliminary experiments before starting the actual study.

The type of immune reaction elicited by the immunization is also affected by the factors described above. As EAE is a typical disease of cellular immunity, Th1 and Th17 cells are key players. For the generation of Th1 and Th17 cells, dendritic cells (DC) and macrophages play important roles [31-34]. Th1 and Th17 cells are originally $CD4^+$ T cells and mainly recruit $CD8^+$ T cells, natural killer (NK) cells, natural killer T (NKT) cells and macrophages, which might be microglial cells in the case of EAE [35-38]. The role of $CD4^+$ T cells and $CD8^+$ T cells in the progression or suppression of EAE is complex because both subsets of T cells contain effector T cells and regulatory T cells. I will summarize the role of T cells in EAE later in this chapter.

EFFECTOR MECHANISM UNDERLYING THE PROGRESSION OF ENCEPHALOMYELITIS

In human MS, the initial event in the pathogenesis of the disease is unknown. In contrast, in EAE, it is known that the exposure of antigenic peptide(s), derived from proteins composing the myelin sheath, to CD4$^+$ T cells initiates the immune response. CD4$^+$ T cells that recognize the antigenic peptide are activated, and they begin to produce a variety of cytokines. In EAE, antigen-presenting cells (APCs) produce interleukin (IL)-12, transforming growth factor (TGF)-β and IL-6 [39, 40]. Thus, APCs promote the differentiation of CD4$^+$ T cells into Th1 and Th17 cells. Interferon (IFN)-γ, which is in turn produced by Th1 cells, activates CD8$^+$ T cells, NK cells and macrophages (microglia). Activated CD8$^+$ T cells and NK cells may damage nerve cells, while activated macrophages (microglia) and CD8$^+$ T cells produce additional amounts of IFN-γ, forming a positive feedback loop [35, 41]. IL-17, which is produced by Th17 cells, induces the expression of cytokines/chemokines, e.g., IL-6, G-CSF, and CXCL1 that are involved in the activation and migration of neutrophils [42].

Hitherto, I simply described the sequence of cellular and molecular events in EAE pathogenesis. However, there are several unresolved questions. First, why do CD4$^+$ T cells respond to peptides derived from self-proteins? One possible answer is that these peptides are hidden antigens [43, 44]. Normally, CD4$^+$ T cells that are able to respond to these hidden antigens do not encounter them, but once CNS cells are damaged and phagocytosed by DCs and macrophages (which are at the same time APCs), these cells are able to present the antigenic peptides to CD4$^+$ T cells. In the case of EAE, activated CD4$^+$ T cells that have been stimulated by synthetic peptides and have clonally expanded may be simply waiting for APCs to present endogenous antigens derived from myelin-producing cells because of spontaneous death or bystander killing by activated CD8$^+$ or NK cells [45]. Second, what kind of antigens do CD8$^+$ T cells recognize in the case of peptide-induced EAE? The injected peptides are antigens for CD4$^+$ T cells. CD8$^+$ T cells must recognize some antigens(s) that are different from those recognized by CD4$^+$ T cells, if they are indeed involved in the progression of EAE [46, 47]. The answer for the second question is difficult because of limited numbers of reports describing the effector CD8$^+$ T cells in EAE progression [48]. As for the role of CD8$^+$ T cells in the course of EAE progression, the majority of studies have described a suppressing role of CD8$^+$ T cells [49-51]. I describe below the detailed role of regulatory/suppressor CD8$^+$ T cells.

SUPPRESSIVE MECHANISMS THAT LIMIT THE PROGRESSION OF ENCEPHALOMYELITIS

The immune mechanisms that promote or suppress encephalomyelitis are largely unknown. However, it is known that there are 2 different types of cells: one promotes immune reactions and the other suppresses them. As described in the previous section, cells that promote encephalomyelitis include CD4$^+$ T cells (Th1 and Th17), a portion of CD8$^+$ T cells, NK cells and macrophages (microglia). Additionally, there are some reports implicating TCRγδ T cells [52-55], which enhance the severity of encephalomyelitis. Cells that suppress encephalomyelitis include various types of cells, such as CD4$^+$ regulatory T cells (Treg) [56], Tr1 [57], Th3 [58], CD8$^+$ regulatory (suppressor) T cells [59, 60] and NKT cells [61].

A complete discussion of the cytokines involved in the progression of autoimmune encephalomyelitis is beyond the scope of this review. The most important may be IFN-γ, which is produced by Th1 cells, and it activates effector cells such as macrophages and microglial cells [41]. IL-12 produced by APCs may be important for the induction of Th1 [62]. Other important cytokines may include inflammatory cytokines such as tumor necrosis factor (TNF)-α [63], IL-6 [64] and IL-1 [65]. IL-2 may be necessary for the proliferation of activated T cell clones [66]. IL-17, produced by Th17 cells, may also play key roles in the progression of some special types of encephalomyelitis [67]. Chemokines may also be important for attracting all the players (cells) to the site of inflammation (CNS) [68]. Cytokines that are mainly involved in the suppression of autoimmune encephalomyelitis include IL-10 [69] and TGF-β (70). IL-10 confers its suppressive activity by reducing the production of IFN-γ [71, 72]. While the suppressive mechanism of TGF-β is not fully understood, suppression may be mediated in part by the induction of CD4$^+$ Treg cells [73]. IL-4 and IL-13, which represent Th2 cytokines, also have suppressive activity against encephalomyelitis by shifting the Th1/Th2 balance in favor of Th2 cells [69, 74, 75].

INVOLVEMENT OF CD4$^+$ REGULATORY T CELLS IN THE PREVENTION/CURE OF ENCEPHALOMYELITIS

There is no doubt that CD4$^+$CD25$^+$Foxp3$^+$ regulatory T cells (Treg) are the most renowned regulatory T cells. A study analyzing the effect of this CD4$^+$ Treg population in EAE by Kumar et al. first appeared in 1996 (56). Since then, more than 250 articles on encephalomyelitis and CD4$^+$ Treg have been published until now (July 2012). The number of these articles dramatically increased after 2004, and continues to increase. This phenomenon is probably related to the discovery of Foxp3, which has a critical role in CD4$^+$ Treg cells [76]. As already described in the previous section, the history of regulatory (suppressor) T cells is complex. The existence of CD4$^+$ T cells that express CD25 (IL-2 receptor α chain) and exhibit strong regulatory activity was first reported by Sakaguchi et al. in 1995 [77]. Of course, this study was not the first to describe T cells with suppressive activity. There were numerous studies on "suppressor T cells" in the 1970s and 1980s [78]. However, research on "suppressor T cells" diminished in the 1990s. There may be several reasons for this, but the most likely is that these cells did not have characteristic markers that could distinguish them from other non-suppressor T cells. In contrast, Sakaguchi's "regulatory T cells" could be distinguished by their expression of CD25 [78]. The shift to "regulatory T cells" (Treg) may have been influenced by the use of cell-sorters. At present, it is accepted that Treg have strong immune-regulatory activity, in encephalomyelitis and in other autoimmune diseases as well [79, 80]. The immune-regulatory activity of Treg has a critical role not only in the prevention of these diseases, but also in their cure [81].

Although animal models of EAE demonstrate an important role of CD4$^+$Foxp3$^+$ Treg in both the prevention and therapy of EAE (79, 81), and observations of patients suffering from MS show diminished activity of these cells [82, 83], the clinical application of this cell population in human autoimmune encephalomyelitis is still distant [84-86]. There may be multiple factors that hinder their application in human diseases. For example, because patients suffering from autoimmune diseases, including MS, usually undergo chronic progression, and they are not expected to die within a short time-frame, both patients and doctors may not feel compelled to try new methods, in contrast to lethal diseases such as cancer, stroke, and heart attack. In addition, because the basic understanding of CD4$^+$Foxp3$^+$ Treg is still poor, there may be few clinicians who recognize the immune-suppressive power, specificity and harmlessness of this cell population. Furthermore, very few drugs that specifically control the activity of CD4$^+$Foxp3$^+$ Treg have been developed to date. A recent report has provided insight into the control of Treg activity [87]. The authors used natalizumab, which is humanized anti-CD49d antibody, in MS patients. The authors anticipated an effect on CD4$^+$ Treg as they express lower levels of CD49d than conventional CD4$^+$ T cells. Their trial demonstrated no significant effect of natalizumab. However, CD8$^+$CD122$^+$ Treg in mice may also express low levels of CD49d (our unpublished observation), suggesting that researchers must consider the role of CD8$^+$ Treg in such trials. Another potential drug that could be effective in stimulating CD4$^+$Foxp3$^+$ Treg, and which may be useful in the prevention and cure of MS, is interferon (IFN)-β [88-91].

Although there are thousands of published articles on the mechanism of suppression by CD4$^+$Foxp3$^+$ Treg, fundamental questions remain unanswered. These include the following: (i) What are the antigen(s) recognized by CD4$^+$Foxp3$^+$ Treg? (ii) Is there antigen specificity in the action of CD4$^+$Foxp3$^+$ Treg? (iii) What are the effector molecule(s) that suppress the target cells? (iv) What are the characteristic criteria of the cells to be regulated? The tentative answers could be as follows: (i) No definite antigens have been identified so far [92]. (ii) Apart from a few experimental conditions, such as in TCR-transgenic mice or in the anti-alloantigen response, antigen specificity has not been observed in the action of CD4$^+$Foxp3$^+$ Treg [93, 94]. (iii) Although some candidates, including IL-10, TGF-β, cytotoxic T-lymphocyte-associated antigen 4 (CTLA-4), and glucocorticoid-induced TNFR-related protein (GITR), have been proposed as effector molecules for Treg [95-98], none has been confirmed with certainty. (iv) Although the proposal that the target of Treg is T cells reacting to self, i.e. the source of autoimmunity, has been put forth by immunologists studying Treg, it has not been proven.

INVOLVEMENT OF CD8$^+$ REGULATORY T CELLS IN THE PREVENTION/CURE OF ENCEPHALOMYELITIS

In comparison to the advances in our understanding of CD4$^+$ Foxp3$^+$ Treg, research on CD8$^+$ regulatory T cells is still in its infancy. Although several investigators have independently published studies on CD8$^+$ regulatory T cells by using different characteristic markers, no effort has been made to identify the various subpopulations systematically. A few of the studies published on CD8$^+$ regulatory T cells are the following: Qa-1-restricted Treg [99], CD8αα [100], CD28$^-$ [101], CD122$^+$ [102], CD45R$^+$ [103], Foxp3$^+$ [104], CD103$^+$ [105],

CD25+ [106], CD11c+ [107], LAP+ [108]. Since it is not the purpose of this chapter to describe in detail the research on CD8+ regulatory T cells, I will discuss only the relationship between encephalomyelitis and CD8+ regulatory T cells.

Before the discovery of CD4+CD25+ Treg, studies on the relationship between CD8+ T cells and encephalomyelitis anticipated an immune-suppressive action of suppressor T cells because the suppressor T cell populations identified were primarily CD8+ rather than CD4+ [109-111]. At the time, cell surface markers to distinguish heterogeneous populations were not available to the same extent as today and cell-sorting techniques required professional skill. Therefore, investigators attempted to establish suppressor T cell clones or suppressor T cell hybridomas for the continuous analysis of suppressor T cells. It was likely that some bias toward CD8+ cells occurred during the process of establishing clones and hybridomas.

After the discovery of CD4+CD25+ Treg, investigators studying CD8+ suppressor T cells realized the importance of distinguishing regulatory T cells from other conventional T cells. These researchers used the various markers mentioned above and discovered T cells with regulatory activity [99-108]. A number of researchers were able to demonstrate a critical role of these cells in EAE. The first evidence of the ability of CD8+ regulatory T cells to suppress EAE was published in 2001 [112], approximately 5 years after evidence for a role of CD4+ Treg [56] (In my opinion, a definitive demonstration of a role for Qa-1-restricted Treg requires markers to narrow the population and allow enrichment of regulatory T cells by cell sorting. "Qa-1 restricted" describes a characteristic of these Treg, but is neither useful as a marker of these Treg nor for enrichment of these cells by cell sorting). CD8+ regulatory T cells that satisfy the new criterion (CD8+CD28-) were first published in 2003 (113). Following this report, CD8+CD122+ Treg (114), CD8αα Treg (115) and CD8+LAP+ Treg [108] were identified.

CONCLUSION

In this chapter, I described the involvement of the immune system, in particular the role of regulatory T cells, in autoimmune encephalomyelitis. Autoimmune encephalomyelitis is observed in humans primarily in the form of multiple sclerosis (MS). It is also observed in animal models of human MS (EAE).

There are 2 major populations in TCRαβ+ T cells—CD4+ T cells and CD8+ T cells. Both populations contain regulatory T cells that effectively suppress other T cells, thereby inhibiting the immune reaction. At present, it appears that CD4+ regulatory T cells are primarily CD4+CD25+Foxp3+ Treg, whereas CD8+ regulatory T cells are composed of many Treg populations with varying cell markers or characteristics. The relationship between CD4+CD25+Foxp3+ Treg and EAE or MS has been intensely studied and trials using Treg to treat MS are ongoing.

In comparison, the application of CD8+ Treg to MS will require more time. Combined therapy targeting CD4+ Treg and CD8+ Treg populations is a novel approach that may lead to a clinical breakthrough because a cooperative effect of CD4+CD25+ Treg and CD8+CD122+ Treg has been identified, even if it is in the murine experimental system [116].

REFERENCES

[1] Report on a case of myoclonic encephalomyelitis of malarial origin. Marinesco MG. *Proc. R. Soc. Med.* 1921;14(Neurol Sect):51-5.

[2] The encephalomyelitis of measles. Greenfield JG. *Proc. R. Soc. Med.* 1929;22(3):297-300.

[3] Encephalomyelitis accompanied by myelin destruction experimentally produced in monkeys. Rivers TM, Schwentker FF. *J. Exp. Med.* 1935;61(5):689-702.

[4] Observations on attempts to produce acute disseminated encephalomyelitis in monkeys. Rivers TM, Sprunt DH, Berry GP. *J. Exp. Med.* 1933;58(1):39-53.

[5] Allergic encephalomyelitis in monkeys in response to injection of normal monkey cord. Morgan IM. *J. Bacteriol.* 1946;51:614.

[6] Allergic encephalomyelitis in monkeys in response to injection of normal monkey nervous tissue. Morgan IM. *J. Exp. Med.* 1947;85(1):131-40.

[7] Prevention of experimental allergic encephalomyelitis in guinea pigs. Ferraro A, Cazzullo CL. *J. Neuropathol. Exp. Neurol.* 1949;8(1):61-9.

[8] Allergic encephalomyelitis in rats and rabbits pretreated with nervous tissue. Waksman BH. *J. Neuropathol. Exp. Neurol.* 1959;18(3):397-417.

[9] Allergic neuritis: an experimental disease of rabbits induced by the injection of peripheral nervous tissue and adjuvants. Waksman BH, Adams RD. *J. Exp. Med.* 1955;102(2):213-36.

[10] Critical relationships between constituents of the antigen-adjuvant emulsion affecting experimental allergic encephalo-myelitis in a completely susceptible mouse genotype. Lee JM. Schneider HA. *J. Exp. Med* 1962;115:157-68.

[11] Experimental autoimmune encephalomyelitis in mice: immunologic response to mouse spinal cord and myelin basic proteins. Bernard CC, Carnegie PR. J. Immunol. 1975;114(5):1537-40.

[12] Minimum structural requirements for encephalitogen and for adjuvant in the induction of experimental allergic encephalomyelitis. Nagai Y, Akiyama K, Suzuki K, Kotani S, Watanabe Y, Shimono T, Shiba T, Kusumoto S, Ikuta F, Takeda S. *Cell Immunol.* 1978;35(1):158-67.

[13] Experimental allergic encephalomyelitis: structural specificity of determinants for delayed hypersensitivity. Hashim GA, Sharpe RD. *Immunochemistry.* 1974;11(10):633-40.

[14] Structure of the human class I histocompatibility antigen, HLA-A2. Bjorkman PJ, Saper MA, Samraoui B, Bennett WS, Strominger JL, Wiley DC. *Nature.* 1987;329(6139):506-12.

[15] The foreign antigen binding site and T cell recognition regions of class I histocompatibility antigens. Bjorkman PJ, Saper MA, Samraoui B, Bennett WS, Strominger JL, Wiley DC. *Nature.* 1987;329(6139):512-8.

[16] A hypothetical model of the foreign antigen-binding site of class II histocompatibility molecules. Brown JH, Jardetzky T, Saper MA, Samraoui B, Bjorkman PJ, Wiley DC. *Nature.* 1988;332(6167):845-50.

[17] Delineation of antigen contact residues on an MHC class II molecule. Peccoud J, Dellabona P, Allen P, Benoist C, Mathis D. *EMBO J.* 1990;9(13):4215-23.

[18] Chronic relapsing experimental autoimmune encephalomyelitis with a delayed onset and an atypical clinical course, induced in PL/J mice by myelin oligodendrocyte glycoprotein (MOG)-derived peptide: preliminary analysis of MOG T cell epitopes. Kerlero de Rosbo N, Mendel I, Ben-Nun A. *Eur. J. Immunol.* 1995;25(4):985-93.

[19] Macrophages in T cell line-mediated, demyelinating, and chronic relapsing experimental autoimmune encephalomyelitis in Lewis rats. Huitinga I, Ruuls SR, Jung S, Van Rooijen N, Hartung HP, Dijkstra CD. *Clin. Exp. Immunol.* 1995;100(2):344-51.

[20] A myelin oligodendrocyte glycoprotein peptide induces typical chronic experimental autoimmune encephalomyelitis in H-2b mice: fine specificity and T cell receptor V beta expression of encephalitogenic T cells. Mendel I, Kerlero de Rosbo N, Ben-Nun A. *Eur. J. Immunol.* 1995;25(7):1951-9.

[21] The N-terminal domain of the myelin oligodendrocyte glycoprotein (MOG) induces acute demyelinating experimental autoimmune encephalomyelitis in the Lewis rat. Adelmann M, Wood J, Benzel I, Fiori P, Lassmann H, Matthieu JM, Gardinier MV, Dornmair K, Linington C. *J. Neuroimmunol.* 1995;63(1):17-27.

[22] Chronic experimental allergic encephalomyelitis in guinea pigs induced by proteolipid protein. Yoshimura T, Kunishita T, Sakai K, Endoh M, Namikawa T, Tabira T. *J. Neurol. Sci.* 1985;69(1-2):47-58.

[23] Monoclonal antibody-induced inhibition of relapsing EAE in SJL/J mice correlates with inhibition of neuroantigen-specific cell-mediated immune responses. Kennedy MK, Clatch RJ, Dal Canto MC, Trotter JL, Miller SD. *J. Neuroimmunol.* 1987;16(3):345-64.

[24] Adoptive transfer of experimental allergic encephalomyelitis in SJL/J mice after in vitro activation of lymph node cells by myelin basic protein: requirement for Lyt 1+ 2- T lymphocytes. Pettinelli CB, McFarlin DE. *J. Immunol.* 1981;127(4):1420-3.

[25] Experimental autoimmune encephalomyelitis mediated by T-cell line. II. Specific requirements and the role of pertussis vaccine for the in vitro activation of the cells and induction of disease. Lando Z, Ben-Nun A. *Clin. Immunol. Immunopathol.* 1984;30(2):290-303.

[26] Genetic control of susceptibility to experimental allergic encephalomyelitis in rats. Gasser DL, Newlin CM, Palm J, Gonatas NK. *Science.* 1973;181(4102):872-3.

[27] Genetic control of the development of experimental allergic encephalomyelitis in rats. Separation of MHC and non-MHC gene effects. Happ MP, Wettstein P, Dietzschold B, Heber-Katz E. *J. Immunol.* 1988;141(5):1489-94.

[28] Studies of experimental allergic encephalomyelitis in old mice. Endoh M, Rapoport SI, Tabira T. *J. Neuroimmunol.* 1990;29(1-3):21-31.

[29] Age-related changes in the development of experimental autoimmune encephalomyelitis. Ditamo Y, Degano AL, Maccio DR, Pistoresi-Palencia MC, Roth GA. *Immunol. Cell Biol.* 2005;83(1):75-82.

[30] Male SJL mice do not relapse after induction of EAE with PLP 139-151. Bebo BF Jr, Vandenbark AA, Offner H. *J. Neurosci. Res.* 1996;45(6):680-9.

[31] The critical role of IL-12 and the IL-12R β2 subunit in the generation of pathogenic autoreactive Th1 cells. Shevach EM, Chang JT, Segal BM. *Springer Semin. Immunopathol.* 1999;21(3):249-62.

[32] Regulation of autoimmune encephalomyelitis by toll-like receptors. Marta M, Meier UC, Lobell A. *Autoimmun. Rev.* 2009;8(6):506-9.

[33] Antigen presentation in the CNS by myeloid dendritic cells drives progression of relapsing experimental autoimmune encephalomyelitis. Miller SD, McMahon EJ, Schreiner B, Bailey SL. *Ann. NY Acad. Sci.* 2007;1103:179-91.

[34] Th17 cell, the new player of neuroinflammatory process in multiple sclerosis. Jadidi-Niaragh F, Mirshafiey A. *Scand J. Immunol.* 2011;74(1):1-13.

[35] The effects of interferon-γ on the central nervous system. Popko B, Corbin JG, Baerwald KD, Dupree J, Garcia AM. *Mol. Neurobiol.* 1997;14(1-2):19-35.

[36] Regulation of experimental autoimmune encephalomyelitis by natural killer (NK) cells. Zhang B, Yamamura T, Kondo T, Fujiwara M, Tabira T. *J. Exp. Med.* 1997;186(10):1677-87.

[37] A synthetic glycolipid prevents autoimmune encephalomyelitis by inducing TH2 bias of natural killer T cells. Miyamoto K, Miyake S, Yamamura T. *Nature.* 2001;413(6855):531-4.

[38] Microglia: intrinsic immuneffector cell of the brain. Gehrmann J, Matsumoto Y, Kreutzberg GW. *Brain Res. Brain Res. Rev.* 1995;20(3):269-87.

[39] Autoimmune inflammation from the Th17 perspective. Furuzawa-Carballeda J, Vargas-Rojas MI, Cabral AR. *Autoimmun. Rev.* 2007;6(3):169-75.

[40] Th17 Cells and autoimmune encephalomyelitis (EAE/MS). Aranami T, Yamamura T. *Allergol. Int.* 2008;57(2):115-20.

[41] Critical influences of the cytokine orchestration on the outcome of myelin antigen-specific T-cell autoimmunity in experimental autoimmune encephalomyelitis and multiple sclerosis. Olsson T. *Immunol. Rev.* 1995;144:245-68.

[42] Expanding the effector CD4 T-cell repertoire: the Th17 lineage. Harrington LE, Mangan PR, Weaver CT. *Curr. Opin. Immunol.* 2006;18(3):349-56.

[43] Autoimmunity in the central nervous system: mechanisms of antigen presentation and recognition. Wucherpfennig KW. *Clin. Immunol. Immunopathol.* 1994;72(3):293-306.

[44] Determinant-regulated onset of experimental autoimmune encephalomyelitis: distinct epitopes of myelin proteolipid protein mediate either acute or delayed disease in SJL/J mice. Tuohy VK, Thomas DM, Haqqi T, Yu M, Johnson JM. *Autoimmunity.* 1995;21(3):203-14.

[45] The role of the antigen-presenting cell in Fas-mediated direct and bystander killing: potential in vivo function of Fas in experimental allergic encephalomyelitis. Thilenius AR, Sabelko-Downes KA, Russell JH. J. Immunol. 1999;162(2):643-50.

[46] The role of CD8+ T cells in multiple sclerosis and its animal models. Goverman J, Perchellet A, Huseby ES. *Curr. Drug Targets Inflamm.* Allergy. 2005;4(2):239-45.

[47] CD8+ T cells in inflammatory demyelinating disease. Weiss HA, Millward JM, Owens T. *J. Neuroimmunol.* 2007;191(1-2):79-85.

[48] Myelin antigen-specific CD8+ T cells are encephalitogenic and produce severe disease in C57BL/6 mice. Sun D, Whitaker JN, Huang Z, Liu D, Coleclough C, Wekerle H, Raine CS. *J. Immunol.* 2001;166(12):7579-87.

[49] Suppression of experimental autoimmune encephalomyelitis by oral administration of myelin basic protein. II. Suppression of disease and in vitro immune responses is mediated by antigen-specific CD8+ T lymphocytes. Lider O, Santos LM, Lee CS, Higgins PJ, Weiner HL. *J. Immunol.* 1989;142(3):748-52.

[50] The CD8 T cell in multiple sclerosis: suppressor cell or mediator of neuropathology? Johnson AJ, Suidan GL, McDole J, Pirko I. *Int. Rev. Neurobiol.* 2007;79:73-97.

[51] The role of CD8 suppressors versus destructors in autoimmune central nervous system inflammation. Zozulya AL, Wiendl H. *Hum. Immunol.* 2008;69(11):797-804.

[52] γδ T cells enhance the expression of experimental autoimmune encephalomyelitis by promoting antigen presentation and IL-12 production. Odyniec A, Szczepanik M, Mycko MP, Stasiolek M, Raine CS, Selmaj KW. *J. Immunol.* 2004;173(1):682-94.

[53] γδ T cells in EAE: early trafficking events and cytokine requirements. Wohler JE, Smith SS, Zinn KR, Bullard DC, Barnum SR. *Eur. J. Immunol.* 2009;39(6):1516-26.

[54] Interleukin-1 and IL-23 induce innate IL-17 production from γδ T cells, amplifying Th17 responses and autoimmunity. Sutton CE, Lalor SJ, Sweeney CM, Brereton CF, Lavelle EC, Mills KH. *Immunity.* 2009;31(2):331-41.

[55] γδ T cells enhance autoimmunity by restraining regulatory T cell responses via an interleukin-23-dependent mechanism. Petermann F, Rothhammer V, Claussen MC, Haas JD, Blanco LR, Heink S, Prinz I, Hemmer B, Kuchroo VK, Oukka M, Korn T. *Immunity.* 2010;33(3):351-63.

[56] Inactivation of T cell receptor peptide-specific CD4 regulatory T cells induces chronic experimental autoimmune encephalomyelitis (EAE). Kumar V, Stellrecht K, Sercarz E. *J. Exp. Med.* 1996;184(5):1609-17.

[57] Tr1 cell-dependent active tolerance blunts the pathogenic effects of determinant spreading. Wildbaum G, Netzer N, Karin N. *J. Clin. Invest.* 2002;110(5):701-10.

[58] IL-4 is a differentiation factor for transforming growth factor-beta secreting Th3 cells and oral administration of IL-4 enhances oral tolerance in experimental allergic encephalomyelitis. Inobe J, Slavin AJ, Komagata Y, Chen Y, Liu L, Weiner HL. *Eur J. Immunol.* 1998;28(9):2780-90.

[59] A suppressor T-lymphocyte cell line for autoimmune encephalomyelitis. Ellerman KE, Powers JM, Brostoff SW. *Nature.* 1988;331(6153):265-7.

[60] T cell vaccination induces T cell receptor Vβ-specific Qa-1-restricted regulatory CD8+ T cells. Jiang H, Kashleva H, Xu LX, Forman J, Flaherty L, Pernis B, Braunstein NS, Chess L. *Proc. Natl. Acad. Sci. USA.* 1998;95(8):4533-7.

[61] A synthetic glycolipid prevents autoimmune encephalomyelitis by inducing TH2 bias of natural killer T cells. Miyamoto K, Miyake S, Yamamura T. *Nature.* 2001;413(6855):531-4.

[62] Prevention of experimental autoimmune encephalomyelitis by antibodies against interleukin 12. Leonard JP, Waldburger KE, Goldman SJ. *J. Exp. Med.* 1995;181(1):381-6.

[63] An antibody to lymphotoxin and tumor necrosis factor prevents transfer of experimental allergic encephalomyelitis. Ruddle NH, Bergman CM, McGrath KM, Lingenheld EG, Grunnet ML, Padula SJ, Clark RB. *J. Exp. Med.* 1990;172(4):1193-200.

[64] Interleukin 6 production in the central nervous system during experimental autoimmune encephalomyelitis. Gijbels K, Van Damme J, Proost P, Put W, Carton H, Billiau A. *Eur. J. Immunol.* 1990;20(1):233-5.

[65] Experimental autoimmune encephalomyelitis is exacerbated by IL-1α and suppressed by soluble IL-1 receptor. Jacobs CA, Baker PE, Roux ER, Picha KS, Toivola B, Waugh S, Kennedy MK. *J. Immunol.* 1991;146(9):2983-9.

[66] Glycosylation processing inhibition by castanospermine prevents experimental autoimmune encephalomyelitis by interference with IL-2 receptor signal transduction.

Walter S, Fassbender K, Gulbins E, Liu Y, Rieschel M, Herten M, Bertsch T, Engelhardt B. *J. Neuroimmunol.* 2002;132(1-2):1-10.

[67] Gene-microarray analysis of multiple sclerosis lesions yields new targets validated in autoimmune encephalomyelitis. Lock C, Hermans G, Pedotti R, Brendolan A, Schadt E, Garren H, Langer-Gould A, Strober S, Cannella B, Allard J, Klonowski P, Austin A, Lad N, Kaminski N, Galli SJ, Oksenberg JR, Raine CS, Heller R, Steinman L. *Nat. Med.* 2002;8(5):500-8.

[68] Inflammation in EAE: role of chemokine/cytokine expression by resident and infiltrating cells. Eng LF, Ghirnikar RS, Lee YL. *Neurochem. Res.* 1996;21(4):511-25

[69] Analysis of cytokine mRNA expression in the central nervous system of mice with experimental autoimmune encephalomyelitis reveals that IL-10 mRNA expression correlates with recovery. Kennedy MK, Torrance DS, Picha KS, Mohler KM. *J. Immunol.* 1992;149(7):2496-505.

[70] Transforming growth factors beta1 and beta2: cytokines with identical immunosuppressive effects and a potential role in the regulation of autoimmune T cell function. Schluesener HJ, Lider O. *J. Neuroimmunol.* 1989;24(3):249-58.

[71] Acceleration of experimental autoimmune encephalomyelitis in interleukin-10-deficient mice: roles of interleukin-10 in disease progression and recovery. Samoilova EB, Horton JL, Chen Y. *Cell Immunol.* 1998;188(2):118-24.

[72] IL-10 is critical in the regulation of autoimmune encephalomyelitis as demonstrated by studies of IL-10- and IL-4-deficient and transgenic mice. Bettelli E, Das MP, Howard ED, Weiner HL, Sobel RA, Kuchroo VK. *J. Immunol.* 1998;161(7):3299-306.

[73] Induction and mechanism of action of transforming growth factor-beta-secreting Th3 regulatory cells. Weiner HL. *Immunol. Rev.* 2001;182:207-14.

[74] Novel genetic regulation of T helper 1 (Th1)/Th2 cytokine production and encephalitogenicity in inbred mouse strains. Conboy IM, DeKruyff RH, Tate KM, Cao ZA, Moore TA, Umetsu DT, Jones PP. *J. Exp. Med.* 1997;185(3):439-51.

[75] IL-4, IL-10, IL-13, and TGF-beta from an altered peptide ligand-specific Th2 cell clone down-regulate adoptive transfer of experimental autoimmune encephalomyelitis. Young DA, Lowe LD, Booth SS, Whitters MJ, Nicholson L, Kuchroo VK, Collins M. *J. Immunol.* 2000;164(7):3563-72.

[76] Control of regulatory T cell development by the transcription factor Foxp3. Hori S, Nomura T, Sakaguchi S. *Science.* 2003 Feb 14;299(5609):1057-61

[77] Immunologic self-tolerance maintained by activated T cells expressing IL-2 receptor α-chains (CD25). Breakdown of a single mechanism of self-tolerance causes various autoimmune diseases. Sakaguchi S, Sakaguchi N, Asano M, Itoh M, Toda M. *J. Immunol.* 1995;155(3):1151-64.

[78] Molecular events in the T cell-mediated suppression of the immune response. Tada T, Hu FY, Kishimoto H, Furutani-Seiki M, Asano Y. *Ann. NY Acad. Sci.* 1991;636:20-7.

[79] Specific T regulatory cells display broad suppressive functions against experimental allergic encephalomyelitis upon activation with cognate antigen. Yu P, Gregg RK, Bell JJ, Ellis JS, Divekar R, Lee HH, Jain R, Waldner H, Hardaway JC, Collins M, Kuchroo VK, Zaghouani H. *J. Immunol.* 2005;174(11):6772-80.

[80] Redirection of regulatory T cells with predetermined specificity for the treatment of experimental colitis in mice. Elinav E, Waks T, Eshhar Z. *Gastroenterology.* 2008;134(7): 2014-24.

[81] Curing CNS autoimmune disease with myelin-reactive Foxp3+ Treg. Stephens LA, Malpass KH, Anderton SM. *Eur. J. Immunol.* 2009;39(4):1108-17.

[82] Decreased FOXP3 levels in multiple sclerosis patients. Huan J, Culbertson N, Spencer L, Bartholomew R, Burrows GG, Chou YK, Bourdette D, Ziegler SF, Offner H, Vandenbark AA. J Neurosci Res. 2005;81(1):45-52.

[83] Natural naive CD4+CD25+CD127low regulatory T cell (Treg) development and function are disturbed in multiple sclerosis patients: recovery of memory Treg homeostasis during disease progression. Venken K, Hellings N, Broekmans T, Hensen K, Rummens JL, Stinissen P. J. Immunol. 2008;180(9):6411-20.

[84] How specificity for self-peptides shapes the development and function of regulatory T cells. Simons DM, Picca CC, Oh S, Perng OA, Aitken M, Erikson J, Caton AJ. *J. Leukoc. Biol.* 2010;88(6):1099-107.

[85] Synthetic glycolipid ligands for human iNKT cells as potential therapeutic agents for immunotherapy. Araki M, Miyake S, Yamamura T. Curr. Med. Chem. 2008;15(23):2337-45.

[86] T-cell vaccination in multiple sclerosis: update on clinical application and mode of action. Hellings N, Raus J, Stinissen P. Autoimmun. Rev. 200;3(4):267-75.

[87] Effects of natalizumab treatment on Foxp3+ T regulatory cells. Stenner MP, Waschbisch A, Buck D, Doerck S, Einsele H, Toyka KV, Wiendl H. *PLoS One.* 2008;3(10):e3319.

[88] Immunoregulatory T cells in multiple sclerosis and the effect of interferon beta and glatiramer acetate treatment on T cell subpopulations. Praksova P, Stourac P, Bednarik J, Vlckova E, Mikulkova Z, Michalek J. *J. Neurol. Sci.* 2012;319(1-2):18-23.

[89] Effect of short-term interferon-β treatment on cytokines in multiple sclerosis: Significant modulation of IL-17 and IL-23. Kürtüncü M, Tüzün E, Türkoğlu R, Petek-Balcı B, Içöz S, Pehlivan M, Birişik O, Ulusoy C, Shugaiv E, Akman-Demir G, Eraksoy M. *Cytokine.* 2012;59(2):400-2.

[90] Dopaminergic Modulation of CD4+CD25+ Regulatory T Lymphocytes in Multiple Sclerosis Patients during Interferon-β Therapy. Cosentino M, Zaffaroni M, Trojano M, Giorelli M, Pica C, Rasini E, Bombelli R, Ferrari M, Ghezzi A, Comi G, Livrea P, Lecchini S, Marino F. *Neuroimmunomodulation.* 2012;19(5):283-292.

[91] IFN-β induces the proliferation of CD4+CD25+Foxp3+ regulatory T cells through upregulation of GITRL on dendritic cells in the treatment of multiple sclerosis. Chen M, Chen G, Deng S, Liu X, Hutton GJ, Hong J. *J. Neuroimmunol.* 2012;242(1-2):39-46.

[92] Myelin basic protein-reactive T cells in multiple sclerosis: pathologic relevance and therapeutic targeting. Zhang J, Raus J. Cytotechnology. 1994;16(3):181-7.

[93] Dendritic cells expand antigen-specific Foxp3+CD25+CD4+ regulatory T cells including suppressors of alloreactivity. Yamazaki S, Inaba K, Tarbell KV, *Steinman RM Immunol. Rev.* 2006;212:314-29.

[94] Biological functions of regulatory T cells. Shevach EM. *Adv. Immunol.* 2011;112:137-76.

[95] Only the CD45RA+ subpopulation of CD4+CD25high T cells gives rise to homogeneous regulatory T-cell lines upon in vitro expansion. Hoffmann P, Eder R, Boeld TJ, Doser K, Piseshka B, Andreesen R, Edinger M. *Blood.* 2006;108(13):4260-7.

[96]   Oral tolerance to myelin basic protein induces regulatory TGF-beta-secreting T cells in Peyer's patches of SJL mice. Santos LM, al-Sabbagh A, Londono A, Weiner HL. *Cell Immunol.* 1994;157(2):439-47.

[97]   CD25+CD4+ regulatory T cells exert in vitro suppressive activity independent of CTLA-4. Kataoka H, Takahashi S, Takase K, Yamasaki S, Yokosuka T, Koike T, Saito T. *Int. Immunol.* 2005;17(4):421-7.

[98]   GITR: a multifaceted regulator of immunity belonging to the tumor necrosis factor receptor superfamily. Nocentini G, Riccardi C. *Eur. J. Immunol.* 2005;35(4):1016-22.

[99]   Inhibition of follicular T-helper cells by CD8+ regulatory T cells is essential for self tolerance. Kim HJ, Verbinnen B, Tang X, Lu L, Cantor H. *Nature.* 2010;467(7313):328-32.

[100] Regulation of immunity by a novel population of Qa-1-restricted CD8αα+TCRαβ+ T cells. Tang X, Maricic I, Purohit N, Bakamjian B, Reed-Loisel LM, Beeston T, Jensen P, Kumar V. *J. Immunol.* 2006;177(11):7645-55.

[101] Specific suppression of human CD4+ Th cell responses to pig MHC antigens byCD8+CD28- regulatory T cells. Ciubotariu R, Colovai AI, Pennesi G, Liu Z, Smith D, Berlocco P, Cortesini R, Suciu-Foca N. *J. Immunol.* 1998;161(10):5193-202.

[102] Essential roles of CD8+CD122+ regulatory T cells in the maintenance of T cell homeostasis. Rifa'i M, Kawamoto Y, Nakashima I, Suzuki H. *J. Exp. Med.* 2004;200(9):1123-34.

[103] Characterization of the CD8+CD45R+(2H4+) suppressor effector cell. Morimoto C, Takeuchi T, Schlossman SF. *Clin. Exp. Rheumatol.* 1989;7 Suppl 3:S3-7.

[104] CD8+Foxp3+ regulatory T cells mediate immunosuppression in prostate cancer. Kiniwa Y, Miyahara Y, Wang HY, Peng W, Peng G, Wheeler TM, Thompson TC, Old LJ, Wang RF. *Clin. Cancer Res.* 2007 Dec 1;13(23):6947-58.

[105] Alloantigen-induced regulatory CD8+CD103+ T cells. Koch SD, Uss E, van Lier RA, ten Berge IJ. *Hum. Immunol.* 2008;69(11):737-44.

[106] Expansion of regulatory CD8+CD25+ T cells after neonatal alloimmunization. Adams B, Dubois A, Delbauve S, Debock I, Lhommé F, Goldman M, Flamand V. *Clin. Exp. Immunol.* 2011;163(3):354-61.

[107] Origins and functional basis of regulatory CD11c+CD8+ T cells. Vinay DS, Kim CH, Choi BK, Kwon BS. *Eur. J. Immunol.* 2009;39(6):1552-63.

[108] Novel CD8+ Treg suppress EAE by TGF-beta- and IFN-gamma-dependent mechanisms. Chen ML, Yan BS, Kozoriz D, Weiner HL. Eur. J. Immunol. 2009;39(12):3423-35.

[109] A suppressor T-lymphocyte cell line for autoimmune encephalomyelitis. Ellerman KE, Powers JM, Brostoff SW. *Nature.* 1988;331(6153):265-7.

[110] Suppression of experimentally induced autoimmune encephalomyelitis by cytolytic T-T cell interactions. Sun D, Qin Y, Chluba J, Epplen JT, Wekerle H. *Nature.* 1988;332(6167):843-5.

[111] Regulatory circuits in autoimmunity: recruitment of counter-regulatory CD8+ T cells by encephalitogenic CD4+ T line cells. Sun D, Ben-Nun A, Wekerle H. *Eur. J. Immunol.* 1988;18(12):1993-9.

[112] CD8$^+$ T cells control the TH phenotype of MBP-reactive CD4$^+$ T cells in EAE mice. Jiang H, Braunstein NS, Yu B, Winchester R, Chess L. *Proc. Natl. Acad. Sci. USA.* 2001;98(11):6301-6.

[113] Regulatory functions of CD8$^+$CD28$^-$ T cells in an autoimmune disease model. Najafian N, Chitnis T, Salama AD, Zhu B, Benou C, Yuan X, Clarkson MR, Sayegh MH, Khoury SJ. *J. Clin. Invest.* 2003;112(7):1037-48.

[114] Essential role of CD8$^+$CD122$^+$ regulatory T cells in the recovery from experimental autoimmune encephalomyelitis. Lee YH, Ishida Y, Rifa'i M, Shi Z, Isobe K, Suzuki H. *J. Immunol.* 2008 Jan 15;180(2):825-32.

[115] Involvement of IFN-γ and perforin, but not Fas/FasL interactions in regulatory T cell-mediated suppression of experimental autoimmune encephalomyelitis. Beeston T, Smith TR, Maricic I, Tang X, Kumar V. *J. Neuroimmunol.* 2010;229(1-2):91-7.

[116] CD8$^+$CD122$^+$ regulatory T cells (Tregs) and CD4$^+$ Tregs cooperatively prevent and cure CD4$^+$ cell-induced colitis. Endharti AT, Okuno Y, Shi Z, Misawa N, Toyokuni S, Ito M, Isobe K, Suzuki H. *J. Immunol.* 2011;186(1):41-52.

In: Encephalitis, Encephalomyelitis and Encephalopathies   ISBN: 978-1-62257-766-8
Editors: Andrew Ruiz and Douglas Fleming   © 2013 Nova Science Publishers, Inc.

Chapter 6

NEUROMYELITIS OPTICA

*Jilpa Patel and Roumen Balabanov**

Rush University Medical Center, Department of Neurological Sciences,
Multiple Sclerosis Center, Chicago IL, US

ABSTRACT

Neuromyelitis optica (NMO), also known as Devic's disease, is a chronic inflammatory disease of the central nervous system. NMO affects optic nerves and spinal cord of patients causing visual loss and myelopathy. Until recently, this disease had a poor prognosis and presented a number of clinical, diagnostic, and management challenges. Over the last decade NMO became a focus of intense research, which led to identification of a disease biomarker and introduction of novel diagnostic criteria. In this review, we discuss the most important clinical and management aspects of the disease. In addition, we analyze the current hypotheses related to the etiology and pathogenesis of NMO. In the conclusion of the review we outline several research directions that may be of future interest.

Keywords: Neuromyelitis optica, Devic's disease, CNS inflammation, aquaporin-4, anti-aquaporin-4 antibody, optic neuritis, myelitis

INTRODUCTION

Neuromyelitis optica (NMO), also known as Devic's disease, is a chronic inflammatory disease of the central nervous system (CNS) affecting the optic nerves and spinal cord of patients. The first account on the disease was credited to Thomas Albutt, who in 1870 described a case of acute non-traumatic myelitis associated with optic neuritis [1]. A decade later in 1880, Wilhelm Erb reported another case of "myelitis transversa dorsalis with neuritis opticorum" [2]. Eugène Devic, a French physician, presented the first review on the disease (16 cases) at the French Congress of Medicine in Lyon in 1894 describing them collectively

---

* Correspondence: Rush University Medical Center, Department of Neurological Sciences, Multiple Sclerosis Center, 1725 W. Harrison, Suite 309, Chicago IL 60612, Tel: 312-942-8011, Fax: 312-942-5523, email: Roumen_Balabanov@rush.edu.

under the term "neuroptico-myélite" [3, 4]. Fernand Gault, a Ph.D. student under Devic's, further expanded this case review into a doctoral thesis [5]. He also coined the term "neuromyélite optic", or neuromyelitis optica, that is currently in use in the International Classification of the Diseases (ICD-9: 340.1; ICD-10:G36). The eponym "Devic's disease" was proposed in 1907 in a review article by Peppo Acchiote [6].

During the 20th century NMO was discussed periodically in a number of reviews and the first unified concept of the disease was established [7-21]. Classically, NMO was defined as a severe inflammatory disease of the CNS characterized by simultaneous or successive involvement of the optic nerves and the spinal cord, while sparing the brain. Clinical course of the disease was viewed as monophasic and often with a fatal outcome. As a nosological entity, NMO was considered to be a rare variant of multiple sclerosis (MS) or acute disseminated encephalomyelitis (ADEM) [5, 9, 16, 17, 21]. Indeed, optic neuritis and transverse myelitis are common clinical presentations of these diseases. In addition, it became apparent that NMO can be associated with certain infectious and connective tissue disorders [22-32]. Initial pathological studies of the disease reported tissue inflammation, demyelination and necrosis at the lesion sites, and hyalinization of the blood vessels, but none of these findings were sufficiently specific or reproducible [11, 14, 16, 17, 19, 33, 34]. The term Devic's syndrome (instead of disease) came into use to reflect this diagnostic ambiguity [16, 27-30].

In 1980s and 1990s, with the introduction of magnetic resonance imaging (MRI) and cerebrospinal fluid (CSF) analysis, two important features contrasting NMO from MS were described: spinal cord lesions are longitudinally extensive spanning several (>3) vertebral segments, and CSF is commonly negative for oligoclonal bands [19, 20]. This was followed in early 2000s, by the discovery of NMO-IgG (anti-aquaporin-4 antibody) and the recognition that NMO is an autoimmune disease mediated by a self-reactive antibody [35-37]. NMO-IgG became a reliable diagnostic biomarker for the disease and new treatment approaches targeting the antibody arm of the immune system were introduced [38, 39]. Most recently, the concept of NMO spectrum disorders was introduced to include not only clinically defined NMO but also other idiopathic inflammatory disorders of CNS, in which NMO-IgG is involved [40].

The goal of this review is to summarize the recent advancements in NMO and to discuss current hypotheses related to its pathogenesis.

CLINICAL PRESENTATION AND NATURAL HISTORY

NMO is a rare sporadic disease of the CNS [11, 19, 20, 41]. Overall disease incidence is unknown but according to some estimates it rounds to about 1:100,000 population [42]. The disease affects predominantly non-Caucasian (African-American, African and Asian) females in their forties [41]. In corroboration, the disease is most common in Africa and Asia, and in countries with tropical climate [16, 26]. Certainly, other demographic groups such as Caucasian males and females, or children can also be affected [41, 43]. Familial cases have been described as well (44, 45).

NMO affects predominantly the optic nerves and spinal cord of patients [1-21]. Optic nerve involvement presents with decreased or complete loss of vision in one or both eyes.

Ocular pain is another prominent symptom. More subtle deficit such as decreased perception of color is a typical early sign. Central scotomas and peripheral visual field defects are common. The optic discs are usually swollen but can be normal in cases of retrobulbar neuritis. Spinal cord involvement presents with paresthesias, sensory loss with a segmental level, gait abnormalities, upper and/or lower extremity weakness that can progress to paraplegia or quadriplegia. Lhermitte's sign (shooting pain in the spine and legs upon neck flexion) is common and indicates cervical cord lesion. Bowel and bladder dysfunction are frequent findings.

Disease symptoms have either acute or subacute onset [19, 20, 41]. They are typically severe and likely to persist without treatment. Optic neuritis tends to be bilateral (simultaneous or sequential) with little spontaneous improvement. Transverse myelitis can be complicated by phrenic nerve paralysis, dysautonomia, paroxysmal tonic spasms, and complete loss of bladder control. Occasionally, spinal cord lesions can extend rostrally and involve brain medulla causing persistent hiccoughs and respiratory failure [46]. Natural course of the disease can take one of the two forms: 1) chronic relapsing-remitting form, accounting for 70-90% of all cases; 2) monophasic form followed by clinical recovery, accounting for the rest [41]. Relapsing-remitting form is associated with female gender, older age at onset, longer optic neuritis-myelitis interval (>3 months), and presence of systemic autoimmunity. The second relapse appears within the first year for 60% and within 3 years for 95% of all patients. Monophasic form is associated with male gender and younger age. Overall, relapsing-remitting form results in worse disease outcome. NMO does not have a secondary progressive phase that is seen in MS, and related neurological disability is a cumulative result of disease relapses [40]. About 50% of all patients would have significant visual or motor impairment, and would require support for walking, within 5 years of disease onset. The five-year mortality rate is 32% with the relapsing-remitting disease and 10% with the monophasic disease. Death is most commonly a consequence of respiratory failure, urosepsis and pulmonary embolism [18-20, 41].

MR imaging and laboratory testing are used for further clinical evaluation. MRI typically detects signal abnormalities in optic nerves and spinal cord, usually in the absence of brain involvement, at least initially [19, 20, 47-49]. T2 signal abnormalities in the optic nerves and/or optic chiasm are common findings; they are also gadolinium-positive during the acute phase of the disease. Spinal cord lesions are characteristically hyperintense on T2- and hypointense on T1-weighted images. They appear centrally-based and longitudinally extensive spanning continuously over 3 vertebral segments (Figure 1). Acutely, the lesions are gadolinium positive and swollen, causing spinal cord enlargement. In time, the swelling diminishes and the gadolinium enhancement becomes less intense, but may remain up to 18 months. Spinal cord atrophy usually follows in 1-2 years as a result of structural damage [49].

CSF studies typically reveal normal opening pressure, clear fluid, increased protein, and pleocytosis (>50 WBC/mm^2) with either lymphocytic or polymorphonuclear cell predominance [19, 20]. Elevated CSF albumin and low serum/CSF albumin ratio reflecting blood-brain barrier breakdown are common findings. Oligoclonal bands are uncommonly detected (<20-30% of patients) and may represent a transient phenomenon associated with marked lymphocytic pleocytosis [50]. Other laboratory testing such as evoked potentials may be of diagnostic significance. Visual evoked potentials (VEP), for instance, can be helpful in detecting subclinical optic neuritis (Figure 1) [20, 51].

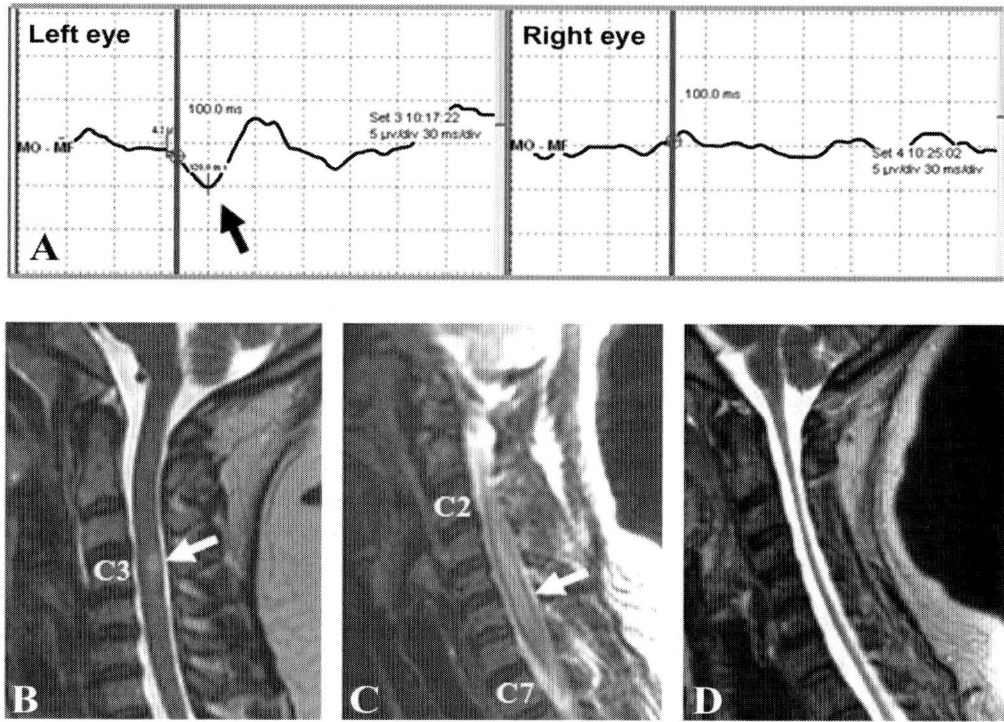

Figure 1. VEP and MRI findings in NMO. A. Testing visual evoked potentials in NMO patients commonly reveals bilateral abnormalities : VEP of left eye demonstrates a delay in conduction velocity of P100 wave from 100 milliseconds (normal response, **red line**) to 127 **milliseconds (patient's** response); VEP of right eye demonstrates complete disappearance of P 100 wave response (courtesy of Thomas Hoeppner, Ph.D., RUMC). B. Spinal cord lesions in MS are typically confined within a single vertebral segment (arrow points to a lesion at C3 level). C. Spinal cord lesions in NMO characteristically spread over several vertebral segments (arrow point to a lesion spanning between C2-C7 levels). D. Diffuse spinal cord atrophy is a typical chronic finding in NMO.

Testing for NMO-IgG (anti-aquapotin-4 antibody) is an essential diagnostic investigation. NMO-IgG is highly sensitive (73%) and specific (91%) for the disease [36]. It is rarely detected in MS (<9% of patients) [36]. Currently, there are two commercial laboratory techniques that are used in the serologic diagnosis of NMO. These include immunostaining of transfected cell lines overexpressing human aquaporin-4 and enzyme-linked immunosorbent assay (ELISA) with a purified protein. Overall, they perform similarly and within the range of the expected sensitivity and specificity [52].

DIAGNOSIS AND DIFFERENTIAL DIAGNOSIS

Diagnosis of NMO is based on specific clinical, imaging, and laboratory criteria (also known as Revised Diagnostic Criteria 2006) (Table 1) [53]. Accordingly, presence of optic neuritis and transverse myelitis are required criteria for the diagnosis. MRI of brain and spinal cord revealing typical findings for the disease are supportive criteria for the diagnosis. Initial MRI of brain should be either normal or demonstrate lesions that are not compatible with MS.

MRI of spinal cord should demonstrate a longitudinally extensive lesion spanning several (>3) vertebral segments. Positive test for NMO-IgG is the final supportive criterion. It is important to mention that the diagnosis of NMO can be established in the absence of NMO-IgG, if the supportive MRI criteria are met. In addition, CSF testing while may be important, is not necessary for the diagnosis. Revised Diagnostic Criteria 2006 are very sensitive and specific (>90% for both) for NMO [53].

A number of clinical presentations have been encountered when only some but not all the diagnostic criteria can be fulfilled; for instance, isolated recurrent optic neuritis or longitudinally extensive transverse myelitis (LETM) (also known as limited forms of NMO). Technically, diagnosis of NMO cannot be established in these cases, even in the presence of NMO-IgG seropositivity. The rate of seropositivity in these cases is about 25% for optic neuritis and 50% for LETM [54-57]. Seropositivity in such cases is associated with 50% risk of recurrence or of developing NMO. Other atypical presentations include association between isolated recurrent optic neuritis, or LETM, and lesions on brain MRI involving the thalamus, hypothalamus, and areas adjacent to the third and fourth ventricles [58, 59]. Cases of co-existent seropositivity of NMO-IgG and anti-nuclear antibody (ANA), or other tests suggestive for connective tissue disorders, can be also cited [60]. A new concept of NMO-spectrum disorders is put forward to address the issues of partiality of clinical presentations and overlap of clinical and laboratory findings (Table 2) [41]. Overall, this concept reflects the biological variation of NMO and, perhaps, the tendency of these patients towards developing of complex autoimmune responses. In practical terms, "spectrum" concept increases the clinical suspicion of NMO-IgG-mediated disease and suggests appropriate therapy.

Differential diagnosis of NMO includes other inflammatory diseases of the CNS with similar clinical presentations. Typically, the list of such diseases includes MS, connective tissue disorders (SLE and Sjögren's syndrome), and CNS infections. Distinction between NMO and MS, almost impossible in the past, now can be done reliably [53, 61]. In contrast to NMO, MS involves the brain very early; wide-spread white matter and cortical lesions are characteristically seen in this disease. In addition, MS lesions in the spinal cord are typically small and localized within the peripheral white matter and do not span over 2 vertebral segments. A longitudinally appearing lesion can be seen in MS but late in the disease as a consequence of accumulation and fusion of multiple small lesions. CSF testing in MS commonly demonstrates positivity for oligoclonal bands (>85%) but normal protein and cell count. NMO-IgG seropositivity is rare in MS (<9 of patients) [36].

Table 1. Revised Diagnostic Criteria for neuromyelitis optica (NMO) [53]

Required criteria:
    Optic Neuritis
    Transverse myelitis
Supportive criteria (two out of three are required):
    Initial brain MRI normal or not compatible with multiple sclerosis (MS)
    Cord MRI T2 lesion > 3 vertebral segments during acute attack
    Positive serology for NMO-IgG (anti-aquaporin-4 antibody)

Table 2. NMO spectrum disorders [41]

Neuromyelitis optica (NMO)
Limited forms of NMO:
    Idiopathic single or recurrent event of longitudinally extensive myelitis
    (>3 vertebral segment spinal cord MRI lesion)
    Bilateral simultaneous or recurrent optic neuritis
Asian optic-spinal multiple sclerosis
Optic neuritis or longitudinally extensive transverse myelitis associated with systemic
    autoimmune disease
Optic neuritis or myelitis associated with characteristic NMO brain lesion pattern
    (hypothalamic, periventricular, brainstem involvement)
Other distinct clinical features in a patient with seropositive for NMO-IgG:
    Intractable vomiting
    Posterior reversible encephalopathy syndrome

Clinically and pathologically, NMO overlaps with the so-called Asian (Japanese) optic-spinal form of MS. In addition, there is strong association of NMO-IgG seropositivity and this disease (58% of patients) [35]. Historically, MS in Asia was divided in Western (conventional) and Asian forms. Asian form of MS was defined as recurrent optic neuritis and transverse myelitis without brain involvement, but it was classified separately from NMO, since the latter was viewed at the time as a monophasic disease [16, 62]. In addition, Asian form of MS accounted for more than 80% of all MS cases, while NMO with a monophasic course was relatively rare [16]. At this point, there is no sufficient evidence to equate NMO to Asian form of MS, but the latter can be viewed as an NMO-spectrum disorder [41].

Distinction between NMO and connective tissues disorders is more difficult, particularly in cases of isolated optic neuritis or transverse myelitis. Historically, NMO has been associated with SLE and Sjögren's syndrome [22-32]. In addition, nearly 30% of all NMO patients test positive for some laboratory markers (ANA or SSA/SSB antibodies) related to these diseases [60]. However, NMO patients rarely develop systemic autoimmunity despite their seropositivity for ANA or SSA/SSB, and SLE or Sjögren's syndrome patients rarely test positive for NMO-IgG in the absence of CNS findings. The possibility of coexistence of NMO and SLE or Sjögren's syndrome (rather than NMO being caused of these disorders) may be considered. The concept of NMO-spectrum disorders can be applied to such cases. "Spectrum" patients are likely to benefit from typical NMO therapies.

Other presentations difficult to distinguish from NMO can be caused by intrinsic spinal cord tumors, syringomyelia, trauma, endocrinopathies, clioquinol intoxication, pulmonary tuberculosis, toxoplasmosis, infectious mononucleosis, tropical myelopathy, human T-lymphotropic virus 1-associated (HTLV-1) myelopathy, and human immunodeficiency virus-1 (HIV-1) [13, 16, 20, 22-27, 63-67]. These can be ruled out by obtaining of a detailed medical history, careful examination, and systemic laboratory testing. Treating the specific causes in such cases can result in clinical improvement.

DISEASE PATHOGENESIS

Julius Dreschfeld and Eugène Devic gave the first pathological descriptions of NMO [3, 68]. Dreschfeld reported on the inflammatory and necrotizing nature of disease lesions, and Devic commented on the fact that the spinal cord lesion of his case extended 4-5cm in length. Subsequent studies provided additional details on the disease pathology. Specifically, lesions appear to be destructive and associated with inflammation, demyelination, tissue necrosis, astrogliosis, and microglial activation [11, 19]. Inflammatory infiltrates comprise of perivascular and parenchymal leukocytes. Spinal cord lesions are central or paracentral and typically involve white and gray matter [19]. Hyalinization of medium-sized arteries in the spinal cord is a common finding and associated with tissue necrosis [11, 14, 33, 34]. Early and acute lesions are characterized by prominent perivascular deposition of immune complexes, complement activation, swelling, and tissue infiltration by neutrophils, and eosinophils [37]. Inflammatory findings may be limited in cases of prior use of steroids and immunosuppressants [16].

Discovery of NMO-IgG provided new insights into disease pathogenesis. NMO-IgG is a self-reactive antibody targeting human aquaporin-4 [69]. Latter belongs to a family of transmembrane proteins that regulate water flow in cells [70]. Aquaporin-4 is a 35kDa protein that is expressed by the CNS astrocytes and astrocytic processes surrounding the small blood vessels or at glia limitans [69]. Localization of aquaporin-4 immediately beyond the basement membrane of blood vessels makes it an accessible target for circulating NMO-IgG. In corroboration, expression of aquaporin-4 appears to be diminished in NMO lesions, particularly in areas of inflammation and immune complex deposition [71, 72]. Such vasculocentric loss of aquaporin-4 is specific for the NMO; in contrast expression of aquaporin-4 is upregulated in MS [71, 72]. Finally, there are *in vitro* data demonstrating that NMO-IgG has the capacity to bind to cultured astrocytes, activate complement, and cause cell death [73]. Overall, it appears that NMO is mediated, at least in part, by a self-reactive antibody that drives an inflammatory reaction into the CNS, which in turn causes tissue injury (Figure 2).

The etiology of NMO remains unknown. High incidence of NMO in the tropics has led to speculations for an infectious cause [74]. There are a number of reports indicating a temporal association between infections and the disease onset [20, 26, 41, 75]. In addition, IgM antibody and Th17 cells mediating host defense against microbial pathogens, are also involved in NMO [37, 76-77]. Positive correlation between *Helicobacter pylori* infection and NMO-IgG seropositivity is suggested as well [78]. Recently, we proposed the hypothesis of cross-immunoreactivity between bacterial aquaporin-Z and human aquaporin-4 proteins [79]. Former is a bacterial water channel regulating cell volume and osmotic stress [70]. In our study we found significant structural homology between these two proteins. Cross-immunoreactivity between aquaporin-Z and aquaporin-4 was ascertained in multiple immune-based assays, and in animal experiments demonstrating that induction of an immune response against aquaporin-Z, can also trigger an autoimmune reaction against aquaporin-4 and CNS inflammation.

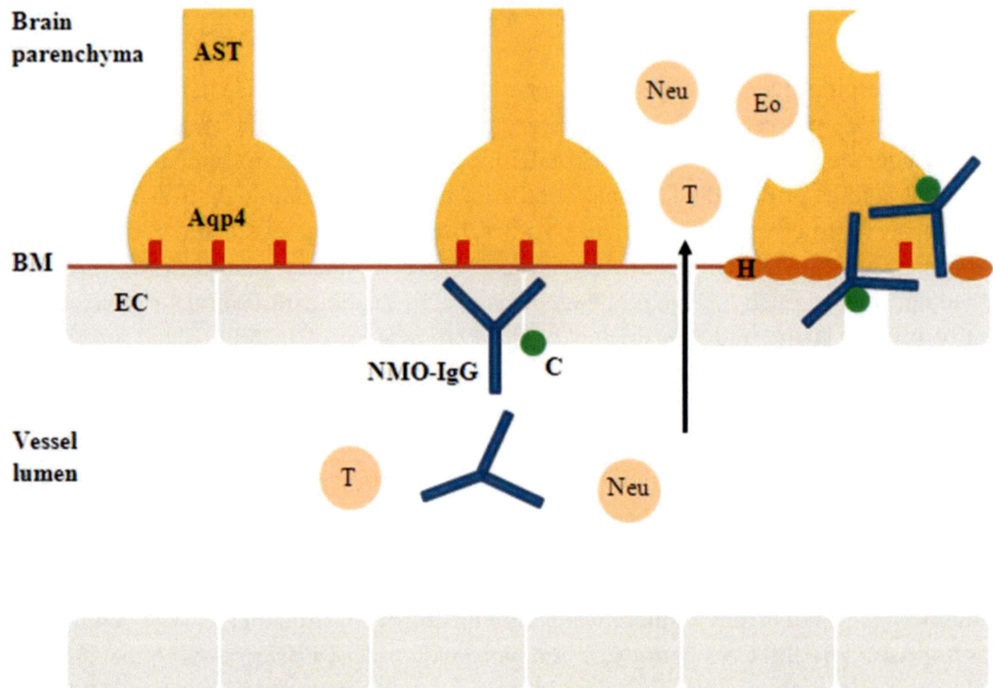

Figure 2. Pathogenesis of NMO. Aquaporin-4 (Aqp4) is expressed by the CNS astrocytes (AST) and localized at their perivascular processes, immediately beyond the basement membrane (BM) and the endothelial cells (EC). The disease is mediated by a self-reactive antibody (NMO-IgG) targeting Aqp4. Complement (C) is recruited and becomes activated by the autoantibody. Cellular inflammation is triggered as well and involves T cells (T), neutrophils (Neu), and eosinophils (Eo). As a result, astrocytes become injured, Aqp4 expression is downregulated and the blood vessel walls accumulate hyaline (H). Ultimately, inflammation leads to loss of function.

The role of genetic factors in NMO is also unknown. There are reports of familial occurrence of the disease but no conclusive evidence is available [44, 45]. There is evidence suggesting that NMO is associated with specific HLA alleles including DR1*801, DP1 501 and DPA1 202, but not with DRB1*1501, the allele that was previously associated with multiple sclerosis [80]. Additionally, NMO is also not associated with mitochondrial DNA mutations implicated in the pathogenesis of Leber hereditary optic neuropathy (LHON) and in multiple sclerosis with prominent optic neuritis [81].

TREATMENT AND MANAGEMENT

Compared to other CNS demyelinating diseases, NMO has a higher disability and mortality rate. In the past, death has been the most common outcome of NMO [7, 11, 18-20, 47]. More recent literature reflects a better prognosis because of the advances in immunotherapy and supportive care. However, most of the new therapeutic approaches originate from small-scale studies and their long-term benefit is uncertain. Treatment of NMO is divided in three categories: rescue treatment of acute disease, prophylactic disease-modification, and symptomatic treatment of disease complications. Rescue treatment is based on the use of steroids and plasma exchange. Its goal is to decrease and stop inflammation, destroy or remove inflammatory cells and molecules, and to allow recovery of injured tissue. Steroid therapy has been recommended and tried with varying success over the years. Typically, treatment is initiated with intravenous methylprednisolone (100-1000mg intravenously once a day for 3 to 5 days), followed by an oral prednisone taper (starting at 60-100mg daily) over a month [16, 18-20]. Steroid-resistant attacks being common in NMO can be treated with plasma exchange, usually 6 to 7 exchanges (1.5 volume each) every other day [38]. In practice, intravenous steroids can be administered first and plasma exchange added after 3 or 4 days as a combination therapy. If effective, steroid/plasma exchange treatment can be applied periodically (every 2 to 3 months) to maintain remission. Disease modification can be achieved by using immunosuppressive agents. The most commonly used immunosuppressants are azathioprine (2-3mg/kg, or 100 to 150mg orally twice daily) or mycophenolate mofetil (1000-1500mg orally twice daily) [82, 83]. They can be started simultaneously with the rescue treatment or immediately after since their effect is delayed. Rituximab (anti-CD20), a monoclonal antibody directed against B-cells (four treatments of 375mg/m^2 one week apart) can be used as well [84]. Other treatment agents with reported clinical benefit include mitoxantrone, methotrexate, and intravenous gamma globulin [85-87]. At this point, there are no studies comparing the efficacy of any of the above-mentioned agents or the benefits of their combinations. In addition, there should be awareness that certain MS therapeutic agents, such as interferon-beta and fingolimod, may worsen NMO symptoms [88, 89]. Finally, any treatment approach should include symptomatic measures such as respiratory support, management of disease-related symptoms (pain, tonic spasms, bowel and bladder dysfunction) and infections. Neurological rehabilitation is likely to be beneficial acutely and in conjunction with the medical therapy.

CONCLUSION

Over the last decade clinical and basic science knowledge of NMO dramatically increased. Collective evidence indicates that NMO is a distinct nosological entity. The concept of NMO-spectrum disorders has growing acceptance and may be included in the future revisions of the International Classification of Diseases. Immunotherapy of NMO is still in its naissance but appears promising and certainly has changed the perception of NMO as an inevitably fatal disease. Disease pathogenesis even though partially understood provides a reliable frame-work for future research. However, despite these advancements a number of important questions remain to be addressed: 1) origin of NMO-IgG is unknown and the possibility of infection-induced cross-reactivity should be investigated; 2) pathogenic processes of NMO-IgG seronegative disease have to be clarified; 3) distribution of lesions in CNS appears to be limited (optic nerves and spinal cord) and the restrictive mechanisms should be identified; 4) there is no accepted animal model of the disease. In addition, a whole host of clinical issues related to standardization of NMO-IgG assays (ELISA vs. immunostaining) and disease monitoring (biomarkers for disease relapse or response to treatment) needs to be addressed. It will be important to understand the significance of NMO in the context of systemic autoimmune or infectious diseases. Finally, collaborative international efforts may be necessary in solving future challenges related to NMO.

REFERENCES

[1]   Albutt, T. On the ophthalmoscopic signs of spinal disease. *Lancet* 1870, 1:76-78.

[2]   Erb, W. Ueber das zusammenvorkommen von neuritis optica und myelitis subacuta. *Arch. Psychiatr. Nervenkr.* 1880, 10:146-157.

[3]   Devic, E. Myélite aiguë dorso-lumbaire avec névrite optique: Autopsie. *Congrès Français du Médicine, Lyon* 1894, 1:434-490.

[4]   Devic, E. Myélite subaiguë compliquée de névrite optique. *Bull. Méd. (Paris)* 1895, 8:1033-1034.

[5]   Gault, F. De la neuromyélite optique aiguë. *Thesis No. 0981. Lyon,* 1894.

[6]   Acchiote, P. Sur un cas de neuromyélite subaiguë ou maladie de Devic. *Rev. Neurol.* 1907, 15:775-777.

[7]   Goulden, C. Optic neuritis and myelitis. *Ophthalmic Rev.* 1914, 34:193-209.

[8]   Beck, G. A case of diffuse myelitis associated with optic neuritis. *Brain* 1927, 50:687-703.

[9]   Ferraro, A. Primary demyelinating processes of the central nervous system: an attempt at unification and classification. *Arch. Neurol. Psychiatry* 1937, 37:1100-1160.

[10]   Putnam, T; Foster, F. Neuromyelitis optica: its relation to multiple sclerosis. *Trans. Am. Neurol. Assoc.* 1942, 68:20-25.

[11]   Stansbury, F. Neuromyelitis optica (Devic's disease): presentation of five cases with pathological study and review of the literature. *Arch. Ophthalmol.* 1949, 42:293-335, 465-501.

[12]   Peters, G. Neuromyelitis optica. In: Lubarsche, O; Henke, F; Rossle, R. (eds.). *Handbuch der speziellen pathologischen anatomie des histologie, Bd. XIII. IIA: Erkrankungen des zentralen nerven systems.* Berlin: Springer; 1958, pp.630-644.

[13]   Burke, D; Cheshire, D. Neuromyelitis optica. A review of the literature and a report of a case, which followed traumatic paraplegia. *Paraplegia* 1968, 6:79-89.

[14]   Cloys, D; Netsky, M. Neuromyelitis optica. In: Vinken, P; Bruyn, G. (eds.). *Multiple sclerosis and other demyelinating diseases. Handbook of clinical neurology,* New York: Elsevier; 1970, vol. 9, pp.426-436.

[15]   Walton, J. Disseminated myelitis with optic neuritis. In: Walton, J. (ed.). *Brain's diseases of the central nervous system.* 8th ed., Oxford University Press; 1977, pp.542-544.

[16]   Kuroiwa, Y. Neuromyelitis optica (Devic's disease, Devic's syndrome). In: Koetsier, J. (ed.), *Demyelinating Diseases. Handbook of clinical neurology.* New York: Elsevier Science; 1985, vol.47, pp.397-408.

[17]   Matthews, W. Neuromyelitis optica. In: Matthews, W. (ed.). *McAlpine's multiple sclerosis,* Edinburgh: Churchill Livingstone; 1985, pp.151-152.

[18]   Whitham, R; Brey, R. Neuromyelitis optica: two new cases and a review of the literature. *J. Clin. Neuroophthalmol.* 1985, 5:263-269.

[19]   Mandler, R; Davis, L; Jeffery, D; Kornfeld, M. Devic's neuromyelitis optica: a clinicopathological study of 8 patients. *Ann. Neurol.* 1993, 34:162-168.

[20]   O'Riordan, J; Gallagher, H; Thompson, A; Howard, R; Kingsley, D; Thompson, E; McDonald, W; Miller, D. Clinical, CSF, and MRI findings in Devic's neuromyelitis optica. *J. Neurol. Neurosurg. Psychiatry* 1996, 60:382-387.

[21] Adams, R; Victor, M; Ropper, A. Multiple sclerosis and allied demyelinative diseases. In: Adams, R; Victor, M; Roper, A. (eds.). *Principles of Neurology.* 6th ed. McGraw Hill; 1997, pp.902-927.

[22] Blanche, P; Diaz, E; Gombert, B; Sicard, D; Rivoal, O; Brezin, A. Devic's neuromyelitis optica and HIV-1 infection. *J. Neurol. Neurosurg. Psychiatry* 2000, 68:795-796.

[23] Chusid, M; Williamson, S; Murphy, J; Ramey, L. Neuromyelitis optica (Devic's disease) following varicella infection. *J. Pediatr.* 1979, 95:737-738.

[24] Corssmit, E; Levertein-van Hall, M; Portegies, P; Bakker, P. Severe neurological complications in association with Epstein-Barr infection. *J. Neurovirol.* 1997, 3:460-464.

[25] Merely, E; Bedim, R; Sola, P; Abruzzi, P; Mansard, G; Fiacre, G; Francine, G. Human herpes virus and human herpes virus 8 DNA sequences in brains of multiple sclerosis patients, normal adults and children. *J. Neurol.* 1997, 244:450-454.

[26] Papais-Alvarenga, R; Miranda-Santos, C; Puccioni-Sohler, M; de Almeida, A; Oliveira, S; Basilio De Oliveira, C; Alvarenga, H; Poser, C. Optic neuromyelitis syndrome in Brazilian patients. *J. Neurol. Neurosurg. Psychiatry* 2002, 73:429-435.

[27] Silber, M; Willcox, P; Bowen, R; Unger, A. Neuromyelitis optica (Devic's syndrome) and pulmonary tuberculosis. *Neurology* 1990, 40:934-938.

[28] April, R; Vansonnenberg, E. A case of neuromyelitis optica (Devic's syndrome) in systemic lupus erythematosus. Clinicopathologic report and review of the literature. *Neurology* 1976, 26:1066-1070.

[29] Kinney, E; Beroff, R; Rao, N; Lay, M. Devic's syndrome and systemic lupus erythematosus: a case report with necropsy. *Arch. Neurol.* 1979, 36:643-644.

[30] Margaux, J; Hayem, G; Meyer, O; Kahn, M. Systematic lupus erythematosus with optical neuromyelitis (Devic's syndrome). A case with a 35-year follow up. *Rev. Rheum. Engl. Ed.* 1999, 66:102-105.

[31] Mochizuki, A; Hayashi, A; Hisahara, S; Shoji, S. Steroid responsive variant of Sjögren's syndrome. *Neurology* 2000, 54:1391-1392.

[32] Inslicht, D; Stein, A; Pomerantz, F; Ragnarsson, K. Three women with lupus transverse myelitis: case reports and differential diagnosis. *Arch. Phys. Med. Rehabil.* 1998, 79:456-459.

[33] Ortiz de Zarate, J; Tamaroff, L; Sica, R; Rodriguez, J. Neuromyelitis optica versus subacute necrotic myelitis. II. Anatomical study of two cases. *J. Neurol. Neurosurg. Psychiatry* 1968, 31:641-645.

[34] Lefkowitz, D; Angelo, J. Neuromyelitis optica with unusual vascular changes. *Arch. Neurol.* 1984, 41:1103-1105.

[35] Lennon, V; Lucchinetti, C; Weinchenker, B. Identification of a marker antibody of neuromyelitis optica. *Neurology* 2003, 60 (suppl 1):A519-520.

[36] Lennon, V; Wingerchuk, D; Kryzer, T; Pittock, S; Lucchinetti, C; Fujihara, K; Nakashima, I; Weinshenker, B. A serum autoantibody marker of neuromyelitis optica: distinction from multiple sclerosis. *Lancet* 2004, 364:2106-2112.

[37] Lucchinetti, C; Mandler, R; McGavern, D; Bruck, W; Gleich, G; Ransohoff, R; Trebs, C; Weinshenker B; Wingerchuk, D; Parisi, J; Lassmann, H. A role for humoral mechanisms in the pathogenesis of Devic's neuromyelitis optica. *Brain* 2002, 125:1450-1461.

[38] Weinchenker, B; O'Brian, P; Petterson, T; Noseworthy, J; Lucchinetti, C; Dodick, D; Pineda, A; Stevens, L; Rodriguez, M. A randomized trial of plasma exchange in acute central nervous system inflammatory demyelinating disease. *Ann. Neurol.* 1999, 46:878-888.

[39] Cree B; Lamb, S; Morgan, K; Chen, A; Waubant, E; Genain, C. An open label study of the effects of rituximab in neuromyelitis optica. *Neurology* 2005, 64:1270-1272.

[40] Wingerchuck, D; Lennon V; Lucchineitti C; Pittock, S; Weinshenker B. The spectrum of neuromyelitis optica. *Lancet Neurol.* 2007, 6:805-815.

[41] Wingerchuk, D; Hogancamp, W; O'Brien, P; Weinshenker, B. The clinical course of neuromyelitis optica (Devic's disease). *Neurology* 1999, 53:1107-1114.

[42] Rivera, J; Kurtzke, J; Booth, V; Corona, T. Characteristics of Devic's disease (neuromyelitis optica) in Mexico. *J. Neurol.* 2008, 255:710-715.

[43] Jeffery, A; Buncic, J. Pediatric Devic's neuromyelitis optica. *J. Pediatr. Ophthalmol. Strabismus* 1996, 33:223-229.

[44] McAlpine, D. Familial neuromyelitis optica: its occurrence in identical twins. *Brain* 1938, 61:430-438.

[45] Ch'ien, L; Medeiros, M; Belluomini, J; Lemmi, H; Whitaker, J. Neuromyelitis optica (Devic's syndrome) in two sisters. *Clin. Electroencephalogr.* 1982, 13:36-39.

[46] Misu, T; Fujihara, K; Nakashima, I; Sato, S; Itoyama Y. Intractable hiccup and nausea with periaqueductal lesions in neuromyelitis optica. *Neurology* 2005, 65:1479-1485.

[47] Fazekas, F; Offenbacher. H; Schmidt, R; Strasser-Fuchs, S. MRI of neuromyelitis optica: evidence for a distinct entity. *J. Neurol. Neurosurg. Psychiatry* 1994, 57:1140-1142.

[48] Filippi, M; Rocca, M. MR imaging of Devic's neuromyelitis optica. *Neurol. Sci.* 2004, Suppl 4:S371-373.

[49] Tashiro, K; Ito, K; Maruo, Y; Homma, S; Yamada, T; Fujiki, N; Moriwaka, F. MR imaging of spinal cord in Devic disease. *J. Comput. Assist. Tomogr.* 1987, 11:516-517.

[50] Piccolo, G; Franciotta, D; Camana., C; Bergamaschi, R; Banfi, P; Sandrini, G; Citterio, A. Devic's neuromyelitis optica: long-term follow-up and serial CSF findings in two cases. *J. Neurol.* 1990, 237:262-264.

[51] Masuhr, F; Bush, M; Wetzel, K; Harms, L; Schielke, E. Relapsing myelitis with pathological visual evoqued potentials: a case of neuromyelitis optica? *Eur. J. Neurol.* 2002, 9:429-432.

[52] Waters, P; McKeaon A; Leite, M; Rajasekharan, S; Lennon V; Villalobos, A; Palace, J; Mandrekar, J; Vincent, A; Bar-Or, A; Pittock, S. Serological diagnosis of NMO: a multicenter comparison of aquaporin-4-IgG assays. *Neurology* 2012, 78:665-671.

[53] Wingerchuk, D; Lennon, V; Pittock, S; Lucchinetti, C; Weinshenker, B. Revised diagnostic criteria for neuromyelitis optica. *Neurology* 2006, 66:1485-1489.

[54] Matiello, M; Lennon, V; Jacob, A; Pittock, S; Lucchinetti, C; Wingerchuk, D; Weinshenker, B. NMO-IgG predicts the outcome of recurrent optic neuritis. *Neurology* 2008, 70:2197-2200.

[55] Jarius, S; Frederikson, J; Waters, P; Paul, F; Akman-Demir, G; Marignier, R; Franciotta, D; Ruprecht, K; Kuenz, B; Rommer, P; Kristoferitsch, W; Wildemann, B; Vincent, A. Frequency and prognostic impact of antibodies to aquaporin-4 in patients with optic neuritis. *J. Neurol. Sci.* 2010, 298:158-162.

[56] Saiz, A; Zuliani, L; Blanco, Y; Tavolato, B; Giometto, B; Graus, F; Spanish-Italian NMO Study Group. Revised diagnostic criteria for neuromyelitis optica (NMO). Application in a series of suspected patients. *J. Neurol.* 2007, 254:1233-1237.

[57] Waters, P; Jarius, S; Littleton, E; Leite, M; Jacob, S; Gray, B; Geraldes, R; Vale, T; Jacob, A; Palace, J; Maxwell, S; Beeson, D; Vincent, A. Aquaporin-4 antibodies in neuromyelitis optica and longitudinally extensive transverse myelitis. *Arch. Neurol.* 2008, 65:913-919.

[58] Pittock, S; Lennon, V; Krecke, K; Wingerchuk, D; Lucchinetti, C; Weinshenker, B. Brain abnormalities in neuromyelitis optica. *Arch. Neurol.* 2006, 63:390-396.

[59] Magaña, S; Matiello, M; Pittock, S; McKeon, A; Lennon, V; Rabinstein, A; Shuster, E; Kantarci, O; Lucchinetti, C; Weinshenker, B. Posterior reversible encephalopathy syndrome in neuromyelitis optica spectrum disorders. *Neurology* 2009, 72:712-717.

[60] Pittock, S; Lennon, V; de Seze, J; Vermersch, P; Homburger, H; Wingerchuk, D; Lucchinetti, C; Zéphir, H; Moder, K; Weinshenker, B. Neuromyelitis optica and non organ-specific autoimmunity. *Arch Neurol.* 2008, 65:78-83.

[61] Polman, C; Reingold, S; Edan, G; Filippi, M; Hartung, H; Kappos, L; Lublin, F; Metz L; McFarland, H; O'Connor, P; Sandberg-Wollheim, M; Thompson. A; Weinshenker, B; Wolinsky, J. Diagnostic criteria for multiple sclerosis: 2005 revisions to the "McDonald Criteria". *Ann. Neurol.* 2005, 58:840-846.

[62] Shibasaki, H; McDonald, I; Kuroiwa, Y. Racial modifications of clinical picture of multiple sclerosis: comparison between Japanese and British patients. *J. Neurol. Sci.* 1981, 49:253-271.

[63] Roberson, F; Ghatak, N; Young, H. Myelopathy presenting as an intrinsic spinal cord tumor. *Surg. Neurol.* 1978, 9:317-321.

[64] Wakui, K; Ito, S; Yabuki, S; Kato, T; Nakano, K. Case of neuromyelitis optica suspected to be toxoplasmosis. *Ganka* 1970, 12:581-601.

[65] Vernant, J; Cabre, P; Smadjia, D; Merle, H; Caubarrère, I; Mikol, J; Poser C. Recurrent neuromyelitis with endocrinopathies: a new syndrome. *Neurology* 1997, 48:58-64.

[66] Roman, G. Tropical myeloneuropathies revisited. *Curr. Opin. Neurol.* 1998, 11:539-544.

[67] Yoshida, Y; Saiga, T; Takahashi, H; Hara, A. Optic neuritis and human T-lymphotropic virus1-associated myelopathy: a case report. *Ophthalmologica* 1998, 212:73-76.

[68] Dreschfeld, J. Acute disseminated myelitis. *B.M.J.* 1894, 1:1174-1177.

[69] Lennon, V; Kryzer T; Pittock, S; Verkman, A; Hinson S. IgG marker of optic-spinal multiple sclerosis binds to the aquaporin-4 water channel. *J. Exp. Med.* 2005, 202:473-477.

[70] Agre, P. The aquaporin water channels. *Proc. Am. Thorac. Soc.* 2006, 3:5-13.

[71] Misu, T; Fujihara, K; Kakita, A; Konno, H; Nakamura, M; Watanabe, S; Takahashi, T; Nakashima, I; Takahashi, H; Itoyama, Y. Loss of aquaporin 4 in lesions of neuromyelitis optica: distinction from multiple sclerosis. *Brain* 2007, 130:1224-1234.

[72] Roemer, S; Parisi, J; Lennon, V; Benarroch, E; Lassmann, H; Bruck, W; Mandler, R; Weinshenker, B; Pittock, S; Wingerchuk, D; Lucchinetti, C. Pattern-specific loss of aquaporin-4 immunoreactivity distinguishes neuromyelitis optica from multiple sclerosis. *Brain* 2007, 130:1194-1205.

[73] Sabater, L; Giralt, A; Boronat, A; Hankiewicz, H; Blanco, Y; Llufriu, S; Alberch, J; Graus, F; Saiz, A. Cytotoxic effect of neuromyelitis optica antibody (NMO-IgG) to astrocytes: an in vitro study. *J. Neuroimmunol.* 2009, 215:31-35.

[74] Cosnett, J. Multiple sclerosis and neuromyelitis optica in tropical and subtropical countries. *Med. Hypotheses* 1981, 7:61-63.

[75] Sellner J; Hemmer, B; Mühlau, M. The clinical spectrum and immunobiology of parainfectious neuromyelitis optica (Devic) syndromes. *J. Autoimmun.* 2010, 34:371-379.

[76] van de Veerdonk, F; Gresnigt, M; Kullberg, B; van der Meer, J; Joosten, L; Netea, M. Th17 responses and host defense against microorganisms: an overview. *B.M.B. Rep.* 2009, 42:776-787.

[77] Li, Y; Wang, H; Long, Y; Lu, Z; Hu, X. Increased memory Th17 cells in patients with neuromyelitis optica and multiple sclerosis. *J. Neuroimmunol.* 2011, 34:155-160.

[78] Wei, L; Minohara, M; Piao, H; Matsushita, T; Masaki, K; Matsuoka, T; Isobe, N; Su, J; Ohyagi, Y; Kira, J. Association of anti-Helicobacter pylori neutrophil-activating protein antibody response with anti-aquaporin-4 autoimmunity in Japanese patients with multiple sclerosis and neuromyelitis optica. *Mult. Scler.* 2009, 15:1411-1421.

[79] Ren, Z; Wang, Y; Duan, T; Liggett, T; Loda, E; Brahma, S; Patel, J; Goswami, R; Grouse, C; Byrne, R; Stefoski, D; Javed, A; Miller, S; Balabanov, R. Cross-immunoreactivity between bacterial aquaporin-Z and human aquaporin-4: Relevance to neuromyelitis optica. *J. Immunol.* 2012 (in press).

[80] Haase, C. Devic's neuromyelitis optica. Disease or variants of multiple sclerosis? *Nervenarzt* 2001, 72:750-754.

[81] Kaman, B; Mandrel, R. Studies of mitochondrial DNA in Devic's disease revealed no pathogenic mutations, but polymorphism also found in association with multiple sclerosis. *Ann. Neurol.* 2001, 51:661-662.

[82] Mandler, R; Ahmed, W; Dencoff, J. Devic's neuromyelitis optica: a prospective study of seven patients treated with prednisone and azathioprine. *Neurology* 1998, 51:1219-1220.

[83] Jacob, A; Matiello, M; Weinshenker, B; Wingerchuk, D; Lucchinetti, C; Shuster, E; Carter, J; Keegan, B; Kantarci, O; Pittock, S. Treatment of neuromyelitis optica with mycophenolate mofetil: retrospective analysis of 24 patients. *Arch. Neurol.* 2009, 66:1128-1133.

[84] Cree, B; Lamb, S; Morgan, K; Chen, A; Waubant, E; Genain, C. An open label study of the effects of rituximab in neuromyelitis optica. *Neurology* 2005, 64:1270-1272.

[85] Weinstock-Guttman, B; Ramanathan, M; Lincoff, N; Napoli, S; Sharma, J; Feichter, J; Bakshi, R. Study of mitoxantrone for the treatment of recurrent neuromyelitis optica (Devic disease). *Arch. Neurol.* 2006, 63:957-963.

[86] Minagar, A; Sheramata, W. Treatment of Devic's with methotrexate and prednisone. *Int. J. MS Care* 2000, 2:39-43.

[87] Baker, J; Metz, L. Devic's neuromyelitis optica treated with intravenous gamma globulin (IVIG). *Can. J. Neurol. Sci.* 2004, 31:265-267.

[88] Palace, J; Leite, M; Nairne, A; Vincent, A. Interferon Beta treatment in neuromyelitis optica: increase in relapses and aquaporin 4 antibody titers. *Arch. Neurol.* 2010, 67:1016-1017.

[89] Min, J; Kim, B; Lee, K. Development of extensive brain lesions following fingolimod (FTY720) treatment in a patient with neuromyelitis optica spectrum disorder. *Mult. Scler.* 2012, 18:113-115.

In: Encephalitis, Encephalomyelitis and Encephalopathies   ISBN: 978-1-62257-766-8
Editors: Andrew Ruiz and Douglas Fleming   © 2013 Nova Science Publishers, Inc.

Chapter 7

VIRAL ENCEPHALOPATHY AND RETINOPATHY IN FARMED FISH

Cherif Nadia
Institut National des Sciences et Technologies de la Mer. Salammbô, Tunisia

ABSTRACT

Viral encephalopathy and retinopathy (VER) in fish is caused by *betanodaviruses* leading to high destructive mortality rates within hatchery-reared larvae and juveniles of a wide variety of marine fish. The disease was also designated viral nervous necrosis (VNN) when first described in 1990. Pathogenesis of VER, in general, is related to the neuro-invasive nature of the virus and subsequent effect on tissues in the brain and retina. The virus localizes in the brain, spinal cord, and retina of the affected fish which exhibit erratic swimming patterns and a range of neurological abnormalities, including vacuolization and cellular necrosis in the central nervous system and retina. Histologically, lesions are observed in the brain, spinal cord and in the eyes of all diseased fish.

Similar to the insect *nodaviruses*, the genome of *betanodaviruses* consists of two single-stranded, positive-sense RNA molecules (RNA1 and RNA2) of about 3.0 and 1.4 kb in length, respectively. RNA1 encodes a non-structural protein of approximately 100 kDa the RNA-dependent RNA polymerase (RdRP) also named protein A, that replicates the viral genome. Whereas RNA2 encodes the capsid protein precursor (CPp) which is about 42 kDa. Phylogenetically, viral isolates were examined into four clusters based on nucleotide sequences of the coat protein gene. The official virus species names are barfin flounder nervous necrosis virus (BFNNV), redspotted grouper nervous necrosis virus (RGNNV), striped jack nervous necrosis virus (SJNNV) and tiger puffer nervous necrosis virus (TPNNV). A novel subtype of *nodavirus* from turbot, *Psetta maxima* (L.), was recently described. Both vertical and horizontal transmissions of the disease have been suggested.

In recent years, great advances have been made in our understanding of teleost immunity, although it is still not as well understood as mammalian immunity. Innate or non-specific immunity is present as the first line of defence against pathogens, whereas the more specific active immunity takes a variable time to develop. At present, there are neither drugs nor vaccines available to prevent VNN in cultured fish. The control of the disease in based on the virus detection in infected animals.

Keywords: Betanodavirus, Encephalopathy, Retinopathy, Aquaculture, Diagnosis, Control

WHAT IS FISH VER?

Encephalopathy may be caused by infectious agents (bacteria, virus, or prion), metabolic or mitochondrial dysfunction, brain tumor or prolonged exposure to toxic elements (including solvents, drugs, radiation, paints, industrial chemicals, and certain metals). Viral encephalopathy and retinopathy (VER) in fish; also reffered to as viral nervous necrosis (VNN) is caused by the infection with a betanodavirus and occurs mainly in larval and juvenile marine finfish leading to devastating neuropathological conditions. It has been reported from all continents, but the majority of reports have come from those regions undertaking intensive culture of marine species. (Yoshikoshi and Inoue 1990, Bellance and Gallet de Saint-Aurin, 1988, Breuil et al., 1991)

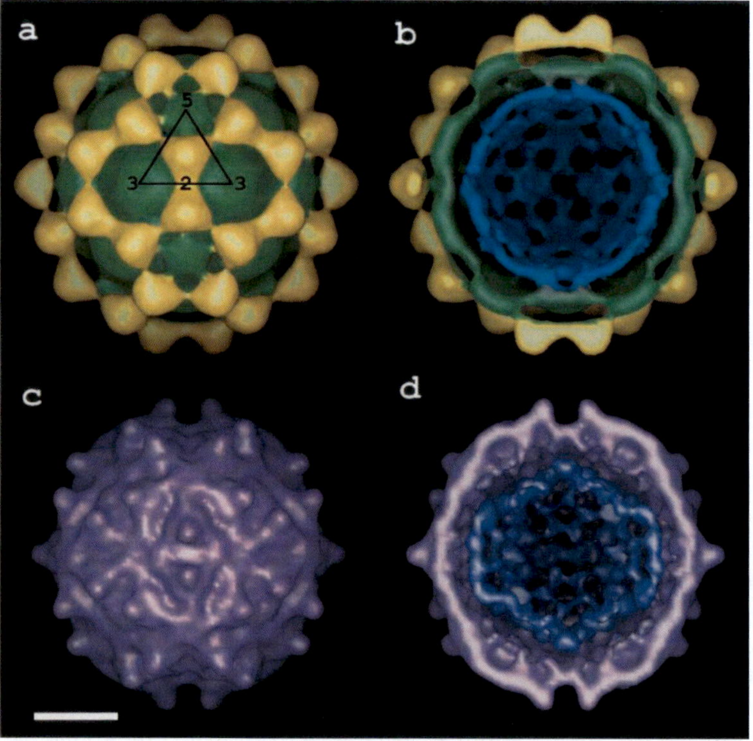

Tang et al. 2002.

Figure 1. CryoEM maps of MGNNV at 23-Å resolution (a) and PaV at 22 Å resolution (c). (b and d) Cutaway views of panels a and c, respectively. Panels a and b are colored radially. The densities for the protrusions (154 to 192 Å), the inner shell of the capsid (112 to 154 Å), and the RNA (112 Å) are gold, green, and blue, respectively. In panel d, the RNA density of PaV is dark purple. In panel a, an icosahedral asymmetric unit is outlined by a triangle, and the positions of the icosahedral five-, three-, and two-fold axes are indicated by numbers. The quasi-two-fold axes are centred between the five- and three-fold axes. Bar, 100 Å..

The Disease Causing Agent

The causative agent of this disease, the nervous necrosis virus, has been well characterized and classified in the Betanodavirus genus, within the family Nodaviridae (Mori et al., 1992; Comps et al., 1994; Nishizawa et al., 1994; Tan et al., 2001). Previously, the *Nodaviridae* family was thought to include only one single genus, which affects insect species (Peducasse, 2000, Thiéry et al., 2004), such as Nodamura virus, Black Beetle virus, Flock House virus and Boolarra virus (Johansen et al., 2002). Recently, based on the genomes organization, Piscine-*Nodavirus* or *Betanodavirus* (Mori et al., 2003, Sommerset and Nerland, 2004) genus has been introduced comprising fish *Nodaviruses*. Moreover, virion morphology, buoyant density, pH stability, capsid structure and bipartite genomic RNA of newly isolated viruses are perfect criteria to classify responsible agents of fish Viral Encephalopathy and Retinopathy within the *Betanodavirus* genus (Frerichs et al., 2000). Fish *Nodaviruses* exhibit close reladness among themselves but are clearly distinct from insect *Nodaviruses* (Munday et al., 2002).

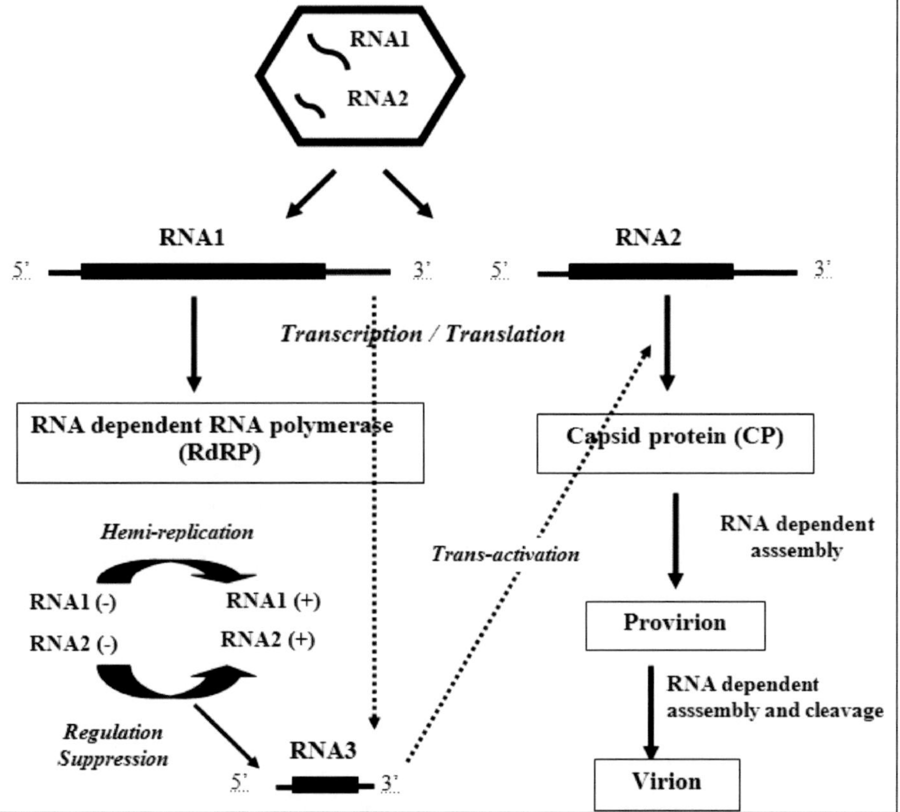

Figure 2. Schematic representation of nodavirus RNA segments. Segment RNA1 (3100 pb) encodes the RNA dependent RNA polymerase, segment RNA2 (1400 pb) encodes the coat or capsid protein and the sub genomic segment RNA3 (400 pb) is transcripted from RNA1 during the viral cycle and encodes protein B2.

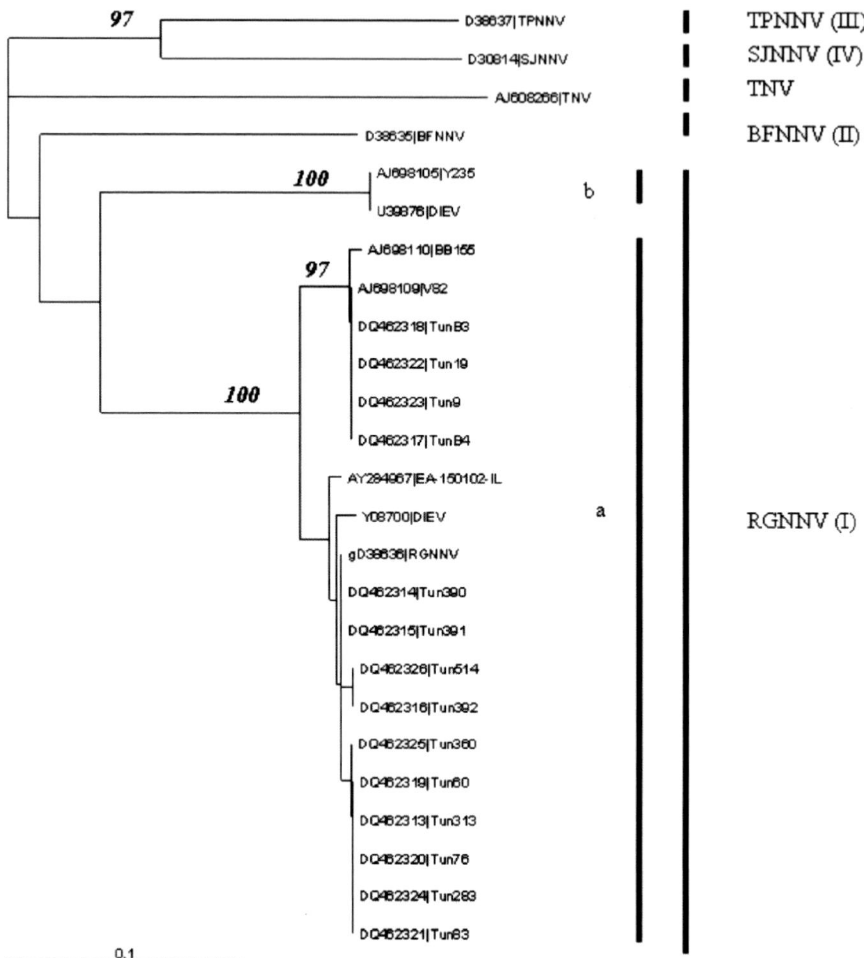

Chérif N. et al., 2009.

Figure 3. Unrooted phylogenetic tree deduced from analysis of the nucleotide sequence (375 nucleotides) of 14 fish betanodaviruses. Tunisian isolates (TunB3, Tun19, Tun9, TunB4, Tun390, Tun391, Tun514, Tun392, Tun360, Tun60, Tun313, Tun76, Tun283 and Tun83) were compared to four reference strains corresponding to the four genotypes (RGNNV-D38636, BFNV-D38635, TPNV-D38637 and SJNNV-D30814) in addition to seven other betanodavirus isolates retrieved from GenBank (AJ608266/TNV, AJ698105/Y23, U39876/DIEV, AJ698106/BB155, AJ698109/V82, AJ286947/EA-105 102 IL, Y08700/DIEV). The lengths of horizontal branches are proportional to the number of nucleotide substitutions and the numerals indicate bootstrap support. The genotypes were named after the definitions made by Nishizawa et al. 1997 (RGNNV, SJNNV, BFNNV, RGNNV) and Thiéry et al. 2004 (I, II, II, IV). The TNV betanodavirus was defined as a Vth genotype.

Fish nodaviruses are icosahedral, non-enveloped viruses with a commonly reported diameter of about 25 nm and a range of 20–34 nm. The virions may be membrane-bound by endoplasmic reticulum or be free in the cytoplasm, and may present as paracrystalline arrays (Glazebrook et al 1990, Breuil et al 1991, Bloch et al 1991, Boonyaratpalin et al 1996, Grotmol et al 1997, Castric et al., 2001, Dannevig et al., 2000)).

The genome consists of two single stranded, positive-sense molecules. The larger genomic segment, RNA1 (3.1 kb), encodes the RNA dependent RNA polymerase (RdRp) of approximately 100 kDa, also named protein A. The smaller segment, RNA2 (1.4 kb), encodes the capsid protein of about 42 kDa. In addition, a subgenomic RNA3 is synthesised during RNA replication from the 3' terminus of RNA1. (Eckerle and Ball, 2002, Chi et al. 2001, Iwamoto et al. 2001, Tan et al. 2001).

Nishizawa and co-workers (1997) have proposed a phyllogenetic analysis tested on a portion of the coat protein gene sequenced from many different fish *Nodavirus* isolates coming from Japanese, Thai, Australian and Italian fish farms. It has contributed to the classification of *Nodavirus* isolates into 4 distinct clusters (Nishizawa et al., 1997) designated SJNNV (striped jack nervous necrosis virus), TPNNV (tiger puffer nervous necrosis virus), RGNNV (red grouper nervous necrosis virus) and BFNNV (barfin flounder nervous necrosis virus), using a partial sequence of RNA2, the T4 region, which is a highly variable region of around 400 nt. Furthermore, Thiery, Cozien, Boisseson, Kerbart-Boscher & Nevarez (2004) detected new subtypes within the RGNNV type. These results demonstrate the high genetic variability of the betanodaviruses.

SYMPTOMS AND COMPLICATIONS

The disease caused by fish nodaviruses invariably involve abnormal swimming behaviour as well as vacuolation and cell necrosis in the central nervous system and the retina (Munday & Nakai 1997). As a result of the lesions, the affected larvae and juveniles exhibit a range of neurological disorders, which result in high mortality rates. Because the virus invades neural tissues that are proliferating, juvenile and larval fish are most severely affected, often suffering mortalities of 100% at about the 10-14 day post-hatching mark. Adult fish are also affected, as some neural cells of teleost fish species continue to proliferate throughout their lives. The disease in older fish is mostly subclinical, with poor weight gain being the only indicator of its presence. However, when these fish are placed into stressful environments, where their immune responses are impaired mortalities have been reported.

There is a great commonality of clinical signs with mass mortality and a variety of neurological abnormalities as follows: abnormalities in the fish's swimming patterns like looping or spiral swimming, reduced co-ordination and/or changes in pigmentation. Other signs include lack of appetite, lethargy and anemia. Affected fish show erratic swimming in circles, on their sides or belly up. Some maintain a vertical position with the head or caudal peduncle above the water surface. Neither external nor internal lesions have been associated to VER infection; nevertheless swim bladder hyperinflation has been often recorded. (Glazebrook et al., 1990, Yoshikoshi and Inoue, 1990; Breuil et al., 1991 Mori et al., 1991; Grotmol et al., 1997, Athanassopoulou et al., 2003).

Histologically, lesions are observed in the brain, spinal cord and in the eyes of all examined fish. Affected brains show pathological changes in the mescencephalon, medulla abolongata and cerebellum (Glazebrook and Campbell 1987; Bellance and Gallet de Saint-Aurin 1988; Glazebrook et al. 1990; Yoshikoshi and Inoue 1990; Munday et al. 1992; Fukuda et al. 1996; Chi et al. 1997; Le Breton et al. 1997; Bovo et al. 1999; Office International des Epizooties 2003).

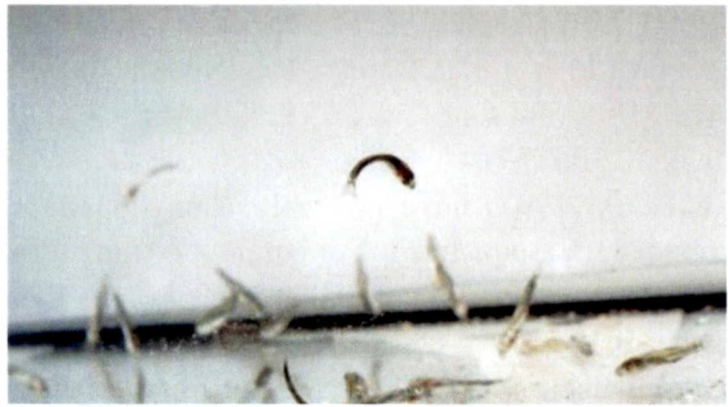

AFSSA Brest, France.

Figure 4. Photo of the appearance of VER clinical signs after 8 days post infection of sea bass fry (< 20g).

Examples of disease signs in an infected animal

Lates calcarifer, uncoordinated darting, corkscrew swimming, pale color, anorexia, wasting;
Dicentrarchus labrax, whirling swim pattern, swim bladder hypernation, anorexia;
Epinephelus akaara, whirling swim pattern;
Pseudocaranx dentex, abnormal swimming behaviour, swimbladder hyperination;
Oplegnathus fasciatus, spiral swimming, dark colour;
Hippoglossus hippoglossus, lethargy, belly-up at rest, abnormal swimming, pale color;
Scophthalmus maximus, spiral and/or looping swim pattern, belly-up at rest, dark color.

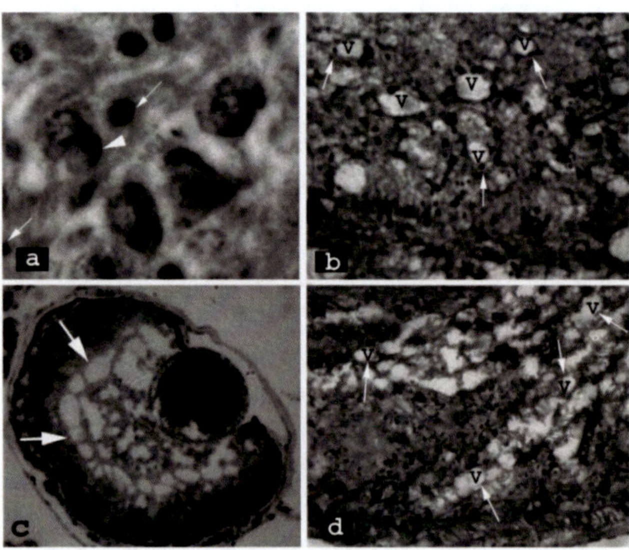

Azad et al., 2006.

Figure 5. Lates calcarifer. Histopathological manifestations (light microscopy, hematoxylin and eosin staining) in VNN affected larvae of Asian seabass at 0 to 40 days post-hatch (dph). (a) Nerve cells in the brain showing pyknotic (arrows) and emarginated nuclei (arrow head) in fish at 6 dph. (b) Highly vacuolated nerve cells (arrows) in the spinal cord in larvae at 6 dph. V = vacuole. (c) Vacuolated (arrows) retinal layers in moribund larvae at 20 dph. (d) Highly vacuolated hepatocytes (arrows) in moribund larvae at 20 dph. V = vacuole.

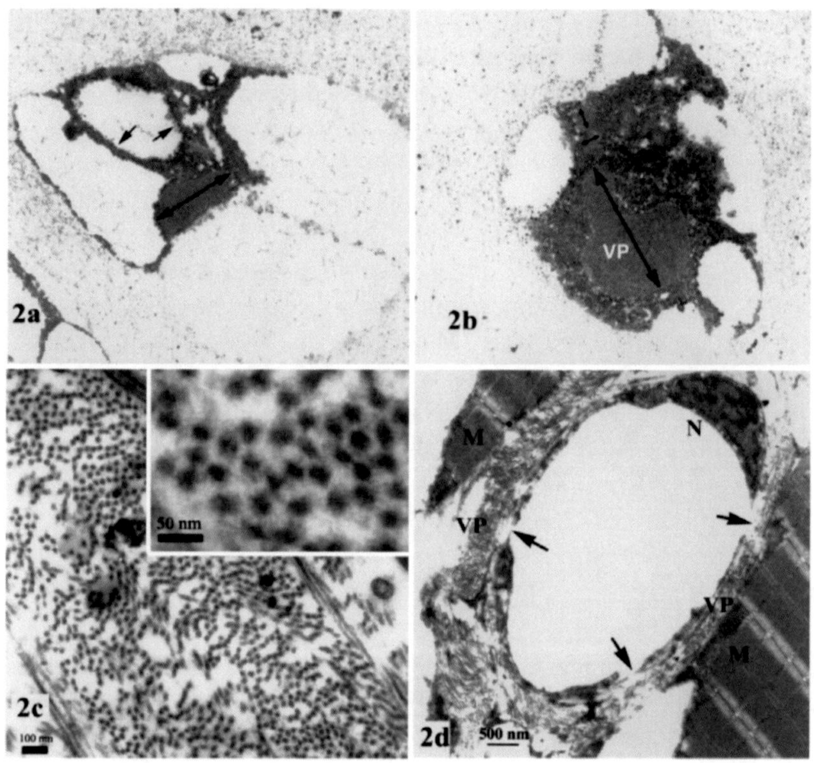

Azad et al., 2005.

Figure 6. Electron micrographs of the central nervous system. (a) Membrane bound viral particles in the cell organelle (arrows) and (b) viral inclusions (double-ended arrows) depicting intracytoplasmic localisation of the virus. (c) Viral particles measuring 28 to 30 nm in the intracellular spaces; (inset) very high magnification of the viral particles. (d) Nerve cell of the spinal cord with emptied cytoplasm and cornered nucleus. Arrows indicate probable exit points of viral particles. VP: viral particles, M: muscle, N: nucleus. Magnification: (a,b) 70 000×.

HOST RANGE OF THE ETHOLOGICAL AGENT

The successful replication of a viral agent in a host is a complex process which consists of a number of interactions, most of them related to the co-evolution of pathogen and host. This co-evolution often leads to a species specificity of the virus and can make interspecies transmission difficult. Therefore, natural host range switches by viruses are rare events. However, when they occur the results can become severe because the viruses may then spread widely through non previously adapted, and therefore immunologically naïve host populations (Bandín and Dopaso, 2011).

Viral nervous necrosis virus infects more than 40 marine fish species from all continents, but the majority of reports have come from those regions undertaking intensive culture of marine species (mazelet 2010). Since the first reported case of *Nodavirus* in the European sea bass, which is the most common affected marine species in the Mediterranean region (Athanassopoulou et al., 2003), a viral disease causing similar lesions of the central nervous system has been described in numerous fish species such as: barramundi (*Lates calcarifer*), turbot (*Scaphthalmus maximus*), grouper (*Epinephelus malabaricus*), and other several cultured species in Japan (Thiéry et al., 1999). In 2001, the virus has also been isolated from cultured asymptomatic sea bream (*Sparus aurata*) (Castric et al., 2001).

The host ranges of SJNNV and TPNNV are limited to striped jack *Pseudocaranx dentex* and tiger puffer *Takifugu rubripes*, respectively. However, recently, SJNNV was found in European sea bass *Dicentrarchus labrax*, sea bream *Sparus aurata* and Senegalese sole *Solea senegalensis* farmed in the Iberian Peninsula, though the samples used were not specified as diseased fish (Thiéry et al. 2004, Cutrín et al.2007). BFNNV has been isolated from some coldwater species, such as halibut *Hippoglossus hippoglossus* and turbot *Scophthalmus maximus*. RGNNV has a broad host range and causes disease among a variety of warm-water fish, particularly groupers and sea bass (Munday et al. 2002). Taken together, these data suggest that the variable region includes the host-specificity determinants of betanodaviruses. (Iwamoto et al. 2004). In addition to fish, NNV was detected by semi-nested PCR in the live food organisms including Artenia sp., Nauplii, the copepod *Tigriopus japonicus*, and the shrimp *Acetesinte medius* (Chi, 2003).

EPIDEMIOLOGY

The use of intensive farming techniques has precipitated numerous outbreaks of viral diseases with high mortalities (Chua et al., 1995; Munday and Nakai, 1997; Muroga, 1997). Relatively little is known about the epidemiology of viral infections in tropical fish. Many of these viruses may be capable of causing latent infections in wild and cultured fish with onset of disease triggered only under poor husbandry and management conditions. The increase in trade and movement of fish amplifies the potential for spread of these viruses through latently infected fish. Among viral infections in cultured marine species, a new disease inducing neurological disorders has appeared since 1985, in a wide variety of hatchery-reared fish (Frerichs et al., 2000, Thiéry et al., 1997). VNN is an acute infectious disease of primarily finfish larvae and fry cultured in seawater. The vertical transmission pattern of the VER from spawners to larvae has been demonstrated (Johnson et al., 2001) for *Pseudocarnax dentex* (Castric et al., 2001, Grotmol and Totland, 2000) and successful control of the disease has been accomplished by the elimination of the virus-carrying brood stock. Interregional trade in live fish and eggs provides a means for the parallel movement of the pathogens.

The virus introduction in the hatchery via gametes or by cohabitation « horizontal transmission » has been proved by Breton et al. in 1997, and by Thiérry et al. in 1999. This transmission pathway has also been suggested due to asymptomatic carriers such as in sea bass. The role of sea bream as a reservoir of *Nodavirus* to infect susceptible species has, in fact, been demonstrated (Castric et al., 2001). Persistent infected brood stock is thought to be a major source of nodavirus, transmitting it to their offspring through virus shed into their gonadal fluids (Grotmol and Totland, 2000).

Phylogenetic and antigenic characterization of new fish *Nodavirus* in Europe and Asia (Sklirits, 2001) displayed that the RGNNV lineage contained isolates from Spain, Portugal, Malta, Italy, France, Thailand, Singapore and Japan. Recently, all *Betanodaviruses* that were isolated from aquatic organisms in Taiwan have also been classified as RGNNV type (Thierry, 2004). This indicates that different lineages are inter-continentally distributed and that they co-circulate within geographic regions (Sklirits, 2001).

Development of the disease is related to the age of the fish, the water temperature, the route of infection and the stress placed on fish in hatchery facilities. Disease develops in young fish both because their immune system is immature and because they still have highly prolific neural cells, which the virus attacks.

A study performed by Skliris et al, 2004 showed a direct correlation between high water temperatures and the development of disease. Clinical signs appeared more rapidly and there was a greater overall mortality rate among fish that had been kept in water temperatures above 25°C. It has also been shown that the genotypic variants have different optimal growth temperatures: 15 to 20°C for BFNNV, 20°C for TPNNV, 20 to 25°C for SJNNV and 25 to 30°C for RGNNV (Mori et al, 2003).

The occurrence of the infection appears to be function of the number of cultured fish in the pond (Munday et al., 2002). High stress in the intensive re-circulating conditions induced by high CO2 and PO4 levels during the summer may have an effect on outbreaks occurrences as well as on the variation of the clinical signs (Athanassopoulouet al., 2003). Natural outbreaks of *Nodavirus* occur in wide range of temperature.

DIAGNOSIS

Rapid and sensitive diagnostic assays for nodavirus are required to identify outbreaks of infection and to screen broodfish that may be carriers (Starkey et al., 2004). The tests that can be used to analyze the presence of nodavirus in a population has been well set out by Munday et al 2002. Available diagnostic tests can be categorized as follows:

1) Demonstration of characteristic lesions in the brain and retina by light microscopy.
2) Demonstration of virions, viral antigens or viral nucleotides.
3) Detection of specific antibodies.
4) Tissue culture of the virus.

Although the virus is neurotrophic, the virus may replicate in other tissues (such as the liver and spleen). Typical histopathological lesions include severe widespread vacuolation throughout the CNS and all retinal layers. These characteristic lesions provide a presumptive diagnosis, but immunofluorescent antibody testing or immunoperoxidase staining is required for confirmation. The location of immunopositive cells detected by immunohistochemistry confirms that the virus favours neural cells which are in the early stages of proliferation and indicates that it enters the CNS along nerves and blood vessels during the viraemic stage of the disease (Johansen et al, 2004 and Tanaka et al, 2004).

Virions of the appropriate size and shape can be rapidly demonstrated using electron microscopy, provided that the concentration of nodavirus in tissues is high enough. This method however, is not confirmatory, even with the use of positive staining, which is able to show more detail than negative staining techniques.

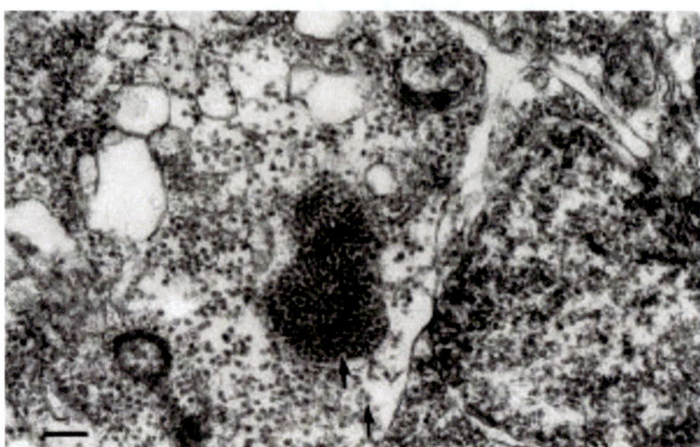

Munday et al, 2002.

Figure 7. Transmission electronmicrograph of betanodavirus particles found in barramundi larvae brain tissue, bar=250nm.

In 1994 PCR amplification of nodavirus RNA was developed (Nishizawa et al, 1994). PCR is the main diagnostic test that is being used by laboratories currently. The sensitivity of this test depends on the nodavirus strain which is being tested, so more specific primers are continuing to be developed (Gagne et al, 2004). Nested RT-PCR is now used as it is 10-100 times more sensitive than the previous RT-PCR methods (Thiery et al, 1999). This test can detect tiny quantities of viral RNA in any tissue and only a minimal amount of tissue is required for testing. Nested RT-PCR is able to diagnose the virus using blood or sperm as well as ovarian and neural tissues. This means is able to pick up latent infection or persistently infected carriers. To expediate the diagnosis in an outbreak situation, cell-culture can be combined with this PCR method (Iwamoto 2001).

The ability to use tissue culture methods was established when it was found that the snakehead cell line (SSN-1) was permissive for isolates of fish nodaviruses (Frerichs et al., 1996). The virus does not lose or change virulence after repeated cell culture (Dannevig et al, 2000) however permissiveness is temperature dependent. The E-11 cell line which has been cloned from the SSN-1 line, is a good alternative line as it exhibits a clear, stable cytopathic effect (CPE) expression and produces high levels of the virus and so can be used for both qualitative and quantitative analyses (Iwamoto et al, 2001).

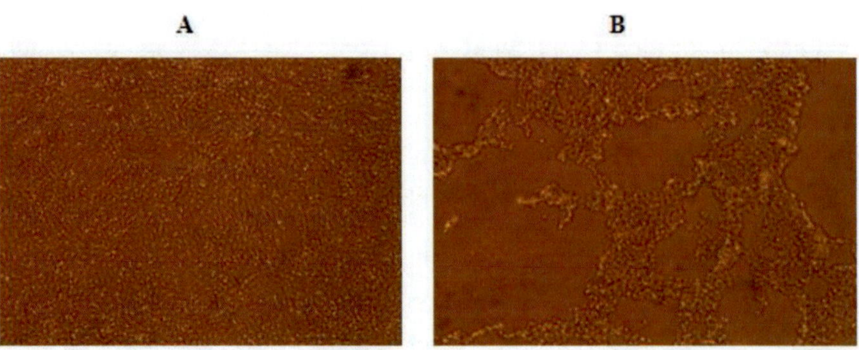

Figure 8. Permissive cell: snakehead cell line (SSN-1). A) normal non-infected cells. B) cells showing CPE caused by RGNNV. (bar=100um) (Cherif N. et al., unpublished data).

Enzyme-linked immunosorbent assays and immunofluorescent antibody tests are the tests involved in the detection of specific nodavirus antibodies. ELISA's can detect specific antibodies in blood and other body fluids. In this way it is able to identify sero-positive broodstock for culling. Rapid testing of multiple samples is another advantage of this test.

Unfortunately this test currently has a variable sensitivity and so it is generally used for epidemiological studies rather than for diagnostic purposes.

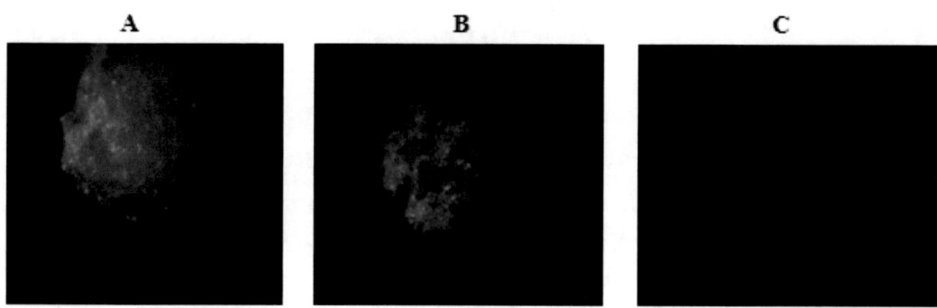

Figure 9. Typical results of IFAT Nodavirus infection after four days post inoculation of fish sample homogenates on a 24-hour SNN-1cells. A: Positive control test. B: Fluorescence observed with tested sea bass sample. C: Negative control.

Immunofluorescent antibody testing is a convenient way to confirm the presence of a nodavirus infection. It is both rapid and economical and the polyclonal anti-VNN serum will detect the full range of nodavirus strains known. However, greater tissue quantities are required than the ELISA test.

CONCLUSION AND CONTROL STRATEGIES

Despite the limited epidemiological knowledge concerning this disease, enough is known for fisheries to be able to implement measures that will reduce the risk to their enterprise. A combination of measures should be used to lessen the risks related to the different forms of transmission.

Studies on vaccination against betanodaviruses have only recently commenced and have focused on using recombinant coat proteins (Tanaka et al 2001, Yuasa et al 2002). These have provided encouraging results and may be suitable for those species in which the disease sometimes expresses itself relatively late (eg some groupers, European sea bass). However, vaccines may need to be tailored for specific situations because not only may one genotype of betanodavirus not protect against another, but one strain of a particular genotype may not protect against another strain (Tanaka et al 2001, Yuasa et al 2002).

Meanwhile, an outbreak of viral encephalopathy and retinopathy (VER) would be a serious threat to the fish farming industry. A number of different control measures could be used to minimize its impact, depending on the circumstances of the outbreak.

The following practices must be considered when implementing any control strategies:

- transportation of live fish between and within freshwater and marine
- operations;

- movement of equipment between farms, river systems and marine sites;
- fish harvesting and transportation to processing plants;
- discharge of processing plant effluent;
- transportation of consumer-ready products; and
- disposal of dead fish.

REFERENCES

Athanassopoulou F, C. Billinis, V. Psychas, and K. Karipoglou. (2003) Viral Encephalopathy and Retinopathy of Dicentrarchus labrax L. farmed in fresh water in Greece. *Journal of fish disease* 26:361-365.

Azad I.S., Shekhar M.S., Thirunavukkarasu A.R. and Jitendran K.P. (2006). Viral Nerve Necrosis (VNN) in the hatchery produced fry of Asian seabass Lates calcarifer: sequential microscopic analysis of histopathology. *Disease of Aquatic Organisms* 73: 123-130.

Azad, I.S., Shekhar, M.S., Thirunavukkarasu, A.R., Poornima, M., Kailasam, M., Rajan, J.J.S., Ali, S.A., Mathew Abraham and Ravichandran, P. (2005). Nodavirus infection causes mass mortalities in hatchery produced larvae of Asian seabass, *Lates calcarifer*, Bloch: first report from India. *Dis. Aquat. Org.*, 63: 113-118.

Bandín I. and Dopazo C. P. (2011). Host range, host specificity and hypothesized host shift events among viruses of lower vertebrates. *Veterinary Research*, 42:67.

Bellance R. and Gallet de Saint-Aurin D (Avril, Mai, Juin, 1988). - L'encéphalite virale du loup de mer. *Caraïbes Médical*, 105-114.

Bloch B, Gravningen K, Larsen JL. (1991) Encephalomyelitis among Turbot Associated with a Picornavirus-Like Agent. *Diseases of Aquatic Organisms*. 10:65-70.

Boonyaratpalin S, Supamattaya K, Kasornchandra J and Hoffman RW (1996). Picorna-like virus associated with mortality and a spongiosus encephalopathy in grouper *Epinephelus malabaricus*. *Diseases of Aquatic Organisms* 26:75–80.

Bovo G, Nishizawa T, Maltese C, Borghesan F, Mulinelli F, Montesi F, De Mas S. (1999) Viral encephalopathy and retinopathy of farmed marine fish species in Italy. *Virus Research*. 63: 143-6.

Breuil, G., Bonami, J. R., Pepin, J. F. & Pichot, Y. (1991). Viral infection (picorna-like virus) associated with mass mortalities in hatchery-reared sea bass (Dicentrarchus labrax) larvae and juveniles. *Aquaculture* 97, 109±116.

Castric J., Thiéry R., Jeffroy J., de Kinkelin P. and Raymond J.C (2001). - Sea bream *Sparus aurata*, an asymptomatic contagious fish host for nodavirus. *Dis. Aqua. Org.*, 47, 33-38.

Chérif N, Thiéry R., Castric J, Biacchesi S, Brémont M,Thabti F, Limem L, Hammami S. (2009). Viral encephalopathy and retinopathy of Dicentrarchus labrax and Sparus aurata farmed in Tunisia. *Vet Res Commun*. Volume 33(4):345-53.

Chi SC, Lo CF, Kou GH, Chang PS, Peng SE, Chen SN. (1997). Mass Mortalities associated with viral nervous necrosis (VNN) disease in two species of hatchery-reared grouper, *Epinephelus fuscogutatus* and *E. akaara* (Temminck and Schlegel). *J Fish Dis* 20: 185-193.

Chi SC, Shieh JR, Lin SJ. (2003). Genetic and antigenic analysis of betanodaviruses isolated from aquatic organisms in Taiwan. *Dis Aquat Organ;* 55: 221-8.

Chua FHC, Loo JJ, Wee JK (1995): Mass mortality in juvenile greasy grouper, Epinephelus tauvina, associated with vacuolating encephalopathy and retinopathy.Edited by: Shariff M, Arthur JR, Subhasinghe P. Diseases in Asian Aquaculture II, Fish Health Section. *Asian Fisheries Society*, Manila; 235-241.

Comps M, Pépin JF, Bonami JR (1994). Purification and characterization of two fish encephalitis viruses (FEV) infecting *Lates calcarifier* and *Dicentrarchus labrax.* *Aquaculture* 123:1-10.

Cutrín JM, Dopazo CP, Thiéry R, Leao P, Olveira JG, Barja JL, Bandín I (2007) Emergence of pathogenic betanodaviruses belonging to the SJNNV genogroup in farmed fish species from the Iberian Peninsula. *J Fish Dis* 30:225–232.

Dannevig, B.H., Nilsen, R. Modahl, I. Jankowska, M. Taksdal, T. Press, C.M. 2000. Isolation in cell culture of nodavirus from farmed Atlantic halibut Hippoglossus hippoglossus in Norway. 43(3): 183-9.

Frerichs G.N., Rodger H.D. and Peric Z., (1996). Cell culture isolation of piscine neuropathy nodavirus from juvenile sea bass, *Dicentrarchus labrax. J. Gen. Virol.* 77, 2067–2071.

Frerichs G. N., Tweedy A., W. G. Starkey, and R. H Richards (2000). Temperature, pH and electrolyte sensivity, and heat, UV disinfectant inactivation of sea bass (Dicentrarchus labrax) neuropathy nodavirus. *Aquaculture* 185:13-24.

Fukuda Y, Nguyen HD, Furuhashi M and Nakai T. (1996). Mass mortality of cultured sevenband grouper, Epinephelus septemfasciatus, associated with viral nervous necrosis. *Fish Pathol* 31: 165-170.

Gagné N, Johnson SC, Cook-Versloot M, MacKinnon AM, Olivier G. (2004). Molecular detection and characterization of nodavirus in several marine fish species from the northeastern Atlantic. *Dis Aquat Org* 62(3):181-189.

Glazebrook JS, Campbell RSF. (1987). Diseases of barramundi (*Lates calcarifer*) in Australia: a review. In: *Management of Wild and Cultured Sea Bass/Barramundi Lates calcarifer*, J.W. Copland and D.I. Grey (ed), ACIAR Press, Canberra, pp. 204-206.

Glazebrook, J.S., Heasman, M.P. and der Beer, S.W. (1990). Picorna-like viral particles associated with mass mortalities in larval barramundi, *Lates calcarifier* (Bloch). *Journal of Fish Diseases.* 13, 245-249.

Grotmol S, Totland GK (2000). Surface disinfection of Atlantic halibut *Hippoglossus hippoglossus* eggs with ozonated sea-water inactivates nodavirus and increases survival of the larvae. *Dis Aquat Org* 39:89–96

Grotmol S, Totland GK, Torud K and Hjeltnes BK (1997). Vacuolating encephalopathy and retinopathy associated with a nodavirus-like agent: a probable cause of mass mortality of cultured larval and juvenile Atlantic halibut *Hippoglossus hippoglossus. Diseases of Aquatic Organisms* 29:85–97.

Iwamoto, T., Y. Okinaka, K. Mise, K. I. Mori, M. Arimoto, T. Okuno, and T. Nakai. 2004. Identification of host-specificity determinants in betanodaviruses by using reassortants between striped jack nervous necrosis virus and sevenband grouper nervous necrosis virus. *Journal of Virology* 78:1256-1262.

Iwamoto, T., Mise, K., Mori, K., Arimoto, M., Nakai, T. & Okuno, T. (2001). Establishment of an infectious RNA transcription system for *Striped jack nervous necrosis virus*, the type species of the betanodaviruses. *J Gen Virol* 82, 2653–2662.

Johnson KN, KL Johnson, R Dasgupta, and T Gratsch (2001). Comparisons among the larger genome segments of six nodaviruses and their encoded RNA replicases. *J.Gen.Virol.* 82:1855-1866.

Johansen R.; Ranheim T.; Hansan M. K.; Taksdal T.; Totland G. K. (2002). Pathological changes in juvenile Atlantic halibut Hippoglossus hippoglossus persistently infected with nodavirus. *Diseases of aquatic organisms,* vol. 50 (3), 161-169.

Le Breton, A., Grisez, L., Sweetman, J., Ollivier, F. (1997). Viral nervous necrosis (VNN) associated with mass mortalities in cage-reared sea bass, Dicentrarcus labrax (L.) *J. Fish Dis.* 20, 145-151.

Mazelet L., Dietrich J., Rolland JL. (2010). New RT-qPCR assay for viral nervous necrosis virus detection in sea bass *Dicentrarchus labrax. Fish and shell fish Immunology.* Volume: 30, Issue: 1, Pages: 27-32.

Mori K, Nakai T, Muroga K, Arimoto M, Mushiake K, Furusawa I (1992). Properties of a new virus belonging to nodaviridae found in larval striped jack(*Pseudocaranx dentex*) with nervous necrosis. *Virology* 187:368-371.

Mori, K., Mangyoku, T. Iwamoto, T. Arimoto, M. Tanaka, S. Nakai, T. 2003. Serological relationships among genotypic variants of betanovirus. *Diseases of Aquatic Organisms* 57: 19-26.

Munday B., Kwang J. and Moody N. (2002). Betanodavirus infection of teleost fish: a review. *J. Fish Dis.,* 25, 127-142.

Munday, B. L., Langdon, J. S., Hyatt, A. & Humphrey, J. D. (1992). Mass mortality associated with a viral-induced vacuolating encephalopathy and retinopathy of larval and juvenile barramundi, *Lates calcarifer* Bloch. *Aquaculture* 103, 197-211.

Munday, B. L. & Nakai, T.(1997). Special topic review: nodaviruses as pathogens in larval and juvenile marine finfish. *World Journal of Microbiology & Biotechnology* 13, 375-381.

Muroga, K., 1997. Viral diseases of cultured marine fish in Japan. *Proceedings of NRIA International Workshop on New Approaches to Viral Aquatic Animal Diseases,* Kyoto, Japan.

Nishizawa, T., Furuhashi, M., Nagai, T. & Muroga, K.(1997). Genomic classification of fish nodaviruses by molecular phylogenetic analysis of the coat protein gene. *Applied and Environmental Microbiology* 63, 1633-1636.

Nishizawa, T., Mori, K., Nakai, T., Furusawa, I. & Muroga, K. (1994). Polymerase chain reaction (PCR) amplification of RNA of striped jack nervous necrosis virus (SJNNV). *Dis Aquat Org* 18, 103–107.

Office International des Epizooties, Viral Encephalopathy and retinopathy. (2003) In: *Manual of Diagnostic Tests for Aquatic Animals, OIE* (ed.) Paris, France. Fourth Edition; 35-41.

Peducasse S. 2000. *Caractérisation du nodavirus, pathogénie et épidémiologie expérimentale de la nodavirose ou de l'encéphalopathie et rétinopathie virales chez le bar juvénile Dicentrarchus labrax* (L.).Th. : Parasitologie : Montpellier, Université Montpellier II : 2000. 181 p.

Sommerset, I. & Nerland, A. H. (2004). Complete sequence of RNA1 and subgenomic RNA3 of Atlantic halibut nodavirus (AHNV). *Dis Aquat Organ* 58, 117–125.

Skliris G. P, J. V Krondiris, D. C Sideris, A. P Shinn, W. G. Starkey, and R. H Richards. (2001) Phylogenetic and antigenic characterization of new fish nodavirus isolates from Europe and Asia. *Virus Research* 75:59-67.

Starkey W. G., R. M. Millar, M. E. Jenkins, J. H. Ireland, K. F. Muir, and R.H Richards (2004). Detection of piscine nodavirus real-time nucleic acid sequence based amplification (NASBA). *Dis.Aquat.Organ* 59:93-100.

Tan, C., Huang, B., Chang, S. F., Ngoh, G. H., Mundy, B., Chen, S. C. & Kwang, J. (2001). Determination of the complete nucleotide sequences of RNA1 and RNA2 from greasy grouper (*Epinephelus tauvina*) nervous necrosis virus, Singapore strain. *J Gen Virol* 82, 647–653.

Tanaka, S., M. Takagi, and T. Miyazaki. 2004. Histopathological studies on viral nervous necrosis of sevenband grouper, Epinephelus septemfasciatus Thunberg, at the grow-out stage. *Journal of Fish Diseases* 27:385-399.

Thiéry R., C Arnauld, and C. Delsert. (1999) Two isolates of sea bass, Dicentrarchus labrax L., nervous necrosis virus with distinct genomes. *Journal of fish disease* 22:201-207.

Thiéry R., J. Cozien, C. Boisséson, S. Kerbart-Boscher, and L. Névarez (2004). Genomic classification of new betanodavirus isolates by phylogenetic analysis of the coat protein gene suggests low host-fish species specificity. *J.Gen.Virol.* 85:3079-3087.

Tanaka S, Mori K, Arimoto M, Iwamoto T, Nakai T. (2001). Protective immunity of sevenband grouper, Epinephelus septemfasciatus (Thunberg), against experimental viral nervous necrosis. *J Fish Dis*;24:15-22.

Yuasa K, Koesharyani I, Roza D, Mori K, Katata M and Nakai T (2002). Immune response of humpback grouper, *Cromileptes altivelis* (Valenciennes) injected with the recombinant coat protein of betanodavirus. *Journal of Fish Diseases* 25:53–56.

Yoshikoshi, K. & Inoue, K.(1990). Viral nervous necrosis in hatchery-reared larvae and juveniles of Japanese parrotfish, *Oplegnathus fasciatus* (Temminck & Schlegel). *Journal of Fish Diseases* 13, 69-77.

In: Encephalitis, Encephalomyelitis and Encephalopathies   ISBN: 978-1-62257-766-8
Editors: Andrew Ruiz and Douglas Fleming   © 2013 Nova Science Publishers, Inc.

Chapter 8

SEPTIC ENCEPHALOPATHY

Yukio Imamura[1]*, *Shota Hori*[2], *Naoya Matsumoto*[3],
Kazuma Yamakawa[3], *Junichiro Nakagawa*[3], *Junya Shimazaki*[3],
Huan Wang[4], *Junji Itou*[5], *Yuki Murakami*[1], *Satoko Mitani*[1],
Hiroshi Ogura[3], *Takeshi Shimazu*[3] and *Akitoshi Seiyama*[2]

[1]Unit for Liveable Cities,
Kyoto University Graduate School of Engineering and Medicine, Kyoto, Japan
[2]Human Health Science, Kyoto University Graduate School of Medicine, Kyoto, Japan
[3]Department of Trauma and Acute Critical Care Center,
Osaka University Hospital, Osaka ,Japan
[4]Institute of Pharmacology, Toxicology and Biochemical Pharmaceutics,
Zhejiang University, Hangzhou, China
[5]Department of Genetics, Cell Biology and Development, University of Minnesota,
MN, US

ABSTRACT

Encephalopathy refers to a syndrome of global brain dysfunction. Septic
encephalopathy shows a devastating neurological symptom. Here we introduce the *septic
encephalopathy*, encephalopathy associated with sepsis. The pathogenesis of septic
encephalopathy originates from the following order: (1) infection, (2) systemic
inflammatory response syndrome (a whole-body inflammatory state), (3) multiple-organ
dysfunction. These processes finally lead to be the symptoms of septic encephalopathy
including mental confusion and delirium. The sequelas provoke the social issue.
Accumulating body of studies suggest the hypothetical molecular mechanisms for patho-
physiology of septic encephalopathy. The sensing of pathogen-associated molecular
patterns such as lipopolysaccharides and peptidoglycans, and damage-associated
molecular patterns such as endogenous DNAs and high mobility group box (HMGB) -1

---

* Correspondence to Yukio Imamura, Unit for Liveable Cities, Kyoto University Graduate School of Engineering
and Medicine, Address: 53 Kawahara-cho, Shogoin, Sakyo-Ku, Kyoto, Japan. Phone: +81-75-751-3970, E-
mail: yimamura-ns@umin.net.

by pattern recognition receptors drives a coordinated immune response. Sepsis is accompanied by a remarkable altered and imbalanced cytokine response (known as a cytokine storm), which burdens onto organs and results in multiple-organ dysfunctions. These processes finally result in septic encephalopathy. On the other hand, brain hemorrhage, edema, and ischemia were also found as complicated symptoms associated with sepsis. Hence, septic encephalopathy includes not only inflammatory symptoms but also neurovascular diseases. These neurovascular involvements may render the septic encephalopathy to be complicated diseases. Conversely, several kinds of trials have been tackled to control the immunological response in sepsis without successful. Recently, however, several lines of evidence suggest the validity that electrical stimulation of vagus nerve on the cervix after onset of sepsis may regulate the over-expressing cytokines and result in better prognosis. Hence, in this chapter, septic encephalopathy is discussed from molecular mechanisms to future therapeutic potential for the patho-physiology, respectively, in the following section: (1) causes, (2) symptoms, (3) potential complications in the future studies.

1. CAUSES

Encephalopathy refers to brain disorders or diseases. The symptoms of encephalopathy can be caused by many different illnesses. For example, dysfunction of mitochondrial DNA (e.g. mitochondrial encephalopathy), excess amount of glycine (e.g. glycine encephalopathy), advance cirrhosis of liver (e.g. hepatic encephalopathy) etc can induce encephalopathy. When it is successful for treating the underlying cause of illnesses with medical intervention, the symptoms of encephalopathy may improve the outcome. Otherwise, encephalopathy will be fatal due to the possible permanent structural changes or irreversible damages to the brain.

In addition, systemic infection (e.g. blood poisoning with bacteria infection) results in encephalopathy. This is called 'septic encephalopathy'. In the worst case senario, 70% of septic patients will be under severe sepsis and the patients with septic encephalopathy (e.g., severe sepsis survivors) are suffering from long-term cognitive impairment[1]. The brain dysfunctions include alterations in memory, attention, concentration and/ or global loss of cognitive function[2]. The pathogenesis of septic encephalopathy is described from sepsis to septic encephalopathy in the following section.

1.1. Sepsis

Our bodies can develop the inflammatory response by the immune system against microbes in the organs including in the blood, urine, lungs and skin and immune responses will often be uncontrollable. This is called **sepsis**. In such a circumstance, lipopolysaccharides (cell wall of Gram-negative bacteria) from bacteria are released as immunological pathogens called pathogen-activated molecular patterns (PAMPs). When the PAMPs binds to pattern recognition receptor (PRR) such as Toll-like receptors (e.g. membrane-bound PRR) and nucleotide oligomerization domain (Nod) -like receptors, anti-bacterial immunological response will be activated in the inflammatory cells. The hypothetical model for various molecular dynamics in the pathogenesis of sepsis is summarized in Figure 1.

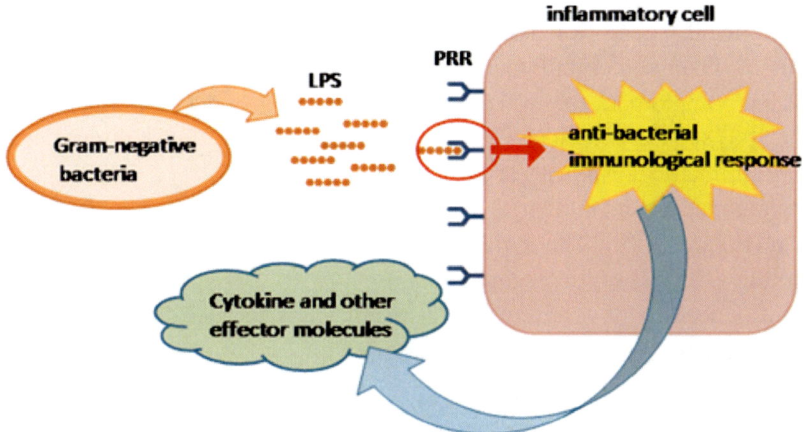

Citation modified from Cohen J, *Nature* 420 (2002) pp 885-891.

Figure 1. Over view of anti-bacterial immunological responses. Lipopolyaccarides from gram-negative bacteria trigger the activation of pattern-recognition receptors on cell surface, which leads to be the production of various cytokines and effecter molecules.

1.2. Systemic Inflammatory Response Syndrome

After cellular injury with PAMPs, damage-associated molecular patterns (DAMPs) are activated. One of an intriguing model for DAMPs suggests that the endogenous DAMPs are released from mitochondria on damaged cells [3]. Both of PAMPs and DAMPs contribute to cause systemic inflammatory response syndromes (e.g. SIRS, a whole body inflammatory state).

High mobility group box (HMGB)-1 protein, a key molecule of DAMPs, is secreted from activated macrophage stimulated with endotoxin[4]. HMGB-1 can interact with toll-like receptor (TLR) and receptor for advanced glycan endproducts (RAGE) receptor (e.g. inflammatory ligand receptors) [5]. HMGB-1 release from cells seems to involve two distinct processes: 1) necrosis, in which case cell membranes are permeabilized and intracellular constitutents may diffuse out of the cell, 2) some form of active or facilitated secretion induced by signaling through the NF-κB (e.g. nuclear factor kappa-light-chain-enhancer of activated B cells), which induces septic shock [6]. Recently, our group found that neutralization of HMGB-1 effectively suppressed the damage in systemic inflammation (e.g. a whole body inflammation) in rat model [7]. Thus, HMGB-1 may be a major target of a therapy for sepsis-induced SIRS.

1.3. Cytokine Storm

The SIRS is a subset of cytokine storm in which is abnormal regulation of various cytokines. Cytokine storms are fatal immune reactions, which are triggered by positive feedback loops between cytokines and immune cells. Recently, it was suggested that complement, a key molecule in host defense against invading microbes, was involved in the process. The complement proteins consist of a number of small proteins generally synthesized in the liver. In a healthy condition, the complements are circulating in the blood stream as an inactive precursor. Once the complement precursors are triggered by the pathological stimuli, the first activated complement (e.g. C1) induces the downstream complement pathways (C1 ->C2 -> ......C5b6789: C1 activates C2, then C2 activates C3..... finally reach to C5b6789) and serve as inflammatory responses [8].

The complement C5a, its receptors and downstream modulator (e.g., HMGB1) enroll the cytokine storm (Figure 2) [9]. The cytokine storm finally leads to be severe sepsis, multiple-organ dysfunction [10] and septic encephalopathy [11]. In these phenomena, the brain will be concurrently influenced by devastating effects of inflammatory mediators such as interleukin-1β, -6, -10, tumor necrosis factor-α, etc with severe septic conditions.

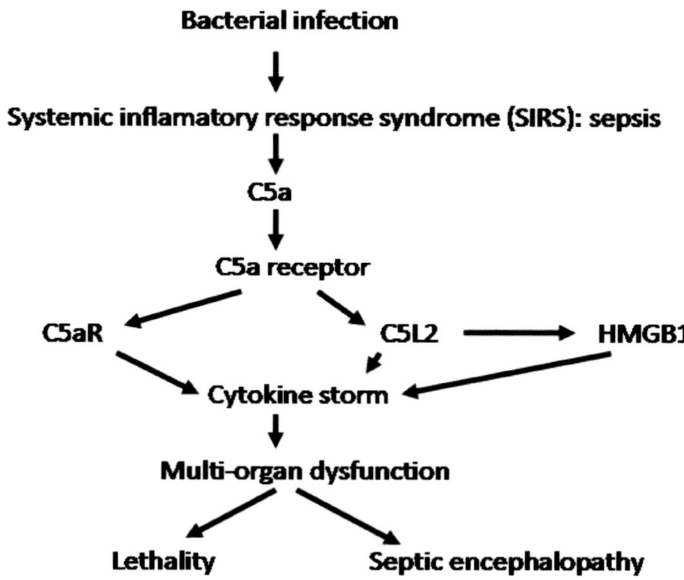

Citation from Ward PA, *The Scientific World JOURNAL* 10 (2010) pp2395–2402.

Figure 2 Sequence of sepsis, complement activation, and lethality. Roles of C5a interacting with its receptors after onset of sepsis induced by CLP in rodents. The downstream effects are the "cytokine storm", together with production of HMGB1 from macrophages, which accentuates the cytokine storm. Ultimately, these events lead to multi-organ dysfunction and lethality.

1.4. Septic Encephalopathy

Severe sepsis survivors are often suffering from septic encephalopathy. Since the symptoms are devastating (e.g. conscious disturbance, derilium etc.), the patho-physiological model of septic encephalopathy has been required to tackle the issue. For a few decades, molecular patho-physiological model of septic encephalopathy has been demonstrated [12]. At first, the molecular components consisting of blood brain barrier, a guardian of brain, are destroyed. The blood brain barrier usually maintains homeostasis in the brain circumstances with a separation of blood from the brain extracellular fluid (CSF) in the central nervous system. It was suggested that the proteases such as matrix metalloproteinases (MMPs), for example MMP-9, with tumor necrosis factor-α during encephalopathy may enroll the dysfunction of the molecules associated with the blood brain barrier [13,14] and thereby increase the permeability of various inflammatory mediators into the brain.

Hence, the molecular mechanisms accounting for the septic encephalopathy pathogenesis have been considered to be originated from 1) dysfunction of blood brain barrier (i.e., increased permeability through the barrier) [15], 2) increased brain inflammatory cytokines through disrupted blood brain barrier[16], 3) enhanced expression of pro-inflammatory cytokines such as tumor necrosis factor-α and interleukins etc trigger neuronal cell death. The neuronal cell death during sepsis may trigger the symptom of septic encephalopathy.

In contrast to the neuronal loss in septic encephalopathy, glial cells seem to show different and unique properties. At first, astrocytes, in their endfeet, were destroyed and swollen, which results in the impairment of function for the blood brain barrier in an animal model of septic encephalopathy. The insults of endothelial cells and pericytes induced by sepsis also participate in this process [16,17]. Second, microglial cells and macrophage, which were induced with the stimulation of inflammatory responses, are increased after an administration of LPS and lasted for more than one month [18]. These phenomena may reveal a long-lasting inflammatory response after septic encephalopathy. These findings also suggest that the immunological reaction affects the expression level of glial cells, which may result in an aberrant brain dysfunction in septic encephalopathy.

In addition, recently, another mechanism for brain dysfunction is suggested. When an increased interleukin-1β binds to interleukin-1 receptor, the receptor activation may induce synaptic plasticity deficiency in septic encephalopathy[19]. Thus, the down-stream signals due to cytokines may trigger brain dysfunction in septic encephalopathy. Furthermore, it was also suggested that sepsis-induced cytokines facilitate an intra-vascular fibrin formation which characterizes neurovascular symptom, disseminated intravascular coagulation[20,21]. Hence, these pathological conditions of septic encephalopathy include potential complicated symptoms such as cerebral ischemic cell death or edema [22-25]. Altogether, these sepsis-related multifacet brain dysfunctions lead to be the symptoms of septic encephalopathy.

2. SYMPTOMS

2.1. Sepsis

The body conditions are defined as SIRS when two of the medical inspections for three days correspond to be as following: (1) hypothermia (< 36 °C) or fever (> 38 °C), (2) higher heart rate (>90/ min), (3) higher respiratory rate (> 20/ min) by hyperventilation, (4) aberrant white blood cell count (< 4000 cells/ mm^3) by leucopenia or > 12000 cells / mm^3 by leukocytosis) [10]. Since the septic patients elevate their inflammatory mediator levels, the measurements of the concentration or the immunodetection for the IL-1beta, IL-6, HMGB-1 etc will also be useful to determine the diagnosis of septic conditions.

2.2. Septic Encephalopathy

In addition to the diagnostic condition during sepsis, septic encephalopathy is able to be diagnosed as an impaired mental state[26]. For example, a group of 69 patients with septic encephalopathy showed the following symptoms with impaired cognitive function: 1) attention, 2) orientation, 3) writing, 4) delirium and 5) coma [27]. In contrast, usual symptoms such as asterixis, tremor and multifocal myoclonus found in other encephalopathies with liver, kidney or endocrine gland failures are rare [27]. Hence, septic encephalopathy is characterized mainly by coma scale scores[28].

2.2.1. Electroencephalogram

Electroencephalogram (EEG) records an electrical activity along scalp. The EEG measures voltage fluctuations resulting from ionic current flows within the neurons of the brain. In neurology, at first, the main diagnostic application of EEG is the case of epilepsy, as epileptic activity can create clear abnormalities on EEG study. Second, the EEG can also be utilized clinically in the diagnosis of coma, encephalopathy and brain death. EEG results are consisted of rhythmic activity. The rhythmic activity is divided into bands by frequency. Depending on the component of rhythmic activities, the EEG results include the components of the wave called α-band for 6-12Hz and β-band for 13-30 Hz frequencies. Since the spatial resolution when EEG recording is performed is dependent on the place and size of the recording electrodes, although EEG has a high temporal resolution (< ms), EEG has a lower spatial resolution than other functional brain imaging such as magnetic resonance imaging (MRI).

Septic encephalopathy can also be determined with EEG [29]. Several lines of pre-clinical trials using rodent model of sepsis indicate that basal brain activity was reduced continuously after induction of sepsis [30,31]. In addition, 15 patients of septic encephalopathy showed that both of α- and β- band frequencies in occipital region (e.g. visual cortex) of the brain (Figure 3) were altered and attention test using sound were aggravated, although not all of the cognitive tests were correlated with EEG results[32]. These findings suggest that an aberrant sensory perception due to septic encephalopathy may possibly be diagnosed with EEG results. However, it is hard to determine the damaged region in the brain only with EEG. Thereby, to correlate the patho-physiology of septic encephalopathy with brain dysfunctional localization, it is necessary to use a brain functional imaging such as functional magnetic resonance imaging (fMRI).

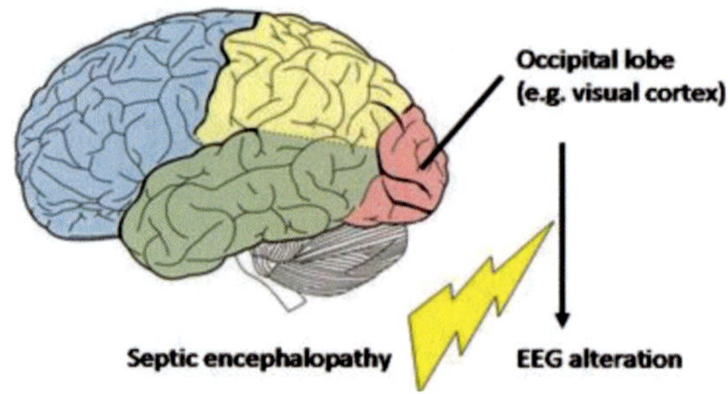

Figure 3. Diagnotic potentials of septic encephalopathy with electroencephalography.
(EEG). Alteration of EEG recording in occipital lobe of the septic brain suggests the potential diagnosis of the septic encephalopathy pathogenesis.

2.2.2. Functional Magnetic Resonance Imaging

Functional magnetic resonance imaging (fMRI) can detect the brain activity which is associated with changes in blood flow. Since the change of blood flow (e.g. hemodynamics) is related to energy use by neuronal cells, fMRI refers to record the map of morphologic alteration and metabolic modulation for neuronal activity in septic encephalopathy. Several lines of studies revealed that no morphological and metabolic changes were found in acute phase of sepsis on a rat model of sepsis [33] or patients [34]. However, in a later phase (e.g. septic encephalopathy), edematous fluid was found in the thalamus or hypothalamus of the brain (Figure 4, red arrows) and the chemical substances such as choline and n-acethylaspartate (e.g., a marker for neuronal energy metabolism) were altered to be increasing neuronal cell loss in cortex and hippocampus [35]. These findings reveal that the cognitive dysfunctions and memory impairments are induced by brain metabolic alteration upon septic condition. Altogether, these findings from EEG and fMRI studies may possibly clarify the patho-physiology of septic encephalopathy in the future studies.

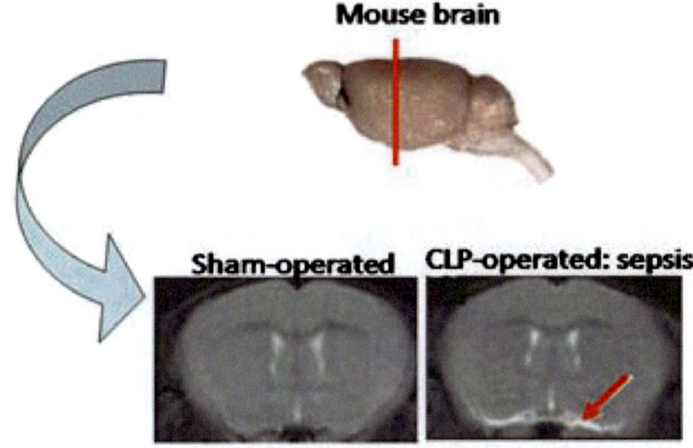

Citation modified from Bozza FA et. al., *J Cereb Blood Flow Metab* 30 (2010) 440-448).

Figure 4. T2-weighted axial MRI of representative brains from a sham-operated (left panel) and a CLP-operated (e.g. a mouse model of sepsis, right panel) mice. Accumulation of edematous fluid is visible as hyperintense area emanating from the blood vessels at the base of the brain (red arrow).

3. POTENTIAL COMPLICATIONS

3.1. Edema

Several lines of review reports suggest the morphological changes in the septic brain[21,36]. Complicated sequela mostly often observed in septic encephalopathy is suggested to be **edema**. For example, an animal model of septic encephalopathy shows vasogenic edema [37,38], followed by impairment of blood brain barrier [19, 39]. The edema was also found in the hippocampus[40]. Since the hippocampus is important for learning and memory, the patho-physiological state with edema may influence on the pathology of memory dysfunctions in septic encephalopathy. These complicated symptoms accompany with the disruption of astrocyte end-feet and swollen, suggesting a potential morphological alteration [37]. Thereby, in addition to the pathological alteration in morphology like edema, various inflammatory cytokines may concomitantly pass through the impaired blood brain barrier and modulate brain dysfunction.

Interleukin-1β, interleukin-6 and tumor necrosis factor-α expressions are increased after onset of sepsis. Especially, interleukin-1β expression levels in the plasma of the septic encephalopathy patients were higher than non-septic encephalopathy patients [41]. Thereby, it is expected that interleukin-1β might be one of the hopeful therapeutic targets for the better prognosis of septic encephalopathy. Especially, the interleukin-1β may develop a novel aspect of the patho-physiology for the synaptic transmission and its plasticity as described in the next section.

3.2. Irregular Synaptic Transmission and Plasticity

The patho-physiology of septic encephalopathy still contains a mystery especially for synaptic function. However, for past decades, several kinds of research reports involving the issue are suggested. For example, the receptors' densities of gamma aminobutyric acid (GABA), which mediates the *inhibitory* synaptic transmission, are increased with the administration of interleukin-1β [42]. On the contrary, the administration of the interleukin-1β suppresses the activities of receptors for α-amino-3-hydroxy-5-methyl-4-isoxazolepropionic acid (AMPA) and N-methyl-d-aspartate (NMDA) [43], which mediates the *excitatory* synaptic transmission for glutamate. NMDA receptors are also well-known to be critical for synaptic plasticity underlying learning and memory [44]. Furthermore, recently, it was suggested that the synaptic plasticity was impaired in septic encephalopathy. Our research groups (Imamura et. al.) (2011) reported that interleukin-1β inhibited the induction of long-term potentiation, a hallmark of synaptic plasticity (e.g. plastic changes of brain activities), in the hippocampus in septic encephalopathy[19]. Hence, these findings may reflect the patho-physiology for the brain dysfunction such as memory deficiency in septic encephalopathy.

3.3. Genetic Involvements

Novel genes for the relevance of septic encephalopathy pathogenesis are suggested. For example, SOX10 gene, which was critical for neural crest and peripheral nervous system development, was mutated in patient with septic encephalopathy [45]. The patient showed more severe injuries with ischemia in septic encephalopathy. It was also reported that mitochondrial DNA haplogroup affected the outcome of septic encephalopathy, showing the importance of mitochondrial dysfunction as one of the pathogenesis of septic encephalopathy [46]. Hence, the genetic variability may also contribute to the vulnerability and outcome for septic encephalopathy.

3.4. Therapeutic Potentials

3.4.1. Anti-Apoptotic Therapy with Pharmaceutical Regents

During septic conditions, apoptotic cell death was found in neuronal cells of the brain. Thereby, the potency of anti-apoptotic therapy has been suggested [47]. For example, the expression level of the inducible nitric oxide synthase (iNOS) was enhanced in the brain from an animal model of sepsis [48] and post-mortem septic patients[49]. The iNOS inhibitor reduced the apoptotic neuronal cell death in septic encephalopathy [48]. In addition, an administration of the iNOS inhibitor improved the behavioral test scores for the cognitive impairment during systemic inflammation in a rodent model of septic encephalopathy [50]. These findings suggest that the inhibition of apoptosis is effective for the treatment of septic encephalopathy. However, in some cases, the validities of anti-apoptotic therapy seem to be partial. The reason why is that since there are some cell death pathways associated with apoptosis, the inhibition of one or two apoptotic pathways sometimes show no anti-apoptotic effects [47]. For instance, the pathways of cysteine-dependent aspartate-directed proteases (caspase)-3, -8 and -9 which play essential roles in apoptosis, necrosis and inflammation [51] employ the property for the caspase-signal crosstalk (Figure 5). This signal crosstalk counteracts the positive effect with anti-apoptotic inhibitor for the therapy. In addition to the therapeutic model for anti-neuronal cell death, the loss of functions of other inflammatory cell types such as B cell, T cell, etc, are also suggested[16,47]. These cell dysfunctions may lead to be the further aberrant immunological responses after the onset of sepsis. Hence, it is hard to regulate the septic brain with a simple cascade and thereby other potential therapeutics for the septic brain are required.

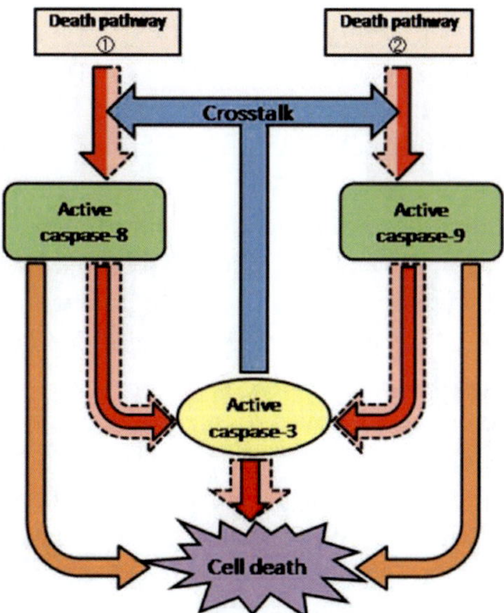

Citation modified from Hotchkiss RS et. al., *Nat Rev Immunol* 6 (2006) pp813-822.

Figure 5. Cross-talk between the two pathways of apoptotic cell death. There is increasing evidence that, in certain cases, the two death pathways can activate each other, via activated caspase-3. These caspases' activations contribute to cell death, respectively.

3.4.2. Possible Suppression of Cytokine Storm

An intriguing hypothetical model for anti-inflammatory pathway to regulate inflammation during sepsis is suggested [52]. α7 subunit of nicotinic acethylcholine receptor may be a key player in anti-inflammatory pathway for the regulation of inflammatory responses

The vagus nerve, tenth cranial nerve regulates heart rate, bronchoconstriction, digestion. Stimulation of the efferent vagus nerve slows heart rate, induces gastric motility. Recently, it was found that the vagus nerve regulated the innate immune response, inhibiting tumor necrosis factor-α production in spleen. Due to the findings, a hypothetical model for the anti-inflammatory pathway is suggested as followed: 1) the vagus nerve stimulation releases the neurotransmitter acetylcholine and the acetylcholine induces an activation of α7 subunit of nicotinic acethylcholine receptor, expressed on the cellular membrane of macrophage and other cells secreting cytokines. 2) binding of acetylcholine to nicotinic acetylcholine receptors activates an intracellular signal transduction which inhibits the release of pro-inflammatory cytokines. 3) ligand receptor signaling may suppress the inflammatory pathway leading to cytokine storm. These models of molecular mechanisms for anti-inflammatory pathways, to date, still include the unclear points, (for example, how to regulate the various mediators from immunological cells, temporally or spatially during systemic inflammation etc.) and warrant further evaluation.

3.4.3. Vagus Nerve Stimulation

To regulate the cytokine storm after the onset of sepsis, several kinds of pre-clinical trials using rodent model of sepsis are performed for pre-clinical trial. For example, the electrical stimulation of vagus nerve with high frequency-repeated voltage pulses (5 mv, 2 ms, 1 Hz, for 5 min at 20 min intervals) ameliorated the aberrant electrical properties and physiological parameters such as heart rate variability in septic rats [53]. In addition, the cholinergic neurotransmitter and its receptor activation are necessary for the inhibition of inflammatory response in a mouse or rat model of sepsis [54-56]. These findings suggest that the vagus nerve stimulation, at least, seems to be effective to inhibit an inflammatory response after sepsis.

How to apply a potential therapy, when the validity will be evaluated in the human, using the vagus nerve simulation against sepsis in clinical settings? One of the hopeful current strategies is subcutaneous implantation of electric pulse generator, which had been already, safely, and effectively applied to the patients with refractory epilepsy (Figure 6). The future development of the non-invasive devise, which can render the electrical pulse stimulation repeatedly on the vagus nerve on cervix, will provide the possible novel medical intervention for sepsis in the intensive care unit.

In conclusion, although there are some future potential therapies for the alleviation of septic encephalopathy with the regulation of inflammatory response after the onset of sepsis, the valid therapeutic method for septic encephalopathy is still not provided. Probably, it is hard to recover the irregular plastic changes of the brain including synaptic plasticity after septic encephalopathy, completely. However, we hope that the recovery of neuronal plasticity with the novel technologies such as the brain nerve stimulation and/ or neurogenesis-induction may lead to be a better outcome of septic encephalopathy in the future.

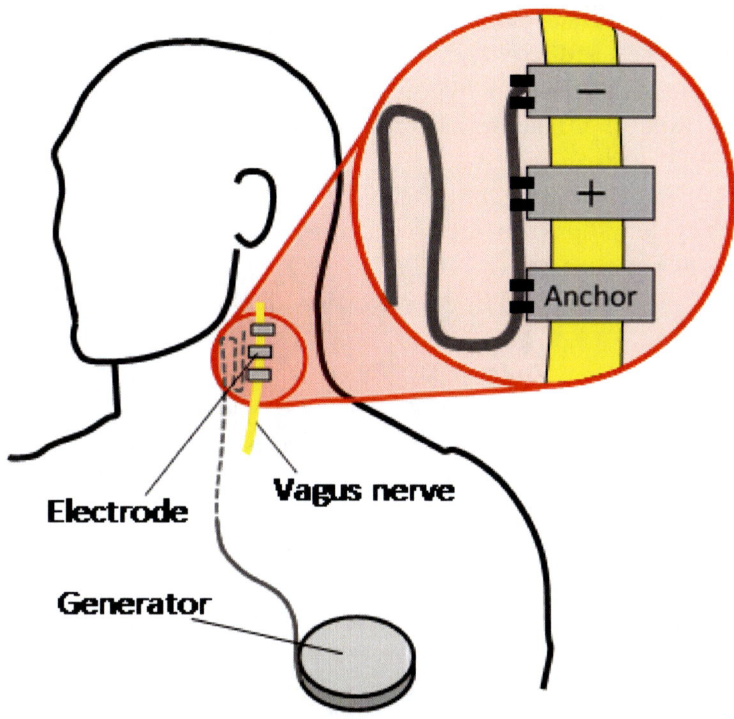

Figure 6. Future potential therapy for sepsis and its encephalopathy with the implanted vagus nerve stimulator.

REFERENCES

[1]   Pytel P, Alexander JJ: Pathogenesis of septic encephalopathy. *Curr Opin Neurol* (2009) 22:283-287.

[2]   Streck EL, Comim CM, Barichello T, Quevedo J: The septic brain. *Neurochem Res* (2008) 33:2171-2177.

[3]   Zhang Q, Raoof M, Chen Y, Sumi Y, Sursal T, Junger W, Brohi K, Itagaki K, Hauser CJ: Circulating mitochondrial DAMPs cause inflammatory responses to injury. *Nature* (2010) 464:104-107.

[4]   Wang H, Bloom O, Zhang M, Vishnubhakat JM, Ombrellino M, Che J, Frazier A, Yang H, Ivanova S, Borovikova L, Manogue KR, Faist E, Abraham E, Andersson J, Andersson U, Molina PE, Abumrad NN, Sama A, Tracey KJ: HMG-1 as a late mediator of endotoxin lethality in mice. *Science* (1999) 285:248-251.

[5]   Sims GP, Rowe DC, Rietdijk ST, Herbst R, Coyle AJ: HMGB1 and RAGE in inflammation and cancer. *Annu Rev Immunol* (2010) 28:367-388.

[6]   Luqman S, Pezzuto JM: NFkappaB: a promising target for natural products in cancer chemoprevention. *Phytother Res* (2010) 24:949-963.

[7]   Shimazaki J, Matsumoto N, Ogura H, Muroya T, Kuwagata Y, Nakagawa J, Yamakawa K, Hosotsubo H, Imamura Y, Shimazu T: Systemic Involvement of HMGB1 and Therapeutic Effect of Anti-HMGB1 Antibody in a Rat Model of Crush Injury. *Shock* (2012) 37(6):634-8.

[8] Bolger MS, Ross DS, Jiang H, Frank MM, Ghio AJ, Schwartz DA, Wright JR: Complement levels and activity in the normal and LPS-injured lung. *Am J Physiol Lung Cell Mol Physiol* (2007) 292:L748-59.

[9] Ward PA: Role of C5 activation products in sepsis. *ScientificWorldJournal* (2010) 10:2395-2402.

[10] Bone RC, Balk RA, Cerra FB, Dellinger RP, Fein AM, Knaus WA, Schein RM, Sibbald WJ: Definitions for sepsis and organ failure and guidelines for the use of innovative therapies in sepsis. The ACCP/SCCM Consensus Conference Committee. American College of Chest Physicians/Society of Critical Care Medicine. *Chest* (1992) 101:1644-1655.

[11] Flierl MA, Stahel PF, Rittirsch D, Huber-Lang M, Niederbichler AD, Hoesel LM, Touban BM, Morgan SJ, Smith WR, Ward PA, Ipaktchi K: Inhibition of complement C5a prevents breakdown of the blood-brain barrier and pituitary dysfunction in experimental sepsis. *Crit Care* (2009) 13:R12.

[12] Cohen J: The immunopathogenesis of sepsis. *Nature* (2002) 420:885-891.

[13] Tsuge M, Yasui K, Ichiyawa T, Saito Y, Nagaoka Y, Yashiro M, Yamashita N, Morishima T: Increase of tumor necrosis factor-alpha in the blood induces early activation of matrix metalloproteinase-9 in the brain. *Microbiol Immunol* (2010) 54:417-424.

[14] Tsao N, Hsu HP, Wu CM, Liu CC, Lei HY: Tumour necrosis factor-alpha causes an increase in blood-brain barrier permeability during sepsis. *J Med Microbiol* (2001) 50:812-821.

[15] Kim KS: Mechanisms of microbial traversal of the blood-brain barrier. *Nat Rev Microbiol* (2008) 6:625-634.

[16] Nishioku T, Dohgu S, Takata F, Eto T, Ishikawa N, Kodama KB, Nakagawa S, Yamauchi A, Kataoka Y: Detachment of brain pericytes from the basal lamina is involved in disruption of the blood-brain barrier caused by lipopolysaccharide-induced sepsis in mice. *Cell Mol Neurobiol* (2009) 29:309-316.

[17] Hofer S, Bopp C, Hoerner C, Plaschke K, Faden RM, Martin E, Bardenheuer HJ, Weigand MA: Injury of the blood brain barrier and up-regulation of icam-1 in polymicrobial sepsis. *J Surg Res* (2008) 146:276-281.

[18] Kondo S, Kohsaka S, Okabe S: Long-term changes of spine dynamics and microglia after transient peripheral immune response triggered by LPS in vivo. *Mol Brain* (2011) 4:27.

[19] Imamura Y, Wang H, Matsumoto N, Muroya T, Shimazaki J, Ogura H, Shimazu T: Interleukin-1beta causes long-term potentiation deficiency in a mouse model of septic encephalopathy. *Neuroscience* (2011) 187:63-69.

[20] ten Cate H: Pathophysiology of disseminated intravascular coagulation in sepsis. *Crit Care Med* (2000) 28:S9-11.

[21] Rittirsch D, Flierl MA, Ward PA: Harmful molecular mechanisms in sepsis. *Nat Rev Immunol* (2008) 8:776-787.

[22] Dempfle CE: Coagulopathy of sepsis. *Thromb Haemost* (2004) 91:213-224.

[23] Levi M, de Jonge E, van der Poll T: Sepsis and disseminated intravascular coagulation. *J Thromb Thrombolysis* (2003) 16:43-47.

[24] Levi M: Pathogenesis and treatment of disseminated intravascular coagulation in the septic patient. *J Crit Care* (2001) 16:167-177.

[25] ten Cate H, Schoenmakers SH, Franco R, Timmerman JJ, Groot AP, Spek CA, Reitsma PH: Microvascular coagulopathy and disseminated intravascular coagulation. *Crit Care Med* (2001) 29:S95-7; discussion S.

[26] Meakins JL, Wicklund B, Forse RA, McLean AP: The surgical intensive care unit: current concepts in infection. *Surg Clin North Am* (1980) 60:117-132.

[27] Young GB, Bolton CF, Austin TW, Archibald YM, Gonder J, Wells GA: The encephalopathy associated with septic illness. *Clin Invest Med* (1990) 13:297-304.

[28] Eidelman LA, Putterman D, Putterman C, Sprung CL: The spectrum of septic encephalopathy. Definitions, etiologies, and mortalities. *JAMA* (1996) 275:470-473.

[29] Young GB, Bolton CF, Archibald YM, Austin TW, Wells GA: The electroencephalogram in sepsis-associated encephalopathy. *J Clin Neurophysiol* (1992) 9:145-152.

[30] Kafa IM, Bakirci S, Uysal M, Kurt MA: Alterations in the brain electrical activity in a rat model of sepsis-associated encephalopathy. *Brain Res* (2010) 1354:217-226.

[31] Lin LC, Chen YY, Lee WT, Chen HL, Yang RC: Heat shock pretreatment attenuates sepsis-associated encephalopathy in LPS-induced septic rats. *Brain Dev* (2010) 32:371-377.

[32] van den Boogaard M, Ramakers BP, van Alfen N, van der Werf SP, Fick WF, Hoedemaekers CW, Verbeek MM, Schoonhoven L, van der Hoeven JG, Pickkers P: Endotoxemia-induced inflammation and the effect on the human brain. *Crit Care* (2010) 14:R81.

[33] Rosengarten B, Walberer M, Allendoerfer J, Mueller C, Schwarz N, Bachmann G, Gerriets T: LPS-induced endotoxic shock does not cause early brain edema formation - an MRI study in rats. *Inflamm Res* (2008) 57:479-483.

[34] Piazza O, Cotena S, De Robertis E, Caranci F, Tufano R: Sepsis associated encephalopathy studied by MRI and cerebral spinal fluid S100B measurement. *Neurochem Res* (2009) 34:1289-1292.

[35] Bozza FA, Garteiser P, Oliveira MF, Doblas S, Cranford R, Saunders D, Jones I, Towner RA, Castro-Faria-Neto HC: Sepsis-associated encephalopathy: a magnetic resonance imaging and spectroscopy study. *J Cereb Blood Flow Metab* (2010) 30:440-448.

[36] Jacob A, Brorson JR, Alexander JJ: Septic encephalopathy: inflammation in man and mouse. *Neurochem Int* (2011) 58:472-476.

[37] Papadopoulos MC, Lamb FJ, Moss RF, Davies DC, Tighe D, Bennett ED: Faecal peritonitis causes oedema and neuronal injury in pig cerebral cortex. *Clin Sci (Lond)* (1999) 96:461-466.

[38] Ari I, Kafa IM, Kurt MA: Perimicrovascular edema in the frontal cortex in a rat model of intraperitoneal sepsis. *Exp Neurol* (2006) 198:242-249.

[39] Tanaka T, Sunden Y, Sakoda Y, Kida H, Ochiai K, Umemura T: Lipopolysaccharide treatment and inoculation of influenza A virus results in influenza virus-associated encephalopathy-like changes in neonatal mice. *J Neurovirol* (2010) 16:125-132.

[40] Kafa IM, Ari I, Kurt MA: The peri-microvascular edema in hippocampal CA1 area in a rat model of sepsis. *Neuropathology* (2007) 27:213-220.

[41] Serantes R, Arnalich F, Figueroa M, Salinas M, Andres-Mateos E, Codoceo R, Renart J, Matute C, Cavada C, Cuadrado A, Montiel C: Interleukin-1beta enhances GABAA

receptor cell-surface expression by a phosphatidylinositol 3-kinase/Akt pathway: relevance to sepsis-associated encephalopathy. *J Biol Chem* (2006) 281:14632-14643.

[42] Winder TR, Minuk GY, Sargeant EJ, Seland TP: gamma-Aminobutyric acid (GABA) and sepsis-related encephalopathy. *Can J Neurol Sci* (1988) 15:23-25.

[43] Coogan A, O'Connor JJ: Inhibition of NMDA receptor-mediated synaptic transmission in the rat dentate gyrus in vitro by IL-1 beta. *Neuroreport* (1997) 8:2107-2110.

[44] Li F, Tsien JZ: Memory and the NMDA receptors. *N Engl J Med* (2009) 361:302-303.

[45] Unzicker A, Pingault V, Meyer T, Rauthe S, Schutz A, Kunzmann S: A novel SOX10 mutation in a patient with PCWH who developed hypoxic-ischemic encephalopathy after E. coli sepsis. *Eur J Pediatr* (2011) 170:1475-1480.

[46] Yang Y, Zhang P, Lv R, He Q, Zhu Y, Yang X, Chen J: Mitochondrial DNA haplogroup R in the Han population and recovery from septic encephalopathy. *Intensive Care Med* (2011) 37:1613-1619.

[47] Hotchkiss RS, Nicholson DW: Apoptosis and caspases regulate death and inflammation in sepsis. *Nat Rev Immunol* (2006) 6:813-822.

[48] Semmler A, Okulla T, Sastre M, Dumitrescu-Ozimek L, Heneka MT: Systemic inflammation induces apoptosis with variable vulnerability of different brain regions. *J Chem Neuroanat* (2005) 30:144-157.

[49] Sharshar T, Annane D, de la Grandmaison GL, Brouland JP, Hopkinson NS, Francoise G: The neuropathology of septic shock. *Brain Pathol* (2004) 14:21-33.

[50] Eckel B, Ohl F, Bogdanski R, Kochs EF, Blobner M: Cognitive deficits after systemic induction of inducible nitric oxide synthase: a randomised trial in rats. *Eur J Anaesthesiol* (2011) 28:655-663.

[51] Alnemri ES, Livingston DJ, Nicholson DW, Salvesen G, Thornberry NA, Wong WW, Yuan J: Human ICE/CED-3 protease nomenclature. *Cell* (1996) 87:171.

[52] Tracey KJ: Reflex control of immunity. *Nat Rev Immunol* (2009) 9:418-428.

[53] Huang J, Wang Y, Jiang D, Zhou J, Huang X: The sympathetic-vagal balance against endotoxemia. *J Neural Transm* (2010) 117:729-735.

[54] Wang H, Yu M, Ochani M, Amella CA, Tanovic M, Susarla S, Li JH, Wang H, Yang H, Ulloa L, Al-Abed Y, Czura CJ, Tracey KJ: Nicotinic acetylcholine receptor alpha7 subunit is an essential regulator of inflammation. *Nature* (2003) 421:384-388.

[55] Rosas-Ballina M, Ochani M, Parrish WR, Ochani K, Harris YT, Huston JM, Chavan S, Tracey KJ: Splenic nerve is required for cholinergic antiinflammatory pathway control of TNF in endotoxemia. *Proc Natl Acad Sci U S A* (2008) 105:11008-11013.

[56] Vida G, Pena G, Deitch EA, Ulloa L: alpha7-cholinergic receptor mediates vagal induction of splenic norepinephrine. *J Immunol* (2011) 186:4340-4346.

In: Encephalitis, Encephalomyelitis and Encephalopathies   ISBN: 978-1-62257-766-8
Editors: Andrew Ruiz and Douglas Fleming   © 2013 Nova Science Publishers, Inc.

Chapter 9

ENCEPHALITIS: CAUSES, INCIDENCE AND TREATMENT-JAPANESE ENCEPHALITIS (JE), THE SPREADING "DISEASE"

[BASED PURELY ON OUR STUDY OF ADULT CASES]

*N. B. S. Sarkari** and Deepak Srivastava*

B.R.D. Medical College, Gorakhpur, India

Encephalitis is defined as inflammation of the brain parenchyma and occasionally involving the leptomeninges. Various viruses more often affect the brain, the commonest being Japanese encephalitis (JE).

The first epidemic of Japanese Encephalitis was recorded in 1871 in Japan and since then it has been a recurrent feature. It was recognized as an Arbovirus infection and caused another major epidemic in Japan in 1924. This virus was isolated in 1935 and named Japanese 'B' and the mosquito transmission was proved in 1938. It is numerically the most important global cause of Arboviral encephalitis with an estimated 30,000 to 50,000 cases and about 15,000 deaths (30 to 50 %) per annum. Similar epidemics of JE have also been reported from Eastern Siberia and various Asian countries. Japanese B is the only virus so far confirmed to cause epidemics in India. The classification of viral encephalitis is as under.

CLASSIFICATION OF VIRAL ENCEPHALITIS

A.   *Arthropod(Arbo Viruses)*
   o   Japanese B encephalitis
   o   Eastern Equine
   o   Western Equine

* Dr. NBS SARKARI, MD. FRCP (London), FRCP (Edin) & FRCP (Glasg,) Former Prof. Head Department of Medicine, B.R.D.Medical College, Gorakhpur, India-273013. E-mail : nbssarkari@gmail.com.

     o St. Louis
     o Russian Spring Summer
     o Venezuela
     o Murray Valley

B. *Enteroviruses*
     o Echo
     o Coxsackie
     o Poliomyelitis

C. *Other Viruses*
     o Herpes Simplex
     o Herpes Zoster-Varicella
     o Mumps
     o Rubella Rubeola
     o Rabies
     o CytomegaloVirus
     o Kyasanur forest Disease
     o Infectious Mononuleosis
     o Post measles subacute sclerosing pan encephalitis

D. *Post Infectious & Post Vaccinal Encephalitis*

JAPANESE ENCEPHALITIS EPIDEMICS IN INDIA

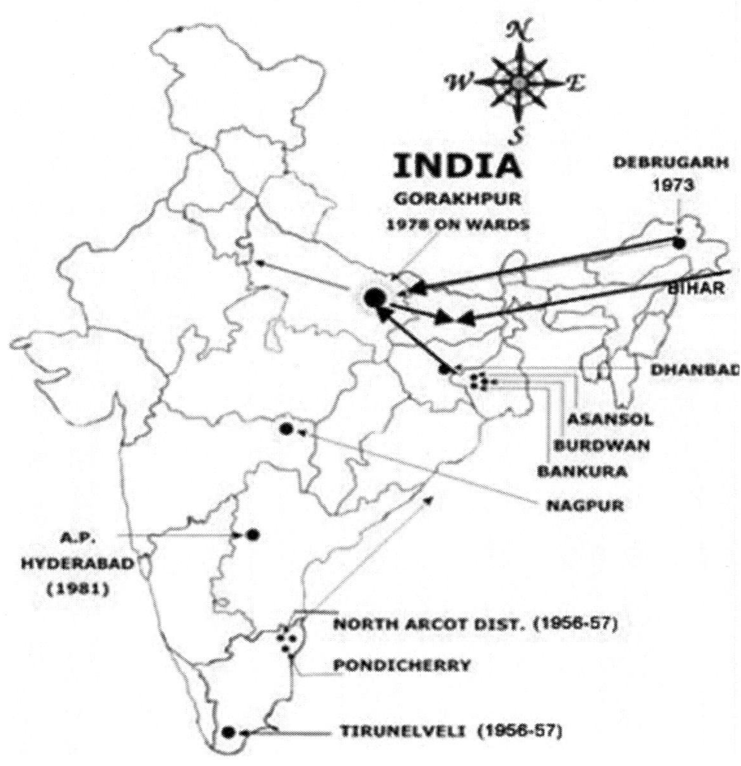

Figure 1. Show spread of JE in INDIA.

The epidemics of JE in India started from the south (1956) and spread to north and east part of India. The major flare up, however, occurred in north east and North West areas of Bengal 1973 & 1976 and now has become an endemic in eastern Uttar Pradesh –Gorakhpur and surrounding areas of western Bihar and Nepal since 1978. Now JE is reported to have spread in many areas of Bihar (Fig.1). This discourse is based on the experience of NBSS right from the very first epidemic of 1978 in Gorakhpur and the follow up of the survivors. All the acute adult cases of 1978 and of subsequent epidemics were hospitalized in the medical wards of BRD Medical College Gorakhpur.

These areas are densely populated; heavy rains and water logging are usual features along with good paddy crops, humid and warm climate with abundant mosquito population. High incidence of JE coincides with heavy rainfall and good paddy crops. The peak incidence (83% cases) is usually from mid Sept to first week of Nov. A sharp decline in the incidence occurs (a) when the paddy crops are harvested (beginning of winter), (b) the draught or (c) heavy floods. During floods the paddy crops are washed away with gushing stream and the villagers leave their dwellings to stay in camps for nearly four to five months. By then the infectivity is markedly reduced.

CLINICAL FEATURES

Patients present with identical features of AES (abrupt onset of altered sensorium preceded by fever, headache, vomiting, and associated with dystonias & convulsions) with cerebrospinal fluid (CSF) findings suggested acute viral involvement of brain. Thorough clinical and full neurological examinations are carried out on admission and recorded on a standard proforma /format so that proper record is kept for future studies. Peripheral blood smears for malarial parasites must be examined in all the cases to exclude malaria. C.S.F. examination should be undertaken soon after admission to confirm the viral picture and also to exclude pyogenic meningitis before the results of serological &/ virological studies are back.

The patients of all age groups are affected including adults i.e. between 15 to 78 years, with M: F ratio of 1.58:1. Pyrexia, headache and vomiting are the common presenting complaints along with altered sensorium (AS). The main symptoms for hospitalization within three days of the onset are AS, convulsions and headache (86% to 96% cases). Some patients may present with status epilepticus but rarely in adults. Altered sensorium may vary from coma (GCS =3) , semi coma (GCS 4-8) in whom there is some grimacing of face, and movement of upper limbs (flexion or extension) on deep painful stimuli and GCS 8-11 who are confused with cloudiness of consciousness and/or drowsy. The GCS score of some patients waxes and wanes with time. The patients, however, with initial consciousness (GCS of 15) may decline to (GCS 5) within 24 to 48. Most of the patients may have expressionless faces with lack of awareness at some stage of hospitalization.

Movement disorders consist of choreoathetoid, bizarre which are irregular with a combination of dystonia, athetosis and tremor making them difficult to classify. Abnormal hypertonic postures of different types consist of ophisthotonus, retraction of neck and pleurothotonus. Decerebrate rigidity, bobbing of eyes (Opsoclonus), pupillary changes and ocular gaze palsies consisting of (a) conjugate deviation (b) oculogyric crisis (c) skew deviation are observed in adults only as very important features of brain stem involvement of JE with waxing and waning character. Papilloedema and Paralytic features i.e. a) monoplegia b) hemiplegia can also be detected in some cases. Cerebellar involvement is rather rare. Convulsions- generalized can be witnessed in about 30% cases at the time of admission. some cases of focal convulsions may also be recorded. Many non neurological features of prognostic importance include abnormal breathing patterns (ABP) pulmonary oedema (PO) upper gastrointestinal haemorrhage (UIGH) and peripheral vascular failure (PVF).

LABORATORY DATA/ DIAGNOSIS

In outbreak situations sero-confirmation is neither required nor it is feasible for any laboratory to confirm all the cases. Only a representative number of positive samples in the beginning of the epidemic are sufficient to clinch the diagnosis. The CSF analysis is rather confirmatory of acute viral involvement of brain. CSF of the patients is clear, colourless and reveals normal or increased CSF: Blood sugar ratio with lymphocytosis in more than75% cases. CSF: blood sugar ratio is rarely reduced and so the CSF protein is seldom raised. Diagnosis of JE is initially made on the basis of clinical features of acute encephalitic syndrome and later immunological sero-confirmation is carried out in CSF/serum by estimation of IgM by using dot enzyme immunoassay/double-sandwich capture ELISA and IgG in serum by Hem-agglutination (HI) test. For serum, 40 units of IgM for JEV (with JEV IgM greater than dengue IgM) are considered positive for JE virus infection. A titer of 1:320 for single sera or a titer of 1:160 for paired sera is diagnostic. An increase from 15 to 30 units of IgM for paired samples is considered evidence of acute JE virus infection. HI antibody titer for IgG 80 in a single sample and titer of 320 in the second sample is considered positive. Similarly isolation of JE virus from CSF and brain can be done in few cases for definite confirmation of the epidemics.

MANAGEMENT

All the patients have to be hospitalized & managed with resuscitative measures, respiratory care. Endotracheal intubation or tracheostomy may be required to help suction of respiratory congestion. The patients of Cheyne Stokes and gasping respiration should be put on ventilator. Cerebral decongestants, antipyretic and continuous cold sponging is carried out. Good & complete nutrition (which should consist of milk, protein powder, pulses, rice extract, thick vegetable soups with butter or ghee, sugar, water and oral rehydration powder) to be administered through Ryle's tube (RT) besides small amounts and IV fluids to keep access to the vein & avoid fluid over load. Anticonvulsants should be administered immediately after admission to the patients of generalized and focal seizures for the total period of hospitalization. Initially as per availability, 10 mg of IV Diazepam or 200 mg IV Phenytoin sodium is administered. Latter all the patients are given Phenytoin 200 mg and Phenobarbitone 120 mg through RT throughout the period of hospitalization. The seizures treated this way do not create much problem since high fever and seizures increase cerebral oedema and deterioration of the G.C.S.

As cerebral decongestant the main drug is Mannitol 20% - 150 ml IV 6 to 8 hourly, along with 30 ml of Glycerol 6 hourly through the RT for one to two weeks. Injection dexamethasone 4 mg IV 8 hourly can be used for 7 days, as a potent cerebral decongestant on the discretion of the treating clinician. It does not produce any obvious deleterious effect like chest infection or increased evidence of UGIH. The possible benefit derived from corticosteroids, when cerebral oedema is clinically significant, appears to out way their potential for possible immunosuppression.

The overall mortality in our series was 511/1199 (43%), and about 63% died within 3 days of hospitalization. Various fatal incidences of acute JE patients have been reported from 8.5% to 76%. No definite reason can be assigned for the high mortality. It may be because of fresh introduction of infection particularly in virgin adult population.

The admission GCS is the most useful predictor of someone, who would die during the acute hospitalization. About 80% of patients with a GCS of 3 die compared to 10% of patients with a GCS of 15. In other patients with a GCS of 4 to 6 and with GCS 8 – 11 it may vary from 20% to 30%. The other important factors which contribute to mortality include decerebrate rigidity, ABP, UGIH, PO and PVF.

Transient global disturbances in such a diffuse brain disease are quite likely in large number of post JE cases.

At the time of discharge about only 2% to3% are without any sequelae and 97% to 98% with various neuropsychiatric deficits. These include

- Psychological disorders,
- Higher Cerebral Dysfunction.
- Speech Disturbances,
- Extra pyramidal feature consisting of a) Hypo kinetic Parkinsonian Feature (b) Hyperkinetic Parkinsonian Feature (c) Dystonic Postures ,
- Pyramidal feature including Paralysis ,
- Hypothalamic Disturbances,
- Cranial Nerve & Eye Changes and Seizures.

Psychological disorders consist of psychotic and nonpsychotic groups. They patients of psychotic group suffer from restlessness, agitation and hype excitability and remain aggressive. Some may have hallucinations, euphoria and emotional instability. Some of them suffer from Psychopathic- anti-social disorder with loss of moral values being a dominant feature in male patients only. This may consist of inappropriate removal of clothes, abusive, speaking indecent words and exhibiting obscene gestures. They have to be prescribed anti psychotic drugs (chlorpromazine with diazepam) and they continue to improve. 98% improve by 5 years and only 2% may be left with mild features without interfering with the routine and activities of daily living (ADL).

Patient with Non psychotic features are Inattentive, depressed or suffer from emotional instability and euphoria. Some may have classical features of depression. They are treated with Amitriptyline and by the ensuing 5 years 99% improve. 1% may have occasional vacant look & remain rather withdrawn without any problem with their jobs.

Higher cerebral dysfunction consists of impairment of intelligence, memory and state of confusion (Confusional state). Confusion clears by six months whereas intelligence and memory take some time to improve and after 5 years all of them become fit for their livelihood.

Speech disturbances: Almost all types of speech disturbances can be detected in the patients at discharge, of course with a lot of overlap with other deficits. These consist of Dysphonia, Dysarthria , Jargon dysphasia, Expressive dysphasia, Nominal dysphasia, Automatic speech, Echolalia, Agraphia, Acalculia, Paraphasia & neologism, mirror writing, Ideo-motor & ideational Apraxia, Constructional Apraxia, Dressing apraxia and Agnosias (visual & tactile). Rapid improvement takes place by 6 months to 5years.

Extra pyramidal features: are associated with all Parkinsonian features, Hyperkinetic movements, Dystonic Postures, Bizarre movements & posture and coarse tremors. Most of the extra pyramidal features clear by one year and almost all of them can resume their normal routine life by 5 years.

Hypothalamic Disturbances transient hypothalamic disturbances in such a diffuse brain disease are quite likely. Almost all types can be detected if observed carefully and consist of Hyper somnolence, Insomnia, Altered sleep rhythm, Increased appetite, Decreased appetite. Increased thirst, Polyuria, Increased libido, Decreased libido, Loss of diurnal variation of temperature, Hyperhydrosis, transient Hypertension, Glycosuria &Hyperglycaemia. All parameters tend to improve rapidly by one year.

Pyramidal features and motor paralysis: Motor paralysis in the form of hemiplegia and monoplegia can be found in about 35% patients though corticospinal signs only without paralysis can also be noted, consisting of generalized hyper reflexia including exaggerated jaw jerk, Hoffman's sign. After 6 months, to 5 years most of them become normal. In the earlier part from 6 months to 1 year they require intermittent help and careful watch particularly during bathing, clothing and some assistance during walking.

Pupillary and Cranial nerve changes: Cranial nerve involvement, pupillary abnormalities including Argyll Robertson pupil and papilloedema can be detected on careful clinical examination. All clear by 6 months.

Seizures: Seizures, focal or generalized, might persist after such a diffuse brain disease. They all need appropriate antiepileptics for 2 to 5 years or even the whole life.

As almost all the neuropsychiatric and neurological deficits clear up by five years, it is indicative of severe neuronal oedema rather than degeneration/ damage.

CONCLUSION

We conclude that during epidemics, where a diagnosis of JE has yet to be confirmed by virological and/or serological tests in only a representative number of samples, the provisional clinical diagnosis of JE can be made with confidence to start early management by features of AES, i.e., (1) abrupt onset of fever, headache, and altered sensorium, (2) dystonias and various movement disorders, (3) bobbing (opsoclonus) of eyes and gaze palsies, (4) with CSF findings suggesting acute viral involvement of CNS, and (5) the presence of minor or gross residual neuropsychiatric and neurological features in the survivors. A large number of them are quite disabled initially and need constant care by family members & also those who require some help intermittently improve with passage of time and eventually return to normal life. Some of them can be left with non-disabling residual features even after 5 years, although they are fit enough for all practical purposes. Practically all of them return to their daily working between 3-5 years, hence the burden on family, society and the exchequer is very negligible. With limited management options, it is suggested to carry out intensive vaccination programmes in endemic areas after detailed surveillance.

PREVENTION: (CONTROL MEASURES)

Pigs are the main store of JEV and possibly the cattle and domestic birds. The migratory birds come to this area during December and January when the temperature falls & paddy has been harvested.

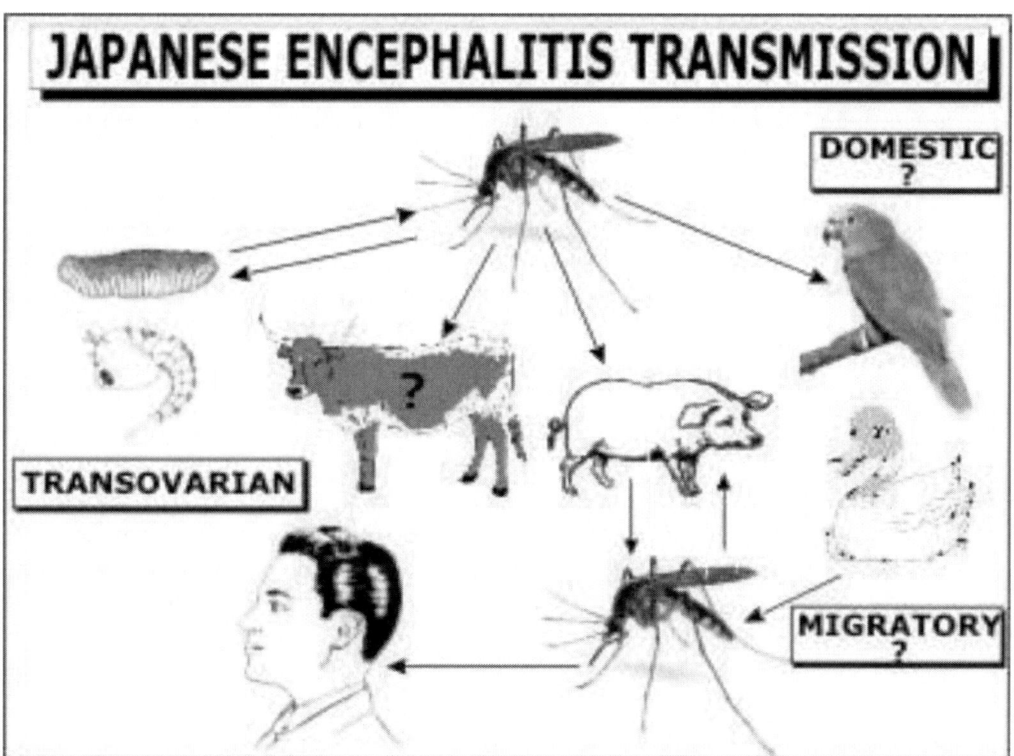

Figure 2. Possible Transmission Cycle.

1. IMMUNISATION OF ANIMALS: Since there is no specific treatment the old maxim is prevention is better than cure. There are mainly three strategies for prevention.
   It is essential to immunise the amplifying hosts- Pigs and swine as done for rabies. All the domestic dogs are immunised to protect them from stray animals and to protect the unfamiliar visitors. It is possibly much easier to detect JEV antibodies and immunise those who do not demonstrate their presence. In the Indian setting it is

easier and cost effective. It should be properly planned with proper surveillance and to take the help of veterinary team as well.

2. VECTOR CONTROL & PERSONAL PROTECTION: The mosquitoes (Culex group) responsible for transmission of the virus should be tackled by insecticide spray. It would me more scientific to detect JEV in the particular mosquito population. Their presence will need intensive and extensive repeated spraying and fogging of the paddy fields, dwellings and the areas of pigs & cattle stay which are usually near the houses of the farmers. Smoke produced because of burning Neem / Mustard cakes in between fogging must be very useful & fruitful for keeping away the vectors. The mosquito repellents not only to be applied by the inhabitants but also over the animals. The use of Mustard and/ or Neem oil over the body of animals and even the inhabitants including children should be very useful and without any side effects. Long clothes to cover most of the body and long shoes extending up to the knees should be put on while working in the water logged paddy fields. The fertilisers/manure should be mixed with Neem/Mustard cakes before being spread in the fields; it will certainly increase the yield besides protecting the field workers. The use of mosquito nets, repellents over the body and in the rooms along with fine door and window nets certainly enhances the protection.

3. VACCINATION: Vaccination of the habitants of endemic areas, children as well as the adults working in the paddy fields and those frequently visiting the villages during the crop season should be carried out.

    There are three types of vaccines available. 1) A mouse brain-derived inactivated vaccine a) Biken vaccine from Japan b) Korean Green Cross. The vaccine is inactivated by protamine sulphate, formaldehyde, and ultra-filtration and purified by ultracentrifugation. 2. Cell cultured-derived inactivated vaccine made in China. One dose provides 80% protection in children but 2 doses with a booster after one to two years offers 95-100% protection. 3. Cell- culture-derived live attenuated vaccine also made in China.

    The primary course of immunization preferably consists of three subcutaneous shots to offer 95 to 100% seroconversion, given 0, day 7-14 and day 30. Single booster may be given after every three years in endemic areas. The effect of vaccination should be monitored by sero-conversion and detection of neutralizing antibodies by regular surveillance.

SUGGESTIONS FOR FURTHER READING

Kabilan L, Rajendran R, Arunachalam N, Ramesh S, SrinivasanS, Philips Samuel P, Dash AP (2004) Japanese encephalitis: an overview. *Indian J Pediatr* 7:609–615.

Rao PN (2001), Japanese encephalitis. *Indian Pediatr.* 38:1252–1264.

Sarkari N. B. S., Thacker A. K. , Barthwal S. P., Mishra V. K., Shiv Prapann, Srivastava Deepak, Sarkari M. (2011) , Japanese encephalitis (JE). Part I: clinical profile of 1,282 adult acute cases of four epidemics. *Journal of Neurology PMID:* 21678123 as supplied by publisher]

Sarkari N. B. S., Thacker A. K. , Barthwal S. P., Mishra V. K., Shiv Prapann, Srivastava Deepak, Sarkari M. (2011) Japanese encephalitis (JE) part II: 14 Years' follow-up of survivors. *Journal of Neurology PMID*: 21681633- as supplied by publisher]

Solomon T (2004) Flavi virus encephalitis. *N Engl. J* Med351:370–378.

Solomon T, Dung MM, Kneen R, Gainsborough M, Vaughn DW, Khanh VT (2000) Japanese encephalitis. *J Neurol. Neurosurg. & Psychiatry* 68:405–415.

Whitley R J& Gnann JW (2002), Viral Encephalitis: familiar infections and emerging Parhogens, *Lancet*; 359:507-14.

INDEX

B

C

D

I

N

O

T

U

V

W

Y